Crown Center
Eleanor Ringle
916-546-3430

PHYSICIAN'S REFERENCE NOTEBOOK

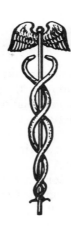

Compiled and Written by
William A. McGarey, M.D.
and Associated Physicians of
The A.R.E. Clinic
in Cooperation with
The Edgar Cayce Foundation

A.R.E.®PRESS • VIRGINIA BEACH • VIRGINIA

A Note to the Reader

The A.R.E. does not present any of the information in this book as prescription for the treatment of disease. Application of medical information found in the Cayce readings should be undertaken only under supervision of a physician.

More in-depth information on certain medical problems is available to A.R.E. members in the Circulating Files. For information on the Files or for a list of suppliers of items found in the Cayce readings, write to: Membership Services, A.R.E., Box 595, Virginia Beach, VA 23451.

2nd Printing, July 1984

Printed in the U.S.A.

CONTENTS

Foreword v
Introduction vii
ACNE 1
AMYOTROPHIC LATERAL SCLEROSIS 6
ANEMIA 14
ANGINA PECTORIS 18
APHONIA 22
APOPLEXY 26
ARTERIOSCLEROSIS 31
ARTHRITIS 39
ASTHMA 55
BALDNESS 60
BREAST CANCER 64
BRONCHITIS 70
CATARACTS 76
COLITIS 80
COLOR BLINDNESS 87
THE COMMON COLD 90
CONSTIPATION 101
CYSTITIS 106
DIABETES 116
DIVERTICULITIS 122
EMPHYSEMA 126
EPILEPSY 132
FLU: Respiratory 148
FLU: Aftereffects 152
FRACTURES AND SPRAINS 158
HEADACHES 164
HEMOPHILIA 168
HEMORRHOIDS 172
HERPES ZOSTER 185
HYDROCEPHALUS 189
HYPERTENSION 194
HYPOGLYCEMIA 198
INDIGESTION AND GASTRITIS 208
KIDNEY STONES 213

LEUKEMIA 223
LEUKOPENIA—LEUKOCYTOSIS. 232
MENOPAUSE 236
MENTAL ILLNESS 244
MIGRAINE HEADACHES. 258
MULTIPLE SCLEROSIS 264
MUSCULAR DYSTROPHY. 278
OBESITY 288
PROSTATITIS. 297
PSORIASIS. 303
PYORRHEA. 312
SCARS AND ADHESIONS 315
SCLERODERMA 322
STUTTERING 329
SYPHILIS 336
TONSILLITIS. 345
ULCERS 350
VARICOSE VEINS 358
APPENDIX. 366
    Acidity—Alkalinity. 366
    Almonds. 369
    Atomidine. 373
    Beef Juice 374
    Castor Oil Pack. 377
    Cough and Hiccough Therapy 378
    Diet: Acid and Alkaline. 382
    Diet for Diabetes. 385
    Diet for Eczema 389
    Eliminants 390
    Epsom Salts Pack 397
    Fasting 398
    General Interest Extracts 406
    Glyco-Thymoline Pack. 409
    Massage 410
    Passion Flower Fusion. 411
    Ventriculin 412
    Why the Patient's Condition Seems to Worsen
       When Treatment Is Given 413
GLOSSARY 414
INDEX 425

FOREWORD

All of the Edgar Cayce physical readings, with few exceptions, were given for individuals with different needs. This probably explains why there are often slight variations in treatment, formula, dosage, manner of application, etc., even between readings on the same subject. Certain methods, products, and formulas, however, were recommended so repeatedly and emphatically that they have almost become specifics for certain types of disorders. Much of the information in *The Physician's Reference Notebook* was the outgrowth of physicians' working with these specifics.

The Edgar Cayce readings, though, should not be viewed as a do-it-yourself doctoring manual. *Any of these suggestions for treatment of disease should be used under the supervision of a professional.*

A.R.E.'s Health Care Professionals Program includes doctors (M.D.s, osteopaths, chiropractors), physical and massage therapists, licensed psychologists, psychiatric social workers and nurses—all A.R.E. members who have agreed to treat clients according to the readings. To use their services A.R.E. members borrow a Circulating File* on a particular ailment and request the names of referred professionals in their locality. The particular member then determines the kind of treatment required and contacts the professional who will help him/her carry out the treatment.

It is well to remember when using *The Physician's Reference Notebook* that so often in the Edgar Cayce readings a patient was told, "either do all of these or none at all!" It is your own physician who should plan a regimen for you which may or may not include various methods suggested in Edgar Cayce's readings for the individuals long ago. That is, some of the recommendations for those other individuals *may not apply to you!* Thus it is imperative that

---

*Circulating Files are collections of verbatim readings and readings extracts selected and arranged by topic. An ongoing research program is constantly adding new subjects to the current collection. Files are available on loan to A.R.E. members.

your own health care professional** study all of the material available and, after diagnosing your condition, prescribe the suitable methods to follow.

Finally, in the concepts of health and healing in the Edgar Cayce readings, one principle that predominates is that the health of the body, mind, and soul are so closely interrelated that it is rarely of value to treat any one of these aspects without also giving some attention to the state of the other two. The reader is reminded that although this volume deals primarily with the physical aspects of health, the mental and spiritual are equally important in a holistic approach to health.

Gladys Davis Turner

** A list of Health Care Professionals in your area is available to A.R.E. members by request from the A.R.E. Membership Department. For membership information write A.R.E., Box 595, Virginia Beach, VA 23451.

INTRODUCTION

Edgar Cayce, over the course of his lifetime, produced a tremendous legacy of information about the human body, its illnesses and means by which health could be achieved once again. Two-thirds of his life's work, more than 9,000 readings, was directed toward individuals who were ill. And, from this extensive source of recorded information, physicians and others who are working with health problems have derived answers that have been meaningful in the lives of their patients.

Cayce talked about the importance of living a life that is in accord with Creative Forces or God. He expounded on the power of the mind and how it may be used creatively. From these readings came the concept that the Spirit is the life, the mind is the builder and the physical is the result.

Yet, Cayce was not one to dwell only on the mind or the value of spiritual qualities. He talked about herbs, about castor oil packs, about inhalants, vitamins and nutrition. He suggested that exercise is of vital importance; that surgery is often life-preserving; that x-rays and x-ray therapy have their useful place in healing; and that the human body is material in its nature and must be given material help.

These readings were usually aimed specifically at individuals rather than at body illnesses. Indeed, often he would describe what was going on inside the body without ever offering what we might call a diagnosis. What he saw was the activity of life forces acting within an ever-changing human organism in such a way that it produced either health or disease. To the unconscious mind of Edgar Cayce, illness was an end-product of disturbed body function that was in all ways interwoven with the mental and spiritual aspects of the total person.

Cayce perceived the individual who experiences a disease process as an eternal being who has lived before and will live again on this plane of existence. Thus, the illness can be a product of present deviation from laws of the human body or it may be a result of karma, the law of cause and effect, from past lifetimes.

From all over the world physicians came to Virginia Beach, attracted by the fascinating way Cayce was able to tune in on any given body and report what was going on inside. Some stayed for a while and a few became interested enough to study this information in depth. The first physician to write a commentary on an illness from the standpoint of the readings was Walter Pahnke, M.D. His work is part of this publication. There have been a number of other writers since, D.O.s and M.D.s, and one commentary on hypoglycemia was written largely by a family nurse practitioner, Edna Germain.

Gradually, over the years, more and more commentaries were written, and became part of a document known as *The Physician's Reference Notebook*. It was made available for members of the Edgar Cayce Foundation's Cooperating Doctors Program. Other commentaries were subsequently written, and they are all drawn together here in book form, which gives information on over 50 conditions of illness in the human body.

The material here is given in such manner that it may be utilized as basic guidance for physicians in treating patients. In this manner, it presents the Cayce material in such a way that a continuing research program can be accomplished.

It should be emphasized, however, that the Edgar Cayce readings were given for individuals and only rarely was a reading intended to give information on a single disease. Multiple sclerosis was one of these. Although difficult to read and understand easily, the language of the Cayce readings was intended for the lay public, rather than for the professional. Thus the information contained in this book can be read and understood and often utilized by almost anyone who wishes to study the material as a student, rather than just as a casual observer.

The commentaries for the most part present functions and therapy as Cayce saw them during the course of his readings. Because of the uniqueness of the language in the readings and the manner in which he "saw" the human body functioning, his approach to understanding the body is accepted as it is given—then, where feasible, correlations are made with information already gained from the scientific study of the body, its ills, and therapy aimed at eradicating these ills.

It is evident that there are a number of very fascinating concepts in these readings which depart rather drastically from generally held concepts in the field of medicine today. These need further study and evaluation.

Because of this approach toward functioning physiology and the relationship Cayce drew between the body, the mind, and the spirit, the idea of holism emerged as a new concept in a 1969 lecture by Dr. James Windsor, and the field of holistic medicine was born.

Much work remains to be done with this material, however. But it does seem to point the observer toward the conclusion that Edgar Cayce was touching on the truth when he offered this information for public use—a truth that conceives of the human being as child of the universe, here on the Earth on an adventure, seeking his way toward both his destiny and his origin, an adventure in consciousness.

William A. McGarey, M.D.
The A.R.E. Clinic, Inc.

THE A.R.E. CLINIC

The A.R.E. Clinic, Inc., in Phoenix, Arizona, offers the best in modern medical care as well as alternative therapies and educational programs. Founded in 1970 by Drs. Bill and Gladys McGarey, the Clinic is a non-profit, tax exempt corporation that initiates formative research into the concepts of holistic healing found in the readings of psychic Edgar Cayce. Patients come from all over the world. Interested persons may contact:

The A.R.E. Clinic, Inc.
4018 North 40th Street
Phoenix, AZ 85018
(602) 955-0551

ACNE

I. Physiological Considerations

Acne is described as an inflammatory disease of the sebaceous glands but more particularly as a chronic inflammatory disease of the sebaceous glands, occurring most frequently on the face, back, and chest. The basic physiological malfunction occurring in the body which gives rise to acne is an imbalance of the eliminating systems of the body, although there are several mechanisms that can play a part in the production of this imbalance. When the eliminations become unbalanced—these being principally through the liver and the kidneys—then the superficial circulation carries a plethora of drosses and metabolic end products which should have been eliminated through the channels of the intestinal tract. This in turn brings about a clogging and a disturbance of the superficial capillary and small lymphatic vessels with subsequent inflammation occurring in the sebaceous glands of the skin.

Some factors causing the eliminative imbalance are incoordination between the deep and superficial circulation, improper diet during the period of menarche (beginning of menses), nervous tensions and suppressions of fears, and glandular reactions and the gradual building of difficulties related to the glands and circulation. Circulatory incoordination is frequently brought about by back injuries, even of a mild nature, which could bring about disturbance of those cerebrospinal centers located in the ganglia of the autonomic nervous system which control the coordination of the deep and the superficial circulations. The deep circulation goes to the organs and functioning portions of the internal part of the body while the superficial circulation supplies the extremities and the peripheral body structures.

In case [78], an injury to the seventh, eighth and ninth dorsals was the primary factor. Perspiration, induced by excitement, originated with the irritation in the dorsal centers. With this irritation any over-excitement makes an extreme call for full circulation (rather than the normal) thus directing too much blood to the superficial circulation. The capillaries and small lymphatics become too full, as it were, producing the excessive perspiration. Inactive eliminations bring impurities to the superficial circulation and thus produce odors which were described as being "obnoxious" and happening in those places where the lymphatic circulation reaches the surface of the body easily. A heavy meal under stress, in this particular case, puts the food in the position of not having adequate blood supply to bring the digestive forces into full action. This brings the external blood in toward the central portions of the body and in this manner causes congestion, especially through those lacteals involved. This produces in turn a reflex which brings about a disturbed elimination with consequent constipation. A capillary uptake of the contents of the large bowel results, and in this manner a loading of the vascular system with substances which should have passed out through the intestines takes place. The skin then attempts to eliminate excessively and this produces the inflammation as a gradual process of time and circumstance. On occasion there may be a thinning of the walls of the intestine which only promotes and intensifies the process.

II. Rationale of Therapy

In approaching therapy, we should remember that the body has a capability of *normal* function:

Thus, we would administer those activities which would bring a normal reaction through these portions, stimulating them to an activity from the body itself, rather than the body becoming dependent upon supplies that are robbing portions of the system to produce activity in other portions, or the system receiving elements or chemical reactions being supplied without arousing the activity of the system itself for a more normal condition.

1968-3

Therapy in the case of acne should be directed at bringing about five principal results:

1. A purification of the vibration of the body forces, which would include a restoration to normal of the thin wall in the intestine.

2. A correction of the cerebrospinal centers and their vibrations,

bringing them back to normal. This would also bring about a coordination of the superficial and deep circulatory systems which is frequently disturbed in acne.

3. A cleansing of the glands of the elimination system such as the liver, kidney, etc.; a balance of these organs and a correction of constipation and difficulties of the lower bowel.

4. A diet in accord with the needs of the circulatory and the elimination systems.

5. Local therapy to aid the skin.

III. Suggested Therapeutic Regimen

1. Acting, in a sense, to purify the vibrations of the body forces and to bring about a change for the better, the following prescription should be followed and all of it used prior to further treatment (aside from diet and local therapy):

> Sulphur, 1 tablespoon
> Rochelle salts, 1 tablespoon
> Cream of tartar, 1 tablespoon

Mix these very thoroughly. Then take a level teaspoonful of this mixture each morning, either in water or dry, before any meal is taken.

2. In order to bring the cerebrospinal control centers, the autonomic, and the sympathetic ganglia to their proper condition, osteopathic therapy should be instituted after the salts have been used but should be given only following a short-wave diathermic treatment to the back for a period of approximately 15 minutes over the upper dorsal area. The combination of these two treatments should be used twice a week for a period of seven weeks, then should be left off for one week, then another cycle should be started using the salts again followed by the physiotherapy and manipulation just described. A third course could be utilized later.

3. A balancing of the glands of the emunctory system—the eliminative organs—could be brought about after the original therapy with the salts has ended. Coca-Cola is suggested as a purifying or clarifying substance for the kidney and bladder. This would be taken more as a medicine than as a soft drink and with water (not carbonated). Various methods of relieving constipation should be utilized—powdered yeast or yeast cake taken daily for ten days and then left off a week would be one such suggested therapy.

The following local treatment and diet may be given to patients. In addition, a combination of oils was suggested in the readings which could be massaged into the skin, perhaps alternating with a medicated cream or lotion: camphorated oil two parts, witch hazel one part, Nujol one part.

Other substances used to bring about a purification of body forces are seen in cases [528] and [78]. Use of these would be up to the judgment of the physician administering the therapy. Atomidine likewise can be used to bring about a glandular balance. These two readings are part of the Circulating File on acne.

Should we not attempt to awaken the inner forces to God's presence? "For, all healing comes from the one source. And whether there is the application of foods, exercise, medicine, or even the knife, it is to bring the consciousness of the forces within the body that aid in reproducing themselves—the awareness of creative or God forces." (2696-1)

William A. McGarey, M.D.

Edgar Cayce readings referenced:
78-2
528-1
1293-2
1576-1
1968-3
4039-1
5092-1

Recommendations

Local Treatment:

1. Wash with prescribed soap twice a day. Rinse off thoroughly and dry. Apply a thin film of medicated cream or lotion.

2. Picking acne lesions is not recommended. Instead take an ice cube, wrap it in a cloth, and freeze the lesion with a corner of the cube for several minutes, two or three times a day. This works best on lesions which have just appeared.

Diet:

1. Take a yeast cake or a packet of dry yeast and blend into eight ounces of tomato or V-8 juice. (You may use other juices if you wish.) A dash of lime juice and Worcestershire sauce adds a little tang in the V-8 mix. Take once a day for 10 days. Then stop for a week and repeat.

2. Obtain some Coca-Cola syrup from a soda fountain. Take one teaspoonful in a glass of *plain* water once or twice a day.

3. No chocolate, sugars, ice cream, pastries, pie, or candy.

4. No carbonated drinks, including diet drinks. No beer or ale.

5. No pork or ham. *Crisp* bacon allowed, however.

6. Limit starches to *one* per meal: bread, rice, potato, spaghetti, corn, etc. No white bread should be eaten.

7. No fried foods. This includes Fritos and potato chips.

8. Vegetables are good for you. Have plenty of salads, vegetable soup, cooked vegetables. Salad dressing is all right.

9. Fruits are fine in season except raw apples, strawberries, and bananas.

10. Meats: Especially recommended are lamb, fish, fowl. *Lean* beef is all right.

11. Milk (skim), eggs, and cheese are allowed.

AMYOTROPHIC LATERAL SCLEROSIS

I. Physiological Considerations

Amyotrophic lateral sclerosis is defined as a degenerative disease of the pyramidal tract and lower motor neurons, characterized by motor weakness and the spastic condition of the limbs associated with muscular atrophy, fibrillary twitching, and final involvement of nuclei in the medulla. It is one of a group of diseases of the motor system of the body, the etiology of which is and continues to be a mystery from the medical standpoint.

The single case included in this file, a 33-year-old man, had symptoms consistent with this definition. His walk was slow and unsteady and he needed crutches. His muscles were twitching and one arm was beginning to atrophy.

In the readings, amyotrophic lateral sclerosis is treated much in the same manner as multiple sclerosis, and the readings give a similar cause in both conditions.

Physiologically, it appears that some factor influences the body's ability to assimilate certain properties through the intestinal tract. In this reading these primary causes are not clarified. Apparently they have something to do with what Cayce in this instance calls karma. In any event, he pictures the lack of assimilation as creating a deficiency of those substances in the bloodstream which will, when they are carried throughout the system, help to replenish and rebuild the nerve and muscle forces which are affected. He sees a necessity for constant rebuilding or regenerating of the cells throughout the body. The nerve cells controlling muscular activity are no exception and he indicates that the lack is so small that it takes a long period of time for disease to manifest.

In the case of multiple sclerosis, the lack was gold. It seems reasonable to assume that here we are also dealing with a lack of gold assimilated in the normal manner through the intestinal tract—through those areas that he often pointed out as being primary in these instances—the lacteals.

The primary deficiency apparently causes, then, a gradual deterioration of anterior horn cells, which then results in deficiency in nerve energies that creates the muscular atrophy. Perhaps this lack contributes to the already present inability of the assimilatory system, by hastening the progress of the disease. The readings described it in one place as a lack of stamina in the nerve and muscle forces of the extremities.

II. Rationale of Therapy

In discussing therapy from this single case, the rationale should be explored to some extent. Much information can be derived from the multiple sclerosis file since Cayce saw so much relationship between the two diseases.

Cayce suggested that, because the disease is of karmic origin, attitudes must be definitely decided upon by the individual—not merely assumed—as to the activities toward divine influences in the body. Where karmic influences are present, Cayce always suggested that attitudes must be definitely changed or no therapeutic results would be seen. He said, "The attitude to be taken should be not merely to be good but to be good for something. The expression of life is of the Divine. The Divine is that influence or force called God. Use same, do not abuse same." (5019-1)

Thus we would see the necessity of mental activity bringing about a change before the physical application of therapy is begun, and this particular portion must be emphasized in each case. One directing the therapy can often not properly assess any changes, but the individual who is ill will know within himself and must face the truth of the statement as seen here in the readings.

Primarily because of the deficiency of gold, the wet cell appliance is used to bring cleansing and healing forces to the body "by the radial activity of the low electrical forces." (5019-1) The gold, then, is given by mouth. It seems reasonable to assume, although not definitely stated in this reading, that gold should be introduced by means of the wet cell appliance in most cases (or perhaps it would have been suggested in a later reading for this particular case had he received a second reading). This would require the clinical appraisal of the condition by the attending physician, and after a two-month period, if there is not progressive improvement, the gold should replace the Atomidine and camphor through the appliance and the Atomidine might then be given by mouth.

In order to introduce at this point a better understanding of the disease process, a complete copy of reading 907-1 follows this commentary. This is on multiple sclerosis specifically but, as already mentioned, probably has a strong bearing on the etiology of amyotrophic lateral sclerosis.

III. Suggested Therapeutic Regimen

Therapy could be divided into five parts, as follows:
1. First things first—mental attitudes
2. Wet cell appliance
3. Massage
4. Gold taken orally
5. Diet

In caring for one's attitudes, not enough can be said. Read Deuteronomy 30 and Exodus 19:5. Then apply these to your life and thinking. Cayce suggested these particularly in all those cases where the trouble was deep-set, and was often seen in association with karma and its physical consequences.

The wet cell with the regular charge was recommended. Two solution jars are to be used: one with Atomidine, one ounce; and distilled water, two ounces. The second contains three ounces of spirits of camphor. These should be alternated, the camphor being used with the attachment at the brachial axis or at the second-third dorsal area of the spine one day; and the Atomidine solution at the fourth lumbar area or the lumbar axis, as Cayce described it, the next day.

Massage should be done gently but thoroughly after the wet cell treatment for a period of 30 to 45 minutes. It should concentrate on the spinal areas but should start at the toes and proceed upward, including all extremities. The sciatic center, the lumbar axis, and the brachial center should be attended to especially, using a mixture of olive oil (two ounces), peanut oil (two ounces), and lanolin (¼ ounce, melted).

Every third day, one drop of each of the following solutions should be added to ½ glass of water and taken immediately: gold chloride solution, one grain per ounce of distilled water; and bromide of soda solution, two grains per ounce of distilled water.

The diet should be low in carbohydrates, and there should be nothing in it containing alcohol. An alkaline-forming diet should be followed rather consistently.

As mentioned earlier, it would be wise to incorporate into the treatment some of the information found in the more extensive Circulating Files on multiple sclerosis. Most often gold chloride was given via the wet cell appliance. In some instances it was also taken orally. Thus, after two months, if regular improvement is not noted, the gold chloride should be started in the solution jar by means of the wet cell appliance. In this instance the attachment of the copper plate should be at the ninth and tenth dorsals in the spine one day, and at the fourth lumbar the next day. When this is begun, Atomidine should be given by mouth in a series that would be best suited to the individual. This would be up to the clinical judgment of the physician. Atomidine has been used in doses of one drop per day for five days, then left off for a period of time, then taken again. It has been given one drop a day for five days, then four drops a day for five days, and then five drops a day for five days. Then it would be left off for a period of one to three weeks, then resumed in the same manner. It has been given beginning with two drops the first day, three drops the second, and so forth on up to ten drops on the ninth day. Then it is decreased one drop per day until the original dose of two drops is reached. Then a rest of several days and the procedure is repeated.

As all of these factors are brought together into a course of therapy, it must be understood that they need to be followed for a long period of time in order to achieve proper results. In nerve lesions and rebuilding of nerve tissue, it is only reasonable to assume that a period of time somewhere between one and three to five years would probably be involved in such a case.

With the rather distressing prognosis to be found in this particular disease, there would be no reason to cease using a program that is constructive in its approach.

Do these, as we have indicated. . .Not as rote, but knowing that within self must be found that which may be awakened to the *building* of that necessary for the body, mentally and physically and spiritually, to carry *its* part in this experience. For the application of any influence must have that which is of

the divine awakening of the activative forces in every atom, every cell of a living body.   **726-1**

William A. McGarey, M.D.

Edgar Cayce readings referenced:
907-1
5019-1

Reading 907-1

Mrs. Cayce: You will have before you the request from Dr. C.G.T. of. . .New York, New York, for a research reading on the disease known as multiple sclerosis. You will consider the following statement from Dr. T.: "The material pathology of multiple sclerosis is a disease of nerve fibres in the spinal cord and brain. The insulating sheaths of these fibres are evidently attacked by some destructive agent which causes them to 'melt away' and be replaced by fibrous tissue." Please answer the following questions.

Mr. Cayce: In giving the true pathological condition, as we find this condition of the spinal cord and of the brain is rather the result of conditions which arise in the assimilating system from the lack of a balance in the hormones of the blood supply.

And it is then a nerve condition, but *impoverished* from the lack of this condition in the bloodstream, or the glandular forces as supply from the system those elements necessary to give the elasticity or that activity which is necessary.

Then this is the source, and the condition in the spinal cord and brain is the effect of that called multiple sclerosis.

The condition, of course, in each individual may be said to be a law unto itself. This, to be sure, is dependent upon that influence from which the activity of the first cell is taken in a body or entity.

Now as the nerve system is that channel through which the atomic energies, or electronic atomic energies pass for activity, there is then the lack of certain elements within the system and in the abilities of the body to produce through the activity of the assimilating system that of *gold.*

Ready for questions.

Q-1. Is this condition produced by an unbalanced diet, or functional failure of glands?

A-1. A combination! For as has just been indicated, in determining the factor as to whether this is a glandular or a diet condition, there must be the *history* of the case itself considered, and the effect there has been upon the parentage as to the sufficient amount of the cellular force *about* each of those atomic forces as go to make up the first cell—or the first foetus itself.

Q-2. If it is a case of unbalanced foods, what should be added?

A-2. This depends upon the progress of it. But as has been

indicated, it is then the effect of gold—the atomic effect of gold that should be added to the system.

Q-3. Which glands are involved?

A-3. Those about the liver and gall duct.

Q-4. What is the nature of the process of the breaking down of the sheaths of these nerve fibres?

A-4. Nerve fibre is both positive and negative, or both white and gray matter, as it passes through the activity of the system. When there is a deficiency of that which supplies to the negative or positive force, there is a drain then that begins upon the system. And as there is the lack of those elements that give stamina or energy to the activity of that portion, it begins first then in those forms of a drain or strain and these *gradually* then take away or they dissolve, or their cells instead of being round in their nature become elongated and gradually pull apart. Thus, the system attempting to build resistance from same causes the losing of the use of any of the energies necessary to replenish same. It's a *wasting* away.

Q-5. Describe the original process which begins in the liver and gall bladder area.

A-5. The cellular force here, or the glandular activity, draws from the spleen, pancreas, and the juices or the excretory functioning of the liver, in the activity of assimilation with the drainage forces from the lacteals.

This, then, lacking in the energies, gradually builds conditions that become hardening forces; which form in that connection between the gall duct, itself, *and* the activity to the larger glands in their assimilation such that a hardening of that portion begins.

Then these gradually act upon the nerve system; by first, as it were, the loss of memory for the moment, then the conditions that may be set up either in the lower portion of the spinal cord or that about the brush end, and those activities gradually increase until they affect or move along the cord itself (in a portion of same) to the brain. And these begin then in the activity upon the use of various portions of the system.

Q-6. Is any outside agent or germ involved in this process?

A-6. We do not find it so. Rather is it the lack of keeping the proper balance about each cell in its division as it increases in its activity.

Q-7. Is this a lack of nerve energy to this particular cell, or a poison which is forming and attacks?

A-7. A poison, naturally. The lack of there being sufficient [nerve energy] makes for a poison to other cells about the original, or the central forces of such activity.

Q-8. What can be done to prevent this disease?

A-8. Keeping a nominal balance of those things in the system that make for keeping the normal balance of the elements or the metals for the system.

Most of these may be tested, especially from the spermatozoa.

Q-9. What is meant by that last statement? Please explain.

A-9. The reproductive glands first become noticed, as to the lack of those elements for reproduction. Then when these are discovered—a lacking in these—there would be the addition then of the gold necessary.

Q-10. Is this best to be given vibratorially, or taken internally?

A-10. Vibratorially is always better for *any* that is a preventive or a destructive force to those influences from within a cellular activity.

Q-11. What general steps should be taken in curing it?

A-11. As has been indicated, or may be drawn from an analysis of that just indicated, there should be the proper distribution. This, of course, depends upon very much the advanced stage of the condition. This is presupposing that it's taken with the first symptoms, see? or the beginning of sterility, or the inactivity from the system as it may be called. The adding then of those vibratory forces as combined with the elements in the diet would be to make for sufficient of gold, silver, and iron in the bloodstream.

Q-12. What suggestions may be given now as to further research readings on this subject through this channel? And explain for Dr. T.'s benefit the source of the information given here.

A-12. This may be taken by first the examinations of that as we have just indicated, and as to how it checks with those conditions existent in the varying stages of that which has been called multiple sclerosis. Then those questions relative to the conditions as they advance, or the effect which has been and is created in the various stages upon individual cases. Then there may be asked for that as would clarify same in the mind of one desirous of making application of information that might be given.

Sources—the universal consciousness.

We are through for the present.

ANEMIA

I. Physiological Considerations

Anemia, as a disease process, does occur as an isolated event; more frequently, however, it is part of clinical conditions which are ill-defined. Wherever there is a languidness, a debilitation, an excessive tiredness that might only loosely be associated with another defined illness, some degree of anemia is usually concomitant.

The readings see an insufficient number or vitality of red blood cells as being closely related to the white blood cells and their makeup, or to assimilation as a whole. Production of new red blood cells occurs mainly within the bone marrow by "coagulation." It is, in effect, the same process that is going on throughout the entire body in the rebuilding process of all cells. Iodine seems to be critical in the process of activating the glands to function normally, and when these glands are given the proper vitamins, the hormones then work with the substances brought through the system via the red cells, the plasma and the white cells to produce structure out of energy. The lymphocytes carry many necessary substances from the Peyer's patches and release this material at the site of construction.

We can visualize how any one of a number of factors might suppress the basic makeup of the bone marrow and result in anemia: decreased intake of iodine, or vitamins, or necessary food substances, as assimilated properties; or any condition within the lymphatics; or circulation which becomes toxic; or any glandular imbalance; or any pathology of the lung.

The thyroid, closely associated with iodine, is frequently an etiologic factor in anemia through malfunction. Faulty eliminations come into play as a factor; the incoordination between the adrenal glands and the lacteal area of the Peyer's patches; catarrhal conditions in the digestive tract affecting assimilation; and the other factors already mentioned.

The vital production of red cells can perhaps be better understood from the standpoint of the readings if we look at several quotations:

First, we find the *blood supply* is deficient in its quality as well as in the quantity; deficient in the red blood count as well as the white, yet the attempts of the body to keep a normal balance prevent...the condition from becoming acute.   726-1

...not as sufficient as of the red blood supply in the system as there should be, though [through?] coagulation; that is, the coordinating of red blood and white blood is good. The rebuilding or the reserve energy in red blood is not sufficient.   4596-1

...this inability of the system to produce proper coagulations through the very infectious forces of the activities of the glandular system, as related to those activities through the glands above the kidneys—as coordinant with the glands about the lacteals...
Q-1. Is there an infection in the bloodstream?
A-1. As has been indicated, rather an incoordination *between* the glandular forces that create the plasm for the blood supply; that is, between the lacteals and the adrenals.   1502-1

When asked what caused the weakness of the body, this answer followed:

...the inability of the forces in the glandular system and the blood supply for creating a greater quantity of blood cells. You see, the red blood cells are made within the bone. Well, the bone doesn't work, because of the shocks to same—the marrow has been in a state lacking proper nutriment.   3193-1

It can be seen that the assimilation through the upper intestinal tract, the normal function of the glands of the system, the integrity of the bone marrow, and the purifying of the system through proper eliminations all contribute in a major fashion to a normal red blood supply.

II. Rationale of Therapy
In approaching therapy, we should remember that the body has a capability of *normal* function:

Thus, we would administer those activities which would bring a normal reaction through these portions, stimulating them to an activity from the

body itself, rather than the body becoming dependent upon supplies that are robbing portions of the system to produce activity in other portions, or the system receiving elements or chemical reactions being supplied without arousing the activity of the system itself for a more normal condition.

1968-3

The basic aims to be taken in seeking a therapeutic result are four in number.

1. The eliminations and assimilations normally are coordinate in their activities; better-than-usual elimination needs to be maintained.

2. The diet should be adequate. This brings all essential food elements to that portion of the body which assimilates them if its health is proper.

3. Assimilation is dependent on the nervous system, the health of the Peyer's patches, and the glandular tissue involved. This needs to be brought to a good level of health.

4. The final step is making sure the bone marrow is functioning properly.

These corrections properly balanced in their application should bring a better functioning production of red cells to the body.

III. Suggested Therapeutic Regimen

Open air, sunshine, and exercise should be a part of each therapeutic regimen, according to the general level of health of the individual.

Diet should include food of an alkaline-reacting nature: vegetables in abundance, fruit and often tuberous vegetables with beef or beef juice (see Appendix), pigs' knuckles or pigs' feet. While these don't sound particularly appetizing, they contribute to blood building. Broiled liver and such meats are recommended, but nothing fried. Fish is suggested, but not shellfish.

Balancing the eliminations with the assimilations may be begun with colonics where necessary. Good eliminations are vitally important to prevent reabsorption of refuse into the bloodstream and subsequent suppression of function in the assimilations of the body.

The assimilations are stimulated as well as brought into a balance with eliminations through the use of manipulations and adjustments. These would vary in their nature, dependent upon the individual and his needs. But often the area of the seventh dorsal to the second lumbar will need special attention. Assimilation is aided sometimes in the presence of excess acidity in the stomach through the use of medication such as Milk of Magnesia or Milk of Bismuth. Ventriculin (see Appendix), with or without iron, and other enzymes also assist when the need is present to improve the assimilation of the upper intestinal tract. Courses of Atomidine are needed wherever glandular malfunction appears. These may be given over five days with two drops in a half glass of water morning and evening. This dosage might be decreased but should not be increased appreciably. The Atomidine should not be taken during a rest period from other therapy.

The bone marrow is best stimulated with infrared lamp treatments 20 to 30 minutes at a time twice a week over the bone structures where red blood cell synthesis is going on. These should be coordinated with the osteopathic adjustments—that is, they should be taken at the same time if possible and taken over a period of five or six weeks with a rest and then another series.

Patience and perseverance seem to be the key words in this particular disease process. As the glandular system becomes more balanced and as the assimilations and eliminations are more perfected in their functioning, the regeneration of the red cells becomes more adequate and the whole individual then comes into a better state of health.

Should we not attempt to awaken the inner forces to God's presence? "For, all healing comes from the one source. And whether there is the application of foods, exercise, medicine, or even the knife, it is to bring the consciousness of the forces within the body that aid in reproducing themselves—the awareness of creative or God forces." (2696-1)

William A. McGarey. M.D.

Edgar Cayce readings referenced:

137-9, 86	3191-1
264-39, 40	3538-1
288-16	4164-1
726-1	4596-1
1503-1	4821-1
1779-1 through 5	5503-1

ANGINA PECTORIS

I. Physiological Considerations

The immediate, apparent physiological cause of the condition we know of as angina pectoris is in nearly all cases an imbalance between the central or deep circulation and the superficial circulation. The latter is the supply of blood to the extremities and the superficial portions of the body, while the central or deep circulation is that which is supplied to the internal organs. In the case of angina the blood supply to the liver, to the lungs, and to the heart are closely related.

The control and the balance achieved between these two circulations are located in the sympathetic ganglia in the upper dorsal region. The control of the blood flow through the liver, the lungs, and the heart lies in a nerve plexus in the aorta. This certainly is also under a higher control from the sympathetic ganglia.

It can be seen that anything which would disturb the balance which is normally achieved between the cerebrospinal and the autonomic nervous systems would in turn cause a disturbance of the circulation if this imbalance had occurred in the upper dorsal area. The disturbance in the case of angina would cause an excess of blood flow to the heart, liver, and lungs particularly with a cessation or a diminished blood flow to the extremities of the body, thus often causing the feet to be cool or cold.

Accumulations or end products of metabolism throughout the circulatory system can create problems in cells throughout the body which in turn cause a lowering of function of what these cells may contribute toward control over the circulation. Undoubtedly other factors must be present, many of which are not known. The cycle of events which lead up to severe angina pectoris associated with congestive failure sometimes is quite extensive.

In case [1071] we see an overactivity mentally and physically causing a disturbed mental association which in turn led to a nervous breakdown. This caused congestions in the eliminative system, particularly engorgement in the transverse and descending colon. This engorgement produced pressures on the heart activity itself. Then these conditions produced assimilative dysfunction with gastric fermentation and an improper flow from the lacteals, the acids of the stomach wall, and the pyloric region apparently involving the pancreas. This disturbance in assimilation then created a kidney malfunction and more specific trouble in the liver. The decrease in liver function then produced an increase in the heart, lung, and liver circulation and an overburdening of these with an increased flow to the brain which produced a numbness of the brain and the lack of proper impulses stemming from the brain tissue. This in turn created more poisons through improper metabolism throughout the system, damaging cells, blood vessels, and lacteals throughout the body so that they in turn could not produce the activities needed to increase the blood flow to the extremities and away from the heart. Apparently these cells throughout the body have an influence on the sympathetic ganglia that basically control or balance the deep and the superficial circulation.

Occasionally a lesion in the brachial area of the spine will cause pressure which produces a weakness to the upper extremities, to the head and the stomach, that results from a cessation of deep blood flow after exercise. In this particular case the blood flow would be away from the heart and to the extremities. In case [5076] there were purpuric areas throughout the body which apparently came about due to the engorgement of the peripheral circulation.

Thus the physiology of angina involves the assimilative and eliminative systems, the circulatory system in maintaining a balance, the nervous systems in their balance between the cerebrospinal and the autonomic and various control centers in the sympathetic nervous system itself. It also involves a close relationship between the liver, lungs, and heart and attributes great importance to the cells of the body itself in maintaining a balance.

II. Rationale of Therapy

The attempt to correct angina pectoris would require first a determination whether the deep circulation was engorged or deficient in the imbalance which undoubtedly exists. Attention must be paid to the intestinal tract, to determine that the toxins—the end products of metabolism—are removed and the elimination is good. A balance should be achieved between the nervous systems, and subluxations of vertebrae should be corrected if present. Assimilation should improve as eliminations are corrected. However, other means might be required if the assimilations are not proper.

It would always be advisable physiologically to bring about the changes in the balance gradually and gently. If these variations from normal are gradually corrected, then the angina will disappear.

III. Suggested Therapeutic Regimen

In all cases a cleansing of the colon—"the poisons *must* be taken away"—should be accomplished. A high colonic once a month perhaps could be taken as the standard with deviations according to what appears to be needed clinically. Eliminations should normally come daily for the patient.

Diet should be a normal one. Whole grain bread should be taken. Basically, white sugar and white flour should not be used. No concentrated vitamins should be added.

Medication: Atomidine was suggested to assist in balancing the circulations and this could be used one drop in a half glass of water daily for five days, leave off for five days and repeat this course three to five times as indicated. After a period of time without the Atomidine, another course of treatment could be instituted. Local therapy for the extremities was recommended—in case [1071] massage of the feet, knees, and entire lower extremities was advised twice a day to increase the circulation in the extremities. The combination used was as follows:

> Olive oil
> Compound tincture of benzoin, equal parts sufficient
> to make two ounces
> Add oil of mustard, 5 drops

The wet cell appliance was suggested for a patient who was *in extremis.* It was not obtained for two weeks, and the patient died before it could be used.

Osteopathic therapy to the brachial area or deep massage was recommended where subluxation had occurred; and for this particular individual it was suggested once a week for 30 weeks or twice a week for 10 weeks in order to restore the subluxation to normal. Short-wave diathermy was suggested prior to the adjustment.

William A. McGarey, M.D.

Edgar Cayce readings referenced:
85-1
1010-22
1071-1
2046-3
5076-1

APHONIA

I. Physiological Considerations

The occurrence of aphonia—or the lack of ability to speak either partially or completely—can be better understood as a physiological process if we briefly explore the makeup of the nervous system. There are basically three nervous systems. The cerebrospinal controls conscious movements and includes in its makeup the frontal portion of the brain and the spinal cord. The autonomic nervous system (Cayce calls this the "sympathetic") supplies various organs functioning at an unconscious level. It may be understood as being the nervous system of the unconscious mind. And the sensory nervous system involves the nerve supply associated with the organs of sense. These are all considered part of one unit collectively.

The three nervous systems have their contact with each other and maintain a balance and a coordination one with the other at all times within that state we call health. Lymphatic patches, apparently within bursae found in certain of the sympathetic ganglia, parallel the various levels of the spinal column. These patches of lymph tissue and fluid become the means by which proper synaptic relationship is maintained between the three nervous systems. Substances of a "globular" nature are manufactured in the Peyer's patches of the small intestine and carried by the lymphocytes to these patches, maintaining coordination between the autonomic and the cerebrospinal nervous systems; and these in turn maintain a balance with the sensory forces of the body.

In aphonia, the centers of association and control are located at the second and third dorsal ganglia, for the most part, with relationships also with the third to the fifth cervical ganglia. The condition of aphonia develops in various manners but nearly always involves these centers just mentioned. Lesions may occur in the patches found in the ganglia, and sometimes may interfere with proper coordination and at other times become actually atrophied. In some instances a general increase of nerve tension throughout the system, often associated with fear, creates lesions in these areas with subsequent overflows of impulses throughout the entire nervous system. "The body gives away, as it were, to feelings over the whole system." This taut condition of the nervous centers results in a circulation through the body which is abnormal or in a sense distorted, and other secondary effects come about involving the lymphatic circulation and the emunctory (excretory) organs. If the conditions are proper, however, the changes in the ganglia bring about an aphonia or a loss of function of the vocal cords because of the incoordination—and at the same time affect sensory organs such as hearing or vision.

Injuries seem to be the cause of aphonia rather frequently—minor injuries which affect the second and third dorsal area in such a manner that the lymph patches concerned with coordination become either atrophic or relatively nonfunctioning.

Poor eliminations can bring about disturbances and sometimes are the primary cause of aphonia; this build-up of wastes within the bloodstream becomes a toxic force and makes it necessary for the body to achieve its own balance after a lapse of time. When this comes about, the throat and larynx area might be disassociated in function from the rest of the body, and the forces there bring about local inflammation in an effort to achieve balance. Fear also is often a concomitant and a contributor.

Psychological causes are mentioned, and in case [294] the following quotation is of interest: "In this manner direct do we find that the variation comes between the natural physical voice and that when in the condition at the present time, for we find the variation is reflected in the manner of speech, for speech is the highest vibration that is reached in the animal kingdom, and in that respect man in his evolution is above that of the other creatures in the creation." (294-11)

Not only is the general circulation involved sometimes in toxic forces and thus in the disturbance, but also the lymphatic, the emunctory, and the hepatic circulations are involved and affected.

II. Rationale of Therapy

In approaching therapy, we should remember that the body has a capability of *normal* functions:

Thus, we would administer those activities which would bring a normal reaction through these portions, stimulating them to an activity from the body itself, rather than the body becoming dependent upon supplies that are robbing portions of the system to produce activity in other portions, or the system receiving elements or chemical reactions being supplied without arousing the activity of the system itself for a more normal condition.

1968-3

Therapy should first be aimed at correcting those conditions which might produce a disturbance in the centers of coordination between the three nervous systems. Then the overtaxed nerve forces of the body as a whole should be relieved, the incoordination which has been a factor in the disease process should be eliminated, and the forces of the body should be coordinated. The diet should be corrected and sufficient stimulus of a medicinal nature should be added to keep the body in a normal force. Some cases that are psychological—where the body is amenable to suggestion—would benefit by suggestive therapy. Attention should be paid to attitudes of mind and to ideals.

III. Suggested Therapeutic Regimen

General therapy should first be aimed at a cleansing of the system with special reference to the hepatic circulation. Castor oil packs and Epsom salt packs were used, as in case [579], where the problem was primarily one of elimination. Hydrotherapy and enemas are useful in this respect.

Osteopathic manipulations and neuropathic manipulations are both recommended, but in differing degrees. Hypersensitive nervous systems must be handled cautiously and gently. Two or three courses of these manipulations, whichever seems most indicated, should be used. A good general diet is suggested except where eliminations are particularly a problem. In this case juices should be taken—probably citrus juices mostly—until cleansing is well on its way.

Where there was a high degree of nervous tension with a "taut condition of nervous centers" (12-1) the following medication was to be used each evening prior to the neuropathic manipulation:

> Muriate of ammonia, 30 grains
> Gum camphor, 20 grains
> Sulfate morphia, 2 grains

Directions: Make 20 pellets. Use one daily each evening.

For this case the prescription was intended to give sufficient stimulus of a medicinal nature to keep the body in natural force. Other medications were not given.

Hypnosis was mentioned but was to be used only as a last resort. Suggestion was used on [294]. Instruction was also given to read the 30th chapter of Deuteronomy and the 14th, 15th, 16th and 17th chapters of John. "Meditate daily upon the use of voice, of mind and of actions in being of material, mental, spiritual aid to others." (12-1) It would be well to stay in the open and be close to nature.

Should we not attempt to awaken the inner forces to God's presence? "For, all healing comes from the one source. And whether there is the application of foods, exercise, medicine, or even the knife, it is to bring the consciousness of the forces within the body that aid in reproducing themselves—the awareness of creative or God forces." (2696-1)

William A. McGarey, M.D.

Note: Cayce used the word "neuropathic" in reference to neuropathic treatments as meaning specific therapy given by a "neuropath," one apparently qualified to massage or treat in a certain manner. *Dorland's Medical Dictionary* gives "neuropathist" as being a neurologist, a specialist in the field of neurology. Neuropath or neuropathic are not defined as referring to any person who treats the nervous system.

Edgar Cayce readings referenced:
12-1
294-11
579-1
2696-1
2929-1
3002-1
3164-1
5708-1

APOPLEXY

Apoplexy—or apoplectic stroke—is medically known to be a sudden collapse with partial or complete paralysis on one side, usually associated with high blood pressure. In the benign form, there is a spasm or a minor hemorrhage in the brain tissue. In the malignant form, on the other hand, there is sudden massive hemorrhage in the brain tissue causing a sudden loss of consciousness and coma.

I. Physiological Considerations

Apoplexy is a disease process primarily involving the whole circulatory system, but including the makeup of the cells and substances within the blood, the flow, the circulation, the pressures within the circulation, and the integrity of the vessel walls. Apparently the control of the circulatory system lies within the sympathetic nervous system throughout its entire length from the coccygeal nerves up to the medulla oblongata. And this control includes not only the balancing or the coordinating between the deep and the superficial circulation, but extends even to the maintenance or control of the platelets or the tendency to form clots; the production of the other formed elements (the white and red cells) within the circulatory system; and the production of those substances which control the integrity of the walls of the veins and the arteries.

In case [1187], a "break" had been brought about in the "cellular force" of the circulatory system, from the area of the lumbar axis of the sympathetic ganglia. This woman, 56 years of age, had been very busy throughout her life doing much heavy work, carrying and moving objects, in addition to bearing eight children. The weakness induced by these activities in the lumbar area contributed in a major manner to this imbalance and a breaking in the functioning of the platelets, or that which might be called the "cellular forces."

Those factors which underlie the creation of this circulatory condition are accumulations of poisons throughout the liver, spleen, and pancreas brought on by poor eliminations; improper diet and assimilation; and overexertion—too much for the body to stand. Incoordination of the deep and superficial circulatory systems is by itself at times a major contributing cause.

As pressures and tensions increase within the body, varying conditions are produced dependent upon the existing health of the body that is involved. There might be swelling or distention or expansion of the arteries (aneurysm); or disturbances of the lower spinal cord centers of the locomotor control which exist in the lumbar area for the legs and in the cervical area for the arms; or weakening of the vessels in the brain with minimal or massive bleeding in the brain tissue.

The increased pressures throughout the vascular system may cause various symptoms, such as shortness of breath or pain in the heart area.

When the pressure occurs through hemorrhage in the brain tissue, brain activity ceases at that level and an incoordination between the higher and the lower areas appears, causing a nonactivity in the locomotor centers. If a clot forms, injury usually takes place sufficient to produce a much more resistant paralysis than if the bleeding is minimal.

It is important to remember, in considering the physiology involved here, that the functioning of the extremities and what are called the locomotor facilities are not completely dependent upon the brain. If the locomotor centers of control are brought back to a balance after a stroke, full function should be restored if the injury to the brain was not severe enough to bring about death. The balance of function between the circulatory system, the sympathetic nervous system and the locomotor centers is a critical factor here.

II. Rationale of Therapy

In approaching therapy, we should remember that the body has a capability of *normal* function:

Thus, we would administer those activities which would bring a normal reaction through these portions, stimulating them to an activity from the body itself, rather than the body becoming dependent upon supplies that are robbing portions of the system to produce activity in other portions, or the

system receiving elements or chemical reactions being supplied without arousing the activity of the system itself for a more normal condition.

1968-3

Therapy for a stroke must be started at the point it is discovered or presented. It is certainly not always possible to determine from external signs and symptoms how extensive bleeding might be or the exact factors that are involved in producing the condition.

Treatment for an acute case of apoplexy without loss of consciousness would need to be approached in a slightly different manner than one which has complete loss of consciousness. Similarly, the individual who has recovered from a stroke and has residual symptoms of paralysis typical of the condition, would need still further changes in procedure. This can be seen by reading case [1187] (5 through 9), a series of readings, in which consciousness was not lost and bleeding was probably not massive. There was some paralysis. Case [1097], on the other hand, had had a stroke seven months earlier and had definite brain damage with paralysis. [1425] illustrates still a third type with sudden loss of consciousness due to hemorrhage, which was described in the reading as being a leakage or seepage from the deeper circulation of the brain.

There are several basic fundamentals of therapy, however, which seem to undergird the therapeutic regimen which might be followed:

1. Keep the circulation from progressing to a more toxic and unbalanced condition.

2. Eliminate poisons that have accumulated in the circulatory system of the body and stimulate eliminations.

3. Remove pressures on the sympathetic centers and the locomotory centers.

4. Aid the body in rebuilding to normal.

If these fundamentals can be kept in mind, progress can be considered in bringing adequate therapy to the individual.

III. Suggested Therapeutic Regimen

Certainly attitudes of mind are important, and if the individual afflicted has no real desire to regain good health and is not willing to be persistent, consistent, and patient, little can be done.

The following are some general measures. The manners in which therapeutic aims are achieved vary in the readings, yet are related. For [592], enemas, tub baths, sweats, and rubs—with a half peanut oil and half olive oil mixture, or half peanut oil and half pine oil—were recommended, the rubs to be applied to the areas affected and to the spine. No further clarification was given in this particular case. However, for [1425], several treatments were advised with more complete directions:

1. Paint over the spine from the second and third cervical areas to the sixth dorsal with a solution made up of laudanum three parts, aconite one part.

2. Then apply hot saturated Epsom salts pack; keep on until it is cold (which would take about 45 minutes). This should be done twice a day.

3. Each day after the packs, osteopathic treatments, especially in the ninth dorsal and the fourth lumbar plexus areas. General osteopathic treatment for eliminations or daily high enemas should be used to remove fecal forces. Water should be at body temperature, half a gallon in amount with salt and soda—one teaspoonful each—added.

The therapy suggested in case [1187] varied from reading to reading and was extremely complicated. It involved enemas, keeping the lower extremities warm, massages, osteopathic treatments, and withholding narcotics. Massaging should be done away from the head toward the extremities.

It would seem that a general therapeutic regimen for acute apoplexy would involve:

1. Enemas as described above, perhaps two or three times the first day and daily thereafter.

2. Osteopathic treatments to bring about a balance in the sympathetics and to stimulate elimination. This should be done gently at first and more vigorously as healing progresses.

3. Balancing of the body as would seem to be best indicated through either painting the skin, followed by Epsom salts hot packs, or massage of the spine and extremities in a general manner as typified by case [1187]. As strength is regained activity should be increased.

Diet: Very light foods should be utilized at first, such as juices, coddled egg and toast or food well cooked, as in a broth. As strength returns, the patient may take simple foods. There should be no fried foods, no pork, no white flour or white sugar substances. Spaghetti, tomatoes, and white bread should never be combined. Fish, fowl, and lamb are the best meats. Cereals should never be taken the same day as citrus fruit juices.

Case [1097] gives a good summary of treatment that was suggested for one paralytic who had not followed prior advice and who wished to regain function of his muscles.

Should we not attempt to awaken the inner forces to God's presence? "For, all healing comes from the one source. And whether there is the application of foods, exercise, medicine, or even the knife, it is to bring the consciousness of the forces within the body that aid in reproducing themselves—the awareness of creative or God forces." (2696-1)

William A. McGarey, M.D.

Edgar Cayce readings referenced:
592-5
1097-7
1103-5
1187-5 through 9
1211-3
1254-1
1407-1
1425-1
3417-1

ARTERIOSCLEROSIS

Arteriosclerosis is presently understood as a condition wherein accumulations or plaques in the walls of arteries impede the blood flow and cause a relative lack of oxygen to the areas supplied by those arteries. These plaques have their origin, it is thought, in the faulty metabolism of cholesterol and other fatty acids.

Since these changes can occur in any part of the arterial vascular system, it can be readily understood that they often play a causative role in cerebrovascular accidents (strokes), myocardial infarcts (heart attacks), and various other conditions where the blood supply is markedly reduced.

From the material in the Edgar Cayce readings, however, an entirely different approach is suggested in considering the etiology and therapy of what we know as arteriosclerosis.

Cayce gave a life reading for a 65-year-old woman who was a highly developed spiritual being. Her reading mentioned that she had been in the Promised Land at the time of Jesus, was taught and even healed by the Master. But the reading dealt mostly with her physical body, because it became evident that the physical must be worked with according to the laws of this environment—no matter how spiritual a person might be. This woman had a degree of arteriosclerosis, and Cayce had much to say about it. For almost everyone, however, the following extract would undoubtedly be important:

These are affectations through the body using up the strength and vitality without taking proper precautions as for the resuscitating of the physical forces through the character of the diet and the manner that the body responds to physical conditions in a material world. . .the physical is in a material world and is subject to the laws of same. . .   **509-2**

Also, in this instance, resuscitation had not been accomplished by directing the material, mental, or spiritual forces for "the recuperation of these conditions."

We would look, then, for causes that affect the activities, the functions, the life support systems of the physical body; and we might suspect that these readings would suggest a treatment program that would tend to precipitate a balancing and a normal function to these same systems.

I. Physiological Considerations

In arteriosclerosis we find causes arising from many sources, as described in the Cayce material. When one abnormal function is aided and abetted by another, symptoms appear, and what we call pathology occurs.

In the case of [509], symptoms had developed over a period of time: sensation of heat in the abdominal area, coldness of hands and feet, fluctuations in the appetite, changes in the way her food tasted, gnawing in the lower portion of the stomach, and a twitching in the lower portion of her jaw near the salivary glands. She also had urinary symptoms and difficulty with her bowels.

According to Cayce's description, however, problems had developed in several areas. First, the adrenal glands were under stress and the woman's emotions had become disturbed. Then, bladder irritations developed, liver-kidney malfunctions appeared, and albumen spilled over in the urine; also irritation in the urethra, then subsequently circulatory disturbances. In the past a lumbosacral "wrench" had not been corrected, which—along with the other developments—produced a gradual hardening of the arterial circulation. This, in turn, caused "prolapsus" of the colon and sphincter muscle irritation. A sequence of events with a group of pathological conditions arose, in the midst of which we find arteriosclerosis.

For a 52-year-old man, [1630], the sequence was different. Improper eliminations and assimilations were the first difficulties here. These were minor and thus neglected; but poisons stemming from eliminatory problems created certain physiological imbalances, disturbing the heart and circulatory forces. Then there arose a general condition with the liver and the eliminating system. Finally, an abnormal blood pressure developed and a slowing and hardening of the arterial circulation, which hindered the circulatory forces among the heart, liver, and kidneys.

Cayce mentioned that a neglected dorsal and cervical subluxation began the whole series of events, creating a need for cathartics. The need was eased temporarily but later a greater disturbance occurred throughout the colon—engorgement in the ascending, transverse and descending colon and a near prolapse of the colon. All these brought about an engorgement of the heart's activity without removing the cause.

An encouraging note came when the reading pointed out that all these difficulties need not be detrimental; the system simply needed adjusting. It went on to state, however, that if the adjustment did not take place, a thinning of the arterial walls would result, causing a seepage, a dripping, or a draining which might bring clotting. This condition, in turn, could cause significant damage to the heart or the brain, depending on where a clot might end up if one were to break off.

A common symptom of heart disease that is associated with arteriosclerosis is dypsnea or shortness of breath. Cayce explained this very disabling symptom thus: When conditions affect the heart's activity, a shortness of breath occurs in certain instances with "the deeper circulation, with the system attempting to adjust itself, drawing away from the superficial circulation." (1630-1) Consciousness of the body's parts is always trying to keep life active in the body.

Perhaps the most important thing about the cause of arteriosclerosis is the multiplicity of factors involved. Diagnosis of such a condition is not difficult for the trained physician. To keep in mind its various causes as well as the symptoms and manifested pathology is to make the "adjustment" of the body more logical and more complete—much as was suggested to [509]:

So, in making the application, physically, mentally or materially, to those things that would bring a better balance, all of the effects as well as the causes. . .are to be taken into consideration. **509-2**

II. Rationale of Therapy

In all approaches to therapy, it should be kept in mind that all healing comes from within, as the Divine within is touched and awakened. The mind has a critical part to play in this process, for it is the mind of the ill person which decides to seek for help and, having made that choice, moves toward the possibility of healing. When disturbances are minimal, we often pay no attention to the warning signals and thus miss the opportune time to correct a problem. On the other hand, when troubles are deep-set, there are usually habit patterns that are involved. These habits tend to continue with a mind of their own and are difficult to alter for the better.

As we find, the disturbances are of a deep-seated nature. And while there may be those suggestions for help or aid, these have reached such proportions that—unless there is a great deal of change in the *mental* attitudes, mental outlook—the applications may only be as *helpful* experiences for the activities being carried on. 1050-1

So the mind has to be activated—not only for deep-seated problems, but also for simple difficulties. And the beginning of arteriosclerosis usually involves a simple problem; however, physical treatments are always a necessity even if they only deal with diet.

The treatments most often recommended to those with arteriosclerosis who came to Mr. Cayce for help are designed to bring about a balancing of the body forces.

1. Osteopathic manipulative treatments were most frequently recommended. These were to be directed toward the lumbosacral area, the mid-dorsal, and the upper dorsal (2nd, 3rd, 4th).

2. The diet must always be corrected. Little starch or sugar; lots of vitamin B-1, found in the yellow foods like corn, squash, carrots, oranges and lemons, for instance; no red meats (fish, fowl or lamb instead are suggested); lots of green foods to create an alkaline-reacting diet; well-balanced meals.

3. Massage was suggested, especially alongside the spine, to aid in balancing the neurological impulses. One oil recommended for massage:

Olive oil (heated), 2 ounces
Tincture of myrrh, 2 ounces
Calamus oil, 10 drops

To [3496] instructions were given to concentrate on the 1st, 2nd, and 3rd cervicals and 6th, 7th, 8th, and 9th dorsals and throughout the lumbosacral area during the massage.

4. Colonics were suggested to aid eliminations and to "reduce the tendencies *and* the plethoric condition through the colon. . ." (1630-1) To a 49-year-old man with a serious problem Cayce suggested osteopathic relaxing treatments to be given after the colonics to remove the strain on the heart. (3454-1)

5. Exercise out in the open was a frequent suggestion for those who developed arteriosclerosis. Walking was the most common exercise

recommended. One man wanted to know if he should have surgery for the prostatic condition he had developed—probably due to many of the same influences that had brought about his arteriosclerosis. His wife asked the question:

Q-3. Will operation on prostate gland relieve his lassitude and excessive tiredness?
A-3. This as we find would prove more detrimental than beneficial under the existent conditions. For the very nature of the condition and the pressure is a part of the ileum plexus disturbance.

Then to remove by operative measures and not to remove the causes would only be to transfer the lethargy of activity of impulse to some other portion of the system. Here, it would be more apt to be upon the kidneys; owing to the effect upon eliminations in these directions.   1684-1

Two other individuals had apparently unassociated problems of a serious nature. One was a 61-year-old woman who was hospitalized for mental problems and diagnosed at that time as having a "softening of the brain" or "breaking down of the brain tissue." The cause was attributed to arteriosclerosis. Her suggested therapy was different. (It followed the pattern given often for mental or neurological problems.) The woman, described in the reading as being spiritually minded, was to be taken home, given nursing care for six to eight months, and was urged to assist in administering her own therapy (wet cell battery, colonics, massages, diet) and to build constructive activities in her experience.

Another woman, 60 years of age, had developed Parkinson's disease, brought on partly by hardening of the arteries. She was having throat and breathing problems. Cayce found that not much could be done for her, for when paralysis agitans "affect[s] more the respiratory system and throat, it will be hard to prevent the separation of physical and spiritual body." (5517-1)

In giving information for these problems—for it must be called more than just *one* problem—Cayce sometimes suggested the use of the radio-active appliance, the wet cell battery, Atomidine, and as little medication as possible. For one man who gave little credence to psychic matters, however, he advised that the present medical regimen be continued—although it had not helped a great deal—and recommended the wet cell battery. But he commented that although the medications were doing their part, more therapy was needed plus a change in this man's attitude. (See 1050-1.)

Warnings and Prevention

Prevention is always better than cure. It takes less time out of one's daily activities than does the cure—which may be lengthy, costly in time and money, and often remarkably difficult to obtain. Prevention can be implemented at any stage: It may be begun before a condition even starts or utilized prior to the most severe complications. At such times, prevention becomes therapy. Thus, it can be seen that therapy and prevention are very closely related—especially if one is dealing with the ongoing, life-giving physiological activities of the human body. It is helpful to remember that it is the human being, with all those God-given qualities included, that is involved—not just a disease.

Such was the case with a 65-year-old man who asked for a physical reading in 1938. His was not an acute case but rather long-standing, somewhat complicated and difficult, but able to be corrected.

In giving that as we find which would be the more beneficial for the body, many conditions which have surrounded and do surround the body must be taken into consideration.

While there are disturbing factors, these conditions have not as yet assumed such proportions that they keep or prevent the body from carrying on in a manner; but not as altogether nor always in the most efficient manner.

For as we find, the disturbing factors are those that are of an insidious nature; that is, hidden; and they affect the organs of the body in such a way and manner that at times they are rather just slow in their reaction, or their activity.

And unless there *are* some measures taken to make the corrections, they may of a sudden cease to perform their functioning—or they may, as it were, spill over; or the pressure that is a part of the disturbing conditions, upon the arteries, may become so intense that the very walls may give way or allow seepages. Thus, through such activities, there would be formed clots that would not only become very disturbing but produce conditions of such natures as to prevent the normal activity in locomotion, or in thought.

1684-1

Cayce found that the blood supply from the heart to the liver was engorged, creating at times excessive arterial pressure and thus slowing the venous return to the liver and lungs. The hepatic circulation—liver, spleen, and kidneys—was suppressed. And there was a "sedentary influence" on the body as a result of the nature of the man's life style, in which he exhibited a greater degree of mental rather than physical activity, resulting in a heaviness and stiffness in the lumbodorsal and sacral areas. Imbalances and accumulation of toxic forces resulted in spite of massages and hydrotherapy that he was already receiving. Suggestions included:

1. Continue the massages and hydrotherapy, but do them regularly.

2. Obtain specific *adjustments* for lesions in the lumbar, sacral, and iliac plexus. Coordinate these with pressures in the secondary cardiac area—2nd, 3rd, and 4th dorsals.

3. Use the radio-active appliance one hour a day, preferably just prior to retiring.

4. Get consistent activity out of doors: walking, golfing, riding, handball, the electric horse, the bicycle—any or all of these would be helpful.

5. The diet should not include fried foods or large quantities of fats that are not easily assimilated.

Cayce gave the man a lengthy reading with much helpful data and finished by suggesting that, "These done, and kept in those manners, we find that many years of useful service and activity may be added. *Without* these—not as premonitions but *warnings*—these must not be so long!" (1684-1)

Arteriosclerosis cannot always be cured nor halted in its progression, simply because we are continually dealing with human beings. Some human beings do not want to pay the price of overcoming their illnesses. One woman, whom Cayce saw as not living more than 30 months, illustrates the fact that attitudes can stop all healing procedures, whether of the body, the mind or the spirit.

This woman, only 58 years old, was being treated for myocarditis, coronary artery arteriosclerosis, and hypertension. Her husband was an osteopath, but she had her own doctor and refused to change even if strongly advised to do so. Cayce saw the need to alter her regimen at the physical level, by having her avoid excitement and by being out of doors with lots of fresh air and restful programs that would lessen the strain on her heart. But he also saw that it was not likely to happen and said, "Rather should the mental body keep a balance." (664-1)

His opening remarks pinpoint the reason for the woman's problem and her resistance to change:

Yes, taking the conditions of this body, [664], as we have here, as a pattern

or example, much might be pointed out as to how the environs of a place, house, room or surroundings are changed or produced by the dwelling there of an individual that radiates even distressed conditions from itself.

664-1

On the other hand, the promise that changes can come about is always there, as exemplified in a reading for a 61-year-old woman: "For we can build with these, if there is the correct application of the appliance and the massages, new brain and nerve tissue." (3496-1) It requires the purpose and desire to be strong, the information to be available, and the steps to be applied—in body, mind, and spirit. And patience, persistence, and consistency.

William A. McGarey, M.D.

Edgar Cayce readings referenced:

509-2
664-1
1050-1
1187-11 through 14
1630-1
1684-1
2538-1, 2
3304-1
3454-1
3496-1
5517-1

ARTHRITIS

Nearly all cases of arthritis fall into one of two general classifications which are relatively easily differentiated, although poorly understood.

Atrophic arthritis—more commonly called rheumatoid—has also been given the name of proliferative arthritis or arthritis deformans. This type of disease process is characterized by inflammatory changes in the synovial membranes of the joints, and in the periarticular structures, and by atrophy and rarification of the bones.* In the early stages there is a migratory swelling and stiffness of the joints with a rather typical fusiform swelling of the proximal interphalangeal joints of the fingers. Later on there is deformity with ankylosis and frequently an ulnar deviation of the fingers as a sign of this disease. Subcutaneous nodules are frequent in these patients, and usually the disease is found beginning in young people, more commonly the male than the female. Present are anemia, chronic emaciation, loss of calcium in the bone structures, and the patient is rather severely and chronically ill.

Hypertrophic arthritis gives an entirely different picture. This has been called more commonly osteoarthritis and is known as degenerative or senescent arthritis. In this disease process there is generally no inflammation and no spreading or migratory type of joint involvement. Rather than a loss of calcium, there is a calcium build-up. An example of this is the so-called Heberden's nodes—a swelling and build-up of calcium about the base of the terminal phalanges of both hands. In osteoarthritis, there are calcific spurs and

---

*See Cecil, R.: *Diseases of the Joints, R. Cecil's Textbook of Medicine,* 5th ed. Philadelphia and London: W.B. Saunders Co., 1942, pp. 1408-1435. See also Robinson, W.D.: *Diseases of the Joints, Cecil and Loebe Textbook of Medicine,* 12th ed. Philadelphia and London: W.B. Saunders Co., 1967, pp. 1390-1420.

there is deformity of the joints, but never ankylosis and rarely, if ever, the ulnar deviation of the fingers such as is found in atrophic arthritis. (There are other types of arthritis not quite so common. The arthritis associated with rheumatic fever, and those found with various inflammatory diseases constitute the majority of this group. Gout might be listed in a separate classification.)

I. Physiological Considerations

Physiological factors in the etiology of rheumatoid arthritis are certainly different from those which bring about the condition we know as osteoarthritis. Thus it would not be surprising to find such a differentiation in the Cayce readings. The severity of the illness, atrophic arthritis, along with its poorer prognosis, would lead one to suspect that the abnormal physiology is of a much deeper origin with much more profound ramifications. If these various factors were not explored to some extent in regard to causation of arthritis in both instances, an understanding of the physiology involved and the therapeutic measures which would become necessary could hardly be obtained.

At the same time, there are certain basic causative factors here which are common to both conditions, and this also might be anticipated. Poor eliminations and the associated condition, inadequate assimilations, seem to be part of the picture in nearly every condition of arthritis, no matter what type it may be. Apparently other abnormal functions within the body contribute to improper eliminations and direct the body down a course which brings either a mild or a serious condition which must be met.

In those cases which Cayce describes, treatment is seldom a simple procedure, even when the individual is not seriously ill. For instance, [4199] was told that her problem originated from tautness of the muscles of the back and the nerves through the autonomic nervous system of the spine, which in turn produced lack of elimination through the skin or through the liver and kidneys. This produced an autointoxication through substances which were picked up in the hepatic circulation; and this in turn created what is described as a "blood force" to the capillaries supplying the bursae and joint spaces of the lower extremities, thus causing a contraction in the lymphatic system of these sacs and hampering the action of the limbs themselves. This described a cause of osteoarthritis.

Another case which was quite similar, [1972], came about through the lack of the activity of the liver as it is related to the gall bladder and its function, in producing "solvents" for assisting in the assimilation of foods for the body. This condition apparently produced an inflammatory reaction which was carried to the centers of locomotion and created an inflammatory reaction in the extremities. Chemical imbalances in the body, lack of iodine in the bloodstream—these are mentioned as etiologic factors. One individual was told that there was a crystallization of most all forms of any foods that have certain potential elements or salts in them. This came about in the joints and tendons, thus creating the arthritic tendency or condition.

Rheumatoid arthritis is often marked by the appearance of subcutaneous nodules. A 57-year-old man, [3363], who was experiencing rheumatoid arthritis as a "meeting of self," was told that the knots or cysts under the skin came about as a result of a "lack of proper distribution of energies that have been used in the body. Not wholly toxic conditions, but producing toxic conditions by their lack of proper elimination." This man, whose disease was obviously karmic in nature, was suffering from lack of proper eliminations throughout his body, which brought about a crystallization of hormones in the circulation of the lymphatics. This created an incoordination between the lymph or superficial circulation and the deeper circulation. All the sympathetic nerves were under stress and strain so that in movements of the body, "these cry out for relief, as it were. . ." There was a lack of proper assimilation as a part of the nerve disorder and disturbance.

In a 53-year-old woman, [5144], whose arthritis had progressed to the point of ankylosis, an unbalanced condition weakened the resistance in the lymphatics and the emuctory circulation through the extremities, especially in the bursae of the body. (Cayce described the bursae as those areas where lymph pockets are gathered in the regular functioning of the body.) Dorland's* describes them as sacs filled with viscid fluid located in tissue where there would otherwise be friction. The joint spaces must also be included in Cayce's description, which is picturesque yet accurate.

Among those with atrophic arthritis, assimilation was proposed as a cause in relationship to a glandular malfunction, as in [5150]. This

*Dorland's Illustrated Medical Dictionary, 24th ed. Philadelphia and London: W.B. Saunders Co., 1957, p. 228.

brought about an infection, creating the arthritis. In another case, there was a lack of the glandular system's ability to reproduce itself. And in still another, the activity of the glands was given as the faulty mechanism and described as a karmic reaction. The glandular disturbance between the liver and the kidneys produced a suppression of elimination and an accumulation in the extremities, which is described as an arthritic tendency in still another case.

Hindered nerve reflexes, depression of the ganglia coming about from poor assimilations and causing improper lymph function, and incoordination of the activity between the liver and the kidneys—all three of these were pointed out as elements in the etiology of arthritis.

From the various functions which are seen to be abnormal, one begins to piece together part of the etiologic mechanisms seen in these psychic readings. Disturbed elimination from any cause, certainly, seems to be the primary abnormality of function. When there are glandular disturbances, it seems more likely that a rheumatoid condition would result, since glandular activity is so closely related to overall organ balance and function; and in the Cayce readings the glands are seen as the mediator of that balancing force which we know as karma. Improper assimilation often comes about before or after the eliminations are disturbed, and the nerve function from the ganglia of the autonomic nervous system is involved in the abnormal physiology.

The readings would likely imply that the development of arthritis is an attempt on the part of the ligaments and the joints themselves to meet the needs of the system which is being poisoned. With the drosses present in the bloodstream, the lymphatics and the lymphocytes with all their resources are unable—in conjunction with the hormones—to bring about a full (what Cayce calls) coagulation or a building up of tissue from energy—a reconstruction, in a sense, of the cells of the body. Thus, the type of arthritis is determined to a great extent by the derangement of function prior to the onset of improper eliminations. It is probably more closely associated with the hormonal disturbance in rheumatoid arthritis; whereas in osteoarthritis the body is better balanced in all of its activities and not subject to such a derangement as comes about in the atrophic manifestation of the disease.

II. Rationale of Therapy

In approaching therapy, we should remember that the body has a capability of normal function:

Thus, we would administer those activities which would bring a normal reaction through these portions, stimulating them to an activity from the body itself, rather than the body becoming dependent upon supplies that are robbing portions of the system to produce activity in other portions, or the system receiving elements or chemical reactions being supplied without arousing the activity of the system itself for a more normal condition.
1968-3

Perhaps the best rational approach to treating arthritis is found in some of the early suggestions given a 40-year-old woman who became case [3244]. Cayce said, ". . .the causes or sources of these conditions are of a very subtle nature. The effects that have been produced in the extremities are hard to cope with." Yet, he said that results would be forthcoming if consistency and persistence were utilized in applying the suggestions which were given. And, he pointed out, the applications which were to be followed would "first meet the conditions, gradually cleanse the system and then begin to renew the energies in the body." (3244-1)

It is highly important that the theory of applying therapy in cycles be followed, since not one reading was given for arthritis wherein a cyclic nature of treatment was not used. The balance of the body as a whole should always be watched carefully for sometimes, by changing a function of elimination without due regard for the ramifications of such an activity, the patient may be put into dire distress. This is particularly true in regard to the Epsom salts baths, the massages, and the Atomidine. The balance within the body is also to be understood if possible. Cayce suggested to [5331] that treatment applied with persistence and consistency may:

. . .make for the coordinating between the eliminations of the sympathetic system, the eliminations which control through the central nerve and blood supply of the organs themselves; that is, the lungs, heart, liver and kidneys, as well as the superficial circulation; these as controlled by the nerves and muscular forces of the sensory or sympathetic system.   5331-1

Medications, particularly sedatives, were not considered valuable in the readings. On the contrary, they would usually cause trouble. An example was the comment made to [3363], a 57-year-old man with rheumatoid arthritis, who was told that aid would require a long period. Unless he was willing to follow the entire therapy program he was told, "do not begin, but keep right on with the injections or the sedatives. . .which are only clogging the body further and will make the body become more and more useless for activity later on."

With these comments in mind, a therapeutic approach would include the following four items:

1. Correct the assimilations. This would include diet, control of digestive abnormalities, and adding beef juice where indicated.

2. Increase eliminations. This might be done with castor oil packs, various eliminants, colonics, and enemas. It would certainly include hydrotherapy, such as ordinary hot baths, Epsom salts baths, fume baths, and any other hydrotherapeutic routine.

3. Improve the nerve supply to the muscles and tendons, and the affected organs through massage, electrical vibrator, and/or osteopathic treatments. Various oils and mixtures are given in the readings, some stimulating in nature and others soothing.

4. Stimulate normal glandular function. This would be done through Atomidine or the wet cell appliance.

The difference in approaching osteoarthritis or rheumatoid arthritis therapeutically is apparent in at least three categories. First, care must be taken that a program is designed for the rheumatoid arthritic which will not disturb the body too greatly. Second, the severe rheumatoid arthritic needs the activities of the wet cell appliance often. Third, because of the deeply ingrained nature of the disease, the rheumatoid would be given a course of therapy perhaps slower in its action but extending over a longer period of time. Osteoarthritis obviously should respond more easily and with less trauma to the patient and the doctor.

III. Suggested Therapeutic Regimen

Undoubtedly, the most consistent routine of therapy for arthritis in the Cayce readings is the combination of Atomidine, Epsom salts baths, and massage. This theme is played over and over again with varying periods of time allotted to the administration of Atomidine; with varying amounts of Epsom salts in the hot bath; and with varieties of oils used for massage.

This triad of therapeutic measures is repeated in cycles with rest periods between, until the body is returned to normal. The condition of the whole body must be kept in mind, of course, and the assimilation and eliminations must be made as proper as possible.

[3009] was a 63-year-old man whose arthritis had been inflam-

matory in previous years but now was classed as chronic. His course
of therapy is interesting because it typifies the suggestions in the
readings. Also, he was told: "Then, at times—just before the period
for the sweats—the condition will apparently be more serious. But
after the third of such sweats we find that improvements should come
to the body, and the disturbance should gradually diminish in the
severity." It is likely that any severe chronic or acute arthritic treated
with these methods will go through periods of stress and pain, and
apparent worsening before conditions actually become improved.
Thus, the suggestions given to this man are of value to consider. The
following are the different steps of therapy:

1. Atomidine, one drop in half a glass of water daily before
breakfast, for three days; then three drops daily for two days; then
four drops daily for two days; then five drops daily for two days.
2. The following day, an Epsom salts bath with 15 pounds of salts
to 50 gallons of water. The water should be as hot as the body can
stand it. An attendant should be used and the body should be
massaged while in the bath where it should remain at least 20 minutes.
3. A rubdown should be given immediately after the body is well
dried off. First, use peanut oil to the limbs and the spine, then use
grain alcohol rub, dipping the hands into the alcohol (85%-90%
proof). This should only be done when the pores are open, such as
after this type of bath.
4. Rest five days before further therapy is started.
5. Then start Atomidine, one drop in half a glass of water daily,
for five days; then five drops daily for five days; then ten drops daily
for two days.
6. Repeat the Epsom salts bath and rubs.
7. Rest another five days, but during this time a peanut oil massage
should be done daily to the spine and to the limbs.
8. After the five-day rest period, repeat the series of Atomidine
and Epsom salts baths, with same instructions.
9. Rest for a longer period then, and use a more consistent amount
of Atomidine prior to the bath in the next cycle and those to follow.
10. Diet should exclude fried foods; any meat should be fish, fowl
and lamb; juices are good, especially vegetable juices; cooked beets
and carrots are especially good; no carbonated drinks.
11. Exercise as much as possible. Keep the daily peanut oil
massage.

Diet and Therapy Procedures

The diet always assumes a rather major proportion in the treatment for arthritis as found in the readings. It seemed to be understood, if not stated, that the diet should be of a laxative nature. Again and again, Cayce advised that celery, lettuce, carrots, and watercress be used often with gelatin as a salad. This, he said, would enhance the values found in all of these vegetables and in the gelatin itself and would be beneficial to the body. For some, figs and dates were suggested to help with the laxative effect of the diet. Vegetable juices especially were found to be helpful. Cooked beets and carrots, and vegetables in large measure were always in order. One meal of green raw vegetables at noon was frequently suggested.

Fish, fowl, and lamb were seen as a primary source of meats; and no fried foods should ever be used. [5331] was told to avoid salt except in kelp and health or sea salts; it is questionable whether any arthritic should ever use much sodium chloride. Starches and sweets together should be avoided. This means no cakes and pastries, or things of that nature. Honey or corn syrup on buckwheat cakes or cornbread or the like would be all right, but not with white bread. Apparently the white flour which is used in cakes and pastries and bread with sweets forms a detrimental combination.

The diet should be well balanced but there should be no starchy foods in the diet. Green leafy vegetables are always excellent, and they should be used in preference to the pod or bulb type of vegetables. Where there is weakness, beef juice should be taken. Wild game is excellent food for the arthritic. A frequent suggestion is to increase the raw vegetables, to decrease the meats, to allow no carbonated drinks, alcohol, or stimulants. Fats should also be avoided. All these factors in the diet should lead toward a better alkalinity, but it must always be remembered that balance is the aim. When there is a balanced diet with the conditions set forth here, the body can assimilate those factors necessary to continue rebuilding cells. Thus assimilation is given proper attention.

Not all the readings on arthritis emphasize eliminants, but there seems to be a consistent understanding that eliminations be made proper. The diet mentioned above assists in this, and sometimes does the whole job. At other times, with a real problem of constipation and accumulation of toxins throughout the system, colonics were suggested prior to any therapy; at other times colonics were suggested during the course of therapy. Eno salts, a teaspoonful in a glass of water before the morning meal for one week, was given as a suggestion to [5197]. Peanut and olive oils absorbed by the body during massages stimulate eliminations. The following prescription was given to [4199] as a substance to excite the mucous or lactic forces to their proper action and carry toxic forces through their proper channel:

> Podophyllin, 1 gr.
> Senna, 2 gr.
> Sanguinaria, 2 gr.
> Sodium bicarbonate, 1 gr.

This dose, in a capsule, was to be repeated in two days. Then, to eliminate those toxic forces from the body, this woman was given a mixture of 15 grains of gold chloride and six grains of sodium bicarbonate in 15 ounces of distilled water, in a dose of five drops four times a day.

Eliminations came about through the fume baths, the showers, and the hot baths, as well as through colonics and cathartics. Fume baths were suggested with witch hazel one time, and then Atomidine the next time. From the information given in the readings, it seems reasonable to assume that it is best not to put too much emphasis on colonics or enemas or cathartics, since this might unbalance the body during convalescence. Epsom salts baths, fume baths, the hot baths, the massages, and the laxative-type diet were emphasized more. Care certainly must be taken in treating a severe arthritic in regard to eliminations as well as to the other parts of the therapy, for "as we find, unless there is great care taken in the administrations for the body, the applications for some portions of the disturbance may be very hard upon other portions of the body." (5144-1)

The oils suggested for use here include peanut oil in the majority of cases. This is used most frequently alone. Often peanut oil and olive oil in equal parts is suggested. Peanut oil, pine oil, and olive oil in equal parts was another variant. For [4199], vinegar was used as a massage across the lumbar area of the back and then to the knees, to be followed by application of hot salt packs—these to be contained in the cloth-like beanbags. They would remain in place until the body is dry. This apparently is also an eliminatory procedure. A rheumatoid arthritic, [3363], was given the following prescription for massage after the Epsom salts bath:

> Usoline or Nujol, 4 ounces
> Olive oil, 2 ounces
> Peanut oil, 2 ounces
> Oil of pine needles, ½ ounce
> Oil of sassafras root, ½ ounce
> Lanolin, liquefied, 1 ounce
> (Shake before applying.)

Olive oil and peanut oil, two ounces each, with one ounce of lanolin was often suggested as a massage oil. [3244], whose assimilations were poor, was told "for the system in attempting to adjust itself to the growing destructive forces has drawn on the vital forces of the body." An oil mixture was given as follows:

> Usoline or Nujol, 4 ounces
> Oil of pine needles, 1 ounce
> Olive oil, 1 ounce
> Peanut oil, 1 ounce
> Lanolin, liquefied, 1 ounce

Perhaps the pine needles provide a stimulant within the body. The Usoline or Nujol is also called Russian white oil.

Two other massage oil mixtures, which bring about a degree of irritation and heat, which is preferable at times, are listed below. These should be used only after the Epsom salts baths.

> Usoline or Nujol, 4 ounces
> Peanut oil, 2 ounces
> Sassafras root oil, ½ ounce
> Oil of pine needles, ½ ounce
> Oil of mustard, ¼ ounce

> Usoline or Nujol, 6 ounces
> Kerosene oil, 1 ounce
> Oil of cedarwood, 2 ounces
> Spirits of camphor, 1 ounce
> Witch hazel, 1 ounce
> Oil of sassafras, 1 ounce
> Oil of mustard, 10 drops

Olive oil and tincture of myrrh in equal parts was another combination. In preparing this, the olive oil should be heated, and then the tincture of myrrh added. The readings do not indicate specifically why one oil is desirable above another. However, peanut oil is the most consistent among all those used.

Atomidine Therapy: Suggested Routines

There were several different routines suggested where Atomidine was concerned. It is always taken in a half glass of water before any food. Apparently, it stimulates the body and prepares it for eliminating toxins through the Epsom salts baths. It appears that the more acute and inflammatory a case of arthritis is, the more careful one should be in using the Atomidine preparatory to the Epsom salts baths. Atomidine routines include:

1. 1 drop in half glass water daily for five days
   5 drops on sixth day
       Three hours after last dose, Epsom salts bath taken with 20 pounds of salts to 40 gallons of water.

With this individual, these measures, Cayce suggested, would be painful; but, if they were kept consistently, results would be seen.

2. 1 drop in half glass water daily for five days
       Rest for two days; then repeat this cycle a second and a third time.
3. 1 drop daily for 10 days
       On the tenth day, 5 drops, followed by the bath.
4. 1 drop daily for five days
       This was followed by an ordinary bath or shower and a massage, then a rest. Repeat cycle a second and a third time. On the fourth series, use 5 drops Atomidine daily for three days, followed by an Epsom salts bath, then an appropriate rest period.
       Continue for a fifth and sixth series
       (Diagnosis: rheumatoid arthritis, case [3363].)
5. 1 drop daily for two days
   2 drops daily for two days
   3 drops daily for two days
   5 drops on seventh day
6. 1 drop daily for three weeks
   Rest period
7. 5 drops daily for five days
   Followed by the bath
8. 1 drop daily for five days
   2 drops daily for five days
   3 drops daily for five days
   4 drops daily for five days
   5 drops daily for five days
   Followed by the bath

It can be seen that the use of Atomidine is certainly varied in the readings and does not follow a particular pattern that can be observed. However, one thing can always be counted on and that is the periodicity or cyclic nature of the therapy, and this should be followed whatever dosage is to be used.

Osteopathic manipulations were recommended occasionally, and in these instances they often eliminated the need for frequent massages. Apparently the manipulation and the massage to a certain extent bring about some of the same changes. Wet cell therapy is at times suggested in very severe cases, at the discretion of the physician.

Suggested Therapy for Osteoarthritis

Probably osteoarthritis and arthritic tendencies (and, questionably, early rheumatoid arthritis) might be grouped together as far as therapy is concerned. A program should be designed to bring the body gradually back to normal. The following—with occasional deviations as might be chosen from prior paragraphs—could serve as an outline for therapy in these cases:

1. Diet. The suggestions already outlined should be followed with consistency and accuracy. This is very important.

2. With a history of constipation, a series of two or three colonics or a series of high enemas taken every three to four days for a period of two weeks, prior to other therapy, is recommended.

3. Atomidine, one drop daily for one week in half a glass of water early in the morning.

4. Rest from therapy for one week.

5. Atomidine, three drops daily for five days, then on the sixth day, 10 drops.

6. That same day, an Epsom salts bath with 20 pounds of Epsom salts to 50 gallons of water. Massage the body over all the joints affected while in the bath. The body should remain in the bath for at least 20 minutes, but should not become overly weak during the process. An ice pack on the head may be of considerable help.

7. Then massage the entire body with an equal mixture of olive oil and peanut oil for 15 to 30 minutes.

8. Rest two weeks from the drops and the bath, while massaging at night three times a week with the oil mixture. This massage should be over the entire body, but particular attention should be paid to those areas involved. Keep the massages regular until therapy is ended.

9. Repeat the entire cycle after this rest period, beginning with three drops of Atomidine (steps 5 through 8).

10. After another rest, repeat the cycle again and continue until the body is back to normal.

Suggested Therapy for Severe Rheumatoid Arthritis

1. The diet should be as has already been outlined. Strict attention should be paid to this part of the therapy.

2. Atomidine in half a glass of water in the morning before breakfast as follows:

> 1 drop each day for five days
> 2 drops each day for five days
> 3 drops each day for five days
> 4 drops each day for five days
> 5 drops each day for five days

3. Following the 25th day of the schedule an Epsom salts bath should be taken, using 20 pounds of Epsom salts to about 50 gallons of hot water, which would mean that the body would be covered thoroughly up to the neck. The affected limbs and joints should be massaged while in the water.

4. After the Epsom salts bath, a thorough massage should be used, applying the combination of oils such as those already described with oil of mustard in them, or one of the more complicated combinations.

5. Rest for a period of two weeks. During this time daily massage should be given to the body, using peanut oil.

6. Colonics or high enemas should be used approximately every 10 days from the beginning of therapy for at least two months. Thereafter, perhaps once a month.

7. After the rest period the whole procedure of Atomidine and baths and massages should be repeated with the rest after that, and the cycle continuing.

8. Osteopathy, two treatments a week during the time of the first series, then according to a cycle that might be established.

9. A wet cell battery may be used in addition to the above therapy. Gold chloride, three grains to three ounces of water, should be used in the solution jar.

It may be advisable, rather than using the Atomidine, to take gold chloride by mouth. The rationale for this has not been established, but it was suggested often as an oral therapy as well as in the wet cell applications. This would need to be decided by the attending physician and may be determined by the response to therapy. If this is to be taken by mouth, then a dropper bottle containing one grain of gold chloride to one ounce of distilled water should be prepared; and an ounce of distilled water to which has been added 10 grains of bicarbonate of soda. From these two solutions, the following amount should be taken daily in half a glass of water: one drop of the gold solution, and two drops of the soda solution.

Mechanisms of Action in Low-Energy Treatment

Throughout the readings Cayce suggested treatment with what he called low electrical energy, and he described the wet cell battery and the impedance device to make this possible. He has suggested both at various places in the treatment of arthritis. One woman, [5623], was told that the impedance device would add to her system, that which "will bring the proper vibration for the system, as to bring resuscitation to the physical forces of the body as come with the active principle of the creative element in the physical body that *produce* the cell in its vibration for the body. Then, this would bring *these* forces as near to the resuscitation *of* the physical body as will be possible in one of the age, and *prevent* the reoccurrence of those conditions for the body."

Cayce says that this energy given by the impedance device is in the nature of radio vibration "as will give to the nerve energy of the nerve systems, both of the cerebrospinal and sympathetic, that proper vibration as will create new energy in the system. These may be materially aided through that of the ultraviolet ray. These will assist only as the vibratory forces are set up, which will be aided through the application of the radio-active appliance carrying that of chloride of gold into the system."

When the device is attached with the lead carrying the gold solution to the umbilical area, Cayce indicated that this would carry "that to the system which creates the proper vibration in the system to resuscitate energy in the glands through which all creative energy must pass in a vibrating body. The activity of that carried in system by the forces as will be applied in that of the ultraviolet will distribute same through the nerve system, so that there will not be centralization, or too much in one place for that of the other, as will give to the system that of the proper vibration." (5623-1)

Should we not attempt to awaken the inner forces to God's presence?

For, all healing comes from the one source. And whether there is the application of foods, exercise, medicine, or even the knife, it is to bring the consciousness of the forces within the body that aid in reproducing themselves—the awareness of creative or God forces.   2696-1

William A. McGarey, M.D.

Edgar Cayce readings referenced:

585-11	3009-1	4199-1	5156-1	5397-1
849-13	3244-1	5077-1	5169-1	5402-1
935-3	3281-1	5120-1	5197-1	5623-1
951-1	3316-1	5144-1	5331-1	
1972-1	3363-1	5150-1	5361-1	

Suggested Diet for Arthritics

1. The following foods should be included in your diet:

a. All kinds of raw vegetables (except cabbage), watercress, chard, mustard greens, kale, carrots, celery, lettuce (leaf or Romaine).

These may be eaten with gelatin. This should be Knox gelatin, taken a minimum of three times per week, but better daily. Use the Knox gelatin recipes; the gelatin may also be taken with tomato juice or other juices.*

b. Black bread (pumpernickle, rye, or whole wheat).

c. Nuts, especially almonds and filberts (raw nuts are better than those roasted and salted).

d. Fish and sea foods, fowl, lamb, wild game, liver, tripe and pigs' knuckles.

e. Vegetable juices, citrus fruit juices at times when cereal is not eaten.

f. Berries, except strawberries; and citrus fruits.

g. Cooked leafy vegetables (except cabbage); pieplant (salsify); parsnips; potato peelings from the baked potato, but not the bulk of it.

h. Jerusalem artichoke once each week (they are a root).

i. Great deal of watercress and beet tops (these especially help the eliminations).

j. Most fruits may be eaten, preferably fresh.

2. The following foods should be avoided:

a. These fruits: apples, bananas, strawberries, tomatoes.

b. These vegetables: cabbage, starchy foods.

c. No fried foods; no fats; no pork of any kind, including bacon.

d. No beef, no veal.

e. No malt drinks; no carbonated water (i.e., in any soft drinks).

f. No alcohol or spices or other stimulants.

---

*Gelatin has been called a catalyst, helping the body make optimal use of the vitamins and other properties of vegetables and fruits.

ASTHMA

I. Physiological Considerations

Asthma, a sometimes explosively sudden constriction of the bronchial passages of the lung causing great respiratory distress, has its origin in neurologic stimuli. These are touched off or released either from lesions that occur as adhesions in the bronchi and the larynx or as pressures exerted on autonomic ganglia and their connections with the cerebrospinal system either with or without spinal subluxations. These pressures exist most commonly in the sixth, seventh, eighth and ninth dorsal especially, although other areas are often involved. Sometimes the first four dorsals may be the originating cause of asthmatic attacks and sometimes those associated with the fourth and fifth cervical. In the latter case, circulatory disturbances with associated lymphatic abnormalities may be expected, causing allergic symptoms through the nose and throat which have been called hay fever. The allergy comes about from lesions in the ganglia areas creating the ability within the tissues to become sensitive to substances in the external environment of the individual.

As indicated, there have been pressures in head and neck and face. These becoming sensitive to the activities of principles about it, the atmosphere, the home environ, the general activities all have their bearing upon the body. It is in a manner, to be sure, an escape from self, but something had better be done about the condition now, else we may have those periods when it will be greater to combat. **3053-1**

The asthmatic attacks come about as a reflex spasm at times from the throat and lungs or bronchi, or from the ganglia themselves, as an overloading of impulses bringing about a spastic condition of the bronchial tree.

These lesions which occur in the larynx and bronchi may be brought into being through previous episodes of pleurisy or acute infection, or through pressure from the ganglia themselves which already have been disturbed. During gestation and in the manner of presentation at birth, certain hindrances prevented segments of ganglia in the lumbar, sacral and in the ninth dorsal from assuming a normal position. Thus this individual had the physical beginnings of asthma at birth. The lack of proper impulse coming from these various autonomic control centers created spasms, or acute asthmatic attacks, and cut off the clarification and purification of the blood through oxidation of a normal nature in the lungs. This, in turn, prevented a normal development of the child. The cell vitality and production were decreased in the bloodstream and the liver; the pancreas and the lymphatic areas of assimilation—Peyer's patches— were affected. Other changes within the body, of course, would come into being through these resultant activities.

In case [5004] asthma began when he was just a boy after a severe bout with the flu when he was delirious with fever. Lesions were formed here in the bronchi and in the larynx as a result of the infection. In still another case, [5360], injury caused a lesion which in turn created disturbing conditions in the bronchial tree. When that part of the body tried to seal itself off, inflammation came about with adhesions developing in the bronchi and the larynx. These, in addition to causing the bouts of asthma, also disturbed the assimilation and the elimination of the body.

Associated conditions, not too often causing the primary asthmatic lesions but often the result of such, include disturbances in the coordination between the superficial and the deep circulation; incoordination of the elimination systems; imbalance of the glandular system; and in case [755] the lesions in the lacteals, the Peyer's patches, which developed an irritation in the nervous system with a reaction which was almost epileptic in its nature. It can be seen that the various systems of function within the body are closely related, and disease syndromes may have their origin in manners that may be only finely differentiated.

Occasionally there will be sensory symptoms associated with the asthma such as dizziness or visual or auditory symptoms of various natures. These have their origin in the same centers of control in the ganglia, bursae where associations of a neurological nature are made between the cerebrospinal and the autonomic nervous system. At these areas the sensory organs are also in close contact; "for there are those connections through the ganglia in the first, second and third dorsal, that connect directly to the organs of the sensory system." (3053-1)

II. Rationale of Therapy

In approaching therapy, we should remember that the body has a capability of normal function:

Thus, we would administer those activities which would bring a normal reaction through these portions, stimulating them to an activity from the body itself, rather than the body becoming dependent upon supplies that are robbing portions of the system to produce activity in other portions, or the system receiving elements or chemical reactions being supplied without arousing the activity of the system itself for a more normal condition.

1968-3

Asthma, when viewed as a condition which has its origin and basis in the nervous system, should then be approached in therapy with the objective of removing the stimulatory factors in the nervous system and correcting those adjunctive, correlated, and resultant imbalances that may prevent a return to normal function.

Since pressures are present in the dorsal and sometimes the cervical ganglia, these should be relieved osteopathically and treatments should be continued long enough to allow continuance of normal nerve function. The eliminations should be restored to normal, and assimilation should be balanced with the elimination. The deep and superficial circulation, which is often disturbed, should be restored to a balance of coordination. The glands of the body should be brought to a balance, and the resistance of the body should be stimulated through the improvement of assimilation and function of the Peyer's patch area of the intestines.

Irritation of an external nature to the respiratory tree should be eliminated so that the other factors involved might be brought to a more normal condition. Dietary adjustments should be made as a portion of the attempt to balance the assimilations of the body.

These factors, applied in a therapeutic regimen, must be done with patience and persistence. The advice given to [1867] was "as we find— these conditions may be *entirely* eliminated. It will require patience, persistence, care, and those precautions as to the diet. . ." (1867-1)

III. Suggested Therapeutic Regimen

Generally, therapy for the asthmatic should be designed to correct the pressures which exist in the various autonomic ganglia segments. Correct the subluxations that may be present. These osteopathic adjustments should be both specific and general and should be done in a cyclic fashion. Dietary precautions should be begun at once, and cleansing of the intestinal tract likewise. Glandular balance should be achieved with Atomidine. Acute attacks and concurrent symptoms should be controlled specifically.

Osteopathic adjustments vary according to the conditions found, of course. Stress should always be placed on correcting subluxations while balancing the lumbar axis with the cervical and the ninth dorsal. The balancing or coordinating is not a simple thing but apparently has much to do with correction of various incoordinations within the body proper.

Diet should be adjusted in all cases. Occasionally, as in case [3053], there will be a deficiency of the acid-forming cells and structures functioning within the body (which may be associated with adrenal deficiency). In these cases an acid-forming diet principally should be suggested. More commonly, however, the elements of a good diet for the asthmatic would be those of severe restriction of sweets (honey allowed only once a day); no white bread, potatoes, tomatoes, dried beans, or rice. All fruits, vegetables, and nuts generally are desirable. Fowl or fish are preferable for protein.

Colonics, where possible, should be given weekly for two or three weeks, then perhaps once monthly; enemas, if colonics are not available.

Atomidine can be given in a series. In case [1413] it was given one drop daily for five days in half a glass of water, then stopped for three days; then two drops daily for five days; then stopped for three days; then one drop daily for five days with a rest, and then two drops with the rest; so continued in this manner.

An interesting therapeutic effect is seen in case [1867]. This eight-year-old was directed to use Calcios, enough to spread on a whole wheat wafer, and take it daily. This would apparently stimulate the hormone activity or the ability of the body to keep the balance between the red blood cells and the leucocytes on the one hand, and the lymphocytes on the other hand. Also, it would eliminate a tendency for inflammation by stimulating the Peyer's patches to work more completely and thus produce resistance to infection. How this is accomplished specifically is not described.

Acute attacks of asthma are controlled in various ways, although it is implied here that as other factors in the therapy are begun, attacks will become progressively less severe. Calcidin, one to five drops in five ounces of warm water, sipped every 15 to 20 minutes, is one suggestion. Atomidine, six drops in a tablespoon of water sipped once every six hours, is another suggestion. In several places special inhalants are suggested to be used in a wide-mouth bottle (a diagram of which can be found in the back of the Circulating File on Asthma.) The inhalant can be prepared as follows: To four ounces of grain alcohol, add in the order named:

> Oil of eucalyptus, 20 minims
> Rectified oil of turpentine, 5 minims
> Compound tincture of benzoin, 15 minims

Bowels should not only be cleansed at the outset of therapy, but daily bowel movements should be continued. Change of climate was suggested occasionally to give the individual less irritating atmospheric conditions.

Should we not attempt to awaken the inner forces to God's presence? "For, all healing comes from the one source. And whether there is the application of foods, exercise, medicine, or even the knife, it is to bring the consciousness of the forces within the body that aid in reproducing themselves—the awareness of creative or God forces." (2696-1)

William A. McGarey, M.D.

Edgar Cayce readings referenced:

674-1, 2	2350-1	3863-1
755-1	2755-1	5236-1
1413-1,3	3053-1,2	5360-1
1467-18	3127-1	5381-1 Supplement
1867-1	3542-1	

BALDNESS

I. Physiological Considerations

   Glandular insufficiency and spinal lesions (subluxation), according
to the Cayce material, are by far the most common causes of hair loss
(baldness) which may be accompanied by nail and even skin changes
(abnormal pigmentation, vitiligo, etc.). Glandular dysfunction—
usually the thyroid, but the thymus and adrenals may also be
involved—may come about through the diet, i.e., insufficient
amounts of necessary elements like calcium, or excesses of others like
potassium. Other causes of glandular dysfunction include insufficient
circulation, stress, infection, toxic chemicals (as found in cosmetics),
general debilitation, etc.

   The most commonly involved gland is the thyroid. It seems that
when some elements necessary for proper thyroid functioning are
missing, toxins which otherwise would have been eliminated are
allowed to accumulate in the system. When this happens, inflammation, congestion, and circulatory disturbances occur, affecting the
scalp and maybe the nails and skin. It is worth noting that the thyroid
to some extent controls the circulation to the scalp, nails and skin,
independent of the mechanism described above. When such disturbances occur, the outcome is hair loss with or without nail and skin
changes, depending on the severity of the condition.

   Impaired circulation from other causes may bring about the same
effects without necessarily involving the thyroid or other glands, but
this is a much less common finding. The exception is spinal subluxation, this being almost equally as frequent as glandular disturbance. It
should be noted, though, that even when spinal subluxation is the
primary condition, the glands often become involved as a result of
impaired circulation through them (the thyroid especially). Hence in
a large majority of cases the glands are either the primary or contributing cause of the condition.

In one or two instances, reference was made to prenatal tendencies as a contributory cause, but no definite information is available on this or on heredity.

II. Rationale of Therapy

The treatments recommended reflect the disease process involved and may be classified as follows:

1. Correction of glandular dysfunction usually includes dietary advice where deficiencies are involved. Atomidine and sometimes glandular extracts (thyroid, adrenals, etc.) are necessary.

2. Osteopathy: Series of treatments to correct spinal subluxation that may be causing circulatory, glandular and other organ system dysfunction as well as hair loss.

3. Others: Treatment of underlying disorders (e.g., avoidance of stress and toxic chemicals, treatment of infections, etc.) as well as complications of basic disease process (e.g., spinal subluxation usually causes widespread effects) which may contribute to or aggravate the hair loss.

Osteopathic adjustments bring about improved circulation to the scalp, nails and skin, thus leading to beneficial changes. When digestive disturbances (assimilations/eliminations) are also present as a result of spinal lesions, toxic accumulations may be substantially eliminated or prevented in the digestive tract, further improving circulation to involved areas. What may be less obvious is that the use of laxatives, colonic enemas, etc., would bring about similar results through elimination of toxins.

These few examples are based on the assumption that the physiology described by Cayce is correct. Intuitively, it seems to make sense to me.

III. Suggested Therapeutic Regimen

Baldness is not a problem treated by the average physician, for there is no recommended medical treatment presently available. The following might be considered a reasonable approach to the average patient, from a study of the Edgar Cayce readings.

1. Correction of glandular deficiency.

    a. *Atomidine:* Various programs were prescribed. There is no given formula for arriving at dosages. One suggestion is as follows:

One drop for seven days, rest five days
Two drops for seven days, rest five days
Three drops for seven days, rest five days
(May repeat this series once or twice.)

b. Thyroid extract in small doses two to three times a week for a few weeks in combination with Atomidine in severe deficiency.

c. Other glandular extracts (replacements), as necessary, e.g., adrenal.

d. Correction of mineral deficiencies and/or excesses (e.g., low calcium, high potassium). Calcios is a good source of calcium (a layer on a cracker taken every other day).

e. Dietary:

1) The skin of Irish potatoes cooked in Patapar paper (to preserve active principles) supplies some essential elements for proper thyroid function. This may be eaten three or more times a week. (Roasted or baked is also good so long as it is not burnt.)

2) Other helpful hints for better thyroid activity include citrus fruit juices—orange juice plus lemon or grapefruit juice plus lime—in combination with Atomidine will act on the thyroid to improve circulation to the scalp. Seafoods were recommended three times a week. Carrots are good.

3) Avoid: fried, greasy foods, fried meats, starches, refined sugars, onions, garlic.

2. Osteopathy: This would be helpful if a history of spinal injury is obtained or when other symptoms and signs warrant this. Even in the absence of the above a few treatments would probably still be beneficial, since circulation to the thyroid, scalp, nails, skin, etc., will be enhanced. The areas manipulated as well as the number of treatments should be considered on an individual basis.

3. Local measures:

a. Crude oil massage to the scalp (one teaspoon) to stay on from one-half hour to 45 minutes. Then cleanse with a 20% grain alcohol solution. Follow this with a massage using white petroleum (Vaseline) into scalp (not too greasy).

An alternative would be a scalp massage with pure hog lard, leaving this on overnight after covering head with an oil cap.

Shampoo in the morning with olive oil shampoo followed by a massage with white Vaseline cut with a little alcohol (one drop grain alcohol to one ounce water). Either may be done once a week.

    b. Violet ray treatment (20-25 times) to scalp, spine, scapula, umbilical area for a total of five to ten minutes on a daily basis. Ultraviolet ray treatments may be used instead, this done every third day, limiting treatment to scalp and spine for three to five minutes for 20-25 treatments.

4. Other: Maintain proper elimination through the use of laxatives, colonic enemas, massages, etc. Diathermy, vibrator, hydrotherapy, radio-active appliance were also recommended in some instances.

A prescription is given in reading 636-1 for restoring hair color. Dosage is half a teaspoon three times a day after meals for ten days with five days rest periods.

Steps 1 and 3 seem to be a must, while 2 and 4 may be utilized at the discretion of the therapist, depending on the case being treated.

Hezekiah U. Chinwah, M.D.

Edgar Cayce readings referenced:

337-24	816-1	Supplement	1566-4	2901-2	4086-1	5013-1
362-1, 2	935-1		1687-1	2998-1	4160-1,2	5339-1
502-1	970-1		1727-2	3497-1	4592-1	5504-1
585-7	1078-1		1904-1	3782-1	4736-1	5609-1
636-1	1120-2		2011-2	3904-1	4877-1	

BREAST CANCER

I. Physiological Considerations

The Edgar Cayce readings on breast cancer describe a limited number of causative or contributory factors in this disease. Reading 2457-4 suggests a prenatal condition manifesting through physical forces and creating a new "element" or activity in the system:

Those conditions as are prenatal in their effect, through the activity of forces made manifest in a physical body, are beginning to become in the manner of producing within the system an element as of its *own* resuscitation, living upon the life *of* the body-physical. That's a very good description of cancer, isn't it? for it *is* malignant in its nature. . . 2457-4

Reading 583-7 gives further insight into cancer in general: ". . .cancerous conditions are where cellular forces have congregated on account of irritation, or poor elimination and irritation following, and the system attempting to relieve same sets up from broken cellular tissue the condition from within which becomes malignant." It appears that cancer is a mis-creative attempt at healing by damaged body cells.

Reading 5045-1 details chemical changes resulting in a decreased number of male hormones, causing hardening in the mammary glands. The remaining readings in this Circulating File suggest poor eliminations, applications for heartburn, toxic forces, lack of proper circulation, catarrhal conditions, adhesions, segregations, strangulations, and centralizations as significant contributing factors to the causation of breast cancer.

Most of the symptoms in these women which were not directly related to the cancer were considered to be sympathetic reflexes. These included fullness and irritation of the organs of the sensory system and respiratory tract, and unspecified effects on the heart's action and the digestive system. Other symptoms noted were torpid liver, engorged spleen, thickened stomach, tendency to colon prolapse, fullness in the locomotaries, general nervous system distress, and weakened optic energies.

II. Rationale of Therapy

Reading 5592-1 seems to give a good general therapeutic approach to breast cancer from the physical perspective—and likely to other malignant processes:

As we would find, in the meeting of the conditions, even in the present, there should not be the necessity—nor *any* reason, will there be added the proper precautions—of an operative case, or operative measures. We would add sufficient to the system as will allow the better clarification of the bloodstream, better pulsation and activity of the heart, and—to be sure—the better eliminating through the alimentary canal; keeping down the acidity in the system in such a way and manner as to allow that that *is* assimilated in the system to become more effective in creating in the plasm of the blood supply the sufficient leucocyte in the white corpuscle as will produce not only better coagulation, but as absorbing of, and destroying of, those tissue and muco-membranes that have become clogged in portions of the glands and in the torso or trunk portion of the body itself, as well as clarifying or clearing the alimentary canal.   **5592-1**

Specific therapies suggested for this woman included animated ash followed by ultraviolet ray, a "less acid" diet, olive oil and Glyco-Thymoline by mouth, monthly colonics, and manipulations of a general massage character.

As for most medical problems covered by the Edgar Cayce readings, diet had a central position of importance in the treatment of breast cancer. Reading 2457-4 suggests to "Feed *all* the food that is of a *nourishing* nature, but not from *meats*. Those of cereals, fruits, vegetables, *and* such—or principally of the nature that are the foods of the hare, the foods of the beef—these are *destructive* forces *to* such as may be seen in the condition attacking system."

Eliminations were stimulated by colonics, Glyco-Thymoline, olive oil and cathartics. The olive oil was to be given "that the muco-membrane in the colon and intestinal area may have more activity or food value for the digestive system itself, as well as aiding the colon in the eliminations and assisting peristaltic movements. . ." (5592-2) Vegetable cathartics were given when necessary, but avoidable "if we will have at least one meal each day of wholly citrus fruit diet, or the pieplant [rhubarb]—as is concentrate—or the fig, or the syrup of same, or those as carry properties that make for the activity of the muco-membranes from the salivary glands to the jejunum, or the activity of same begins, or to the action of the glands that make for separations in the system—or lacteals. We will find these should carry those sufficient, when the colonics have removed those pressures as produce those in the system of *mucus* in intestinal tract." (5592-1)

Animated ash with ultraviolet ray is a particularly novel and exciting approach to cancer therapy. The ash produced from burning bamboo in a partial vacuum is taken orally and focused on the "centers from which those activities of the nerve impulse and blood supply receive their impulses in their activity through the system." (5592-1)

Five minutes after the ash has been taken, apply the ultraviolet light for one and a half to two minutes, at least thirty-eight to forty inches from the body, over the lower cervical and upper dorsal area. Preferably use the quartz light, or mercury quartz light. This is the heavier of such machines. Should this redden the body too much, then we would use the green light or glass *between* the body and the ultraviolet, which will prevent so much irritation to the superficial circulation and such strong light. . .Or the light may be moved some more distance away from the body.

The light taken after the ash will cause the action of the ash of the carbon to clarify through the releasing of oxygen in the bloodstream, by being centralized in the portions of the lungs thus affected, and in the tissue adjacent to same.   511-1

Local therapy included grape, beet, and plaintain poultices, and Anidex ointment. Anidex was prepared by mixing two grains of animated ash to one ounce of Iodex. This ointment was to be massaged into the breast and axilla on alternate days to assist in the drying of tissues and the drawing off of refuse forces.

Other treatments included medications for analgesic, antiemetic, and tonic purposes; fume baths; male hormone injections; beef juice; manipulative therapy; and x-ray, "*deep* therapy for. . .*loosening* oxygen for the bone structure." (2457-4) Exotic therapies included atropine and electrical treatments, and a serum to be produced from "the 'wolve' [tendon] in the beef or the hare, at this season, and injections made in that region where the blood supply to the system is most effective." (2457-4) Surgery and radium implants were suggested for patients in extreme circumstances.

Warnings

The readings from the breast cancer file give warnings about the use of drugs, surgery, and radiation in specific cases of cancer therapy.

Drugs: "To give only hypnotics or narcotics is to gradually allow the body to lose its resistance or ability for resuscitation." (511-1)

Surgery: "To operate under the existent condition would prevent proper coagulation in tissue. . ." (511-1)

The medical readings consistently recommend building up the "coagulation" abilities and body resistances before submitting the body to operative procedures. And it is often suggested that if these can be reactivated, healing may be stimulated and surgical intervention may not be necessary or advisable.

X-ray: "To add the high vibrations of the x-ray in this particular condition would not be well. While there are such applications where emanations of the radial activity of radium or the high vibrations would become destructive to a condition of this nature, we find that this condition in this body arises from other sources. For with the accumulations centralized here, the high vibrations would only produce a burn (which would be more destructive than the condition is itself) or disseminate same through the system where it would simply take on the form of other conditions, such as brittleness of the bone, softening in other portions of cartilaginous forces, and make of the body a cripple." (683-3) ". . .x-ray—that destroys tissue, but not being enabled to eliminate that destroyed, tends to come back upon itself after certain radiations." (3370-1)

Healing

Spiritual: "For ye know deep in thyself that all healing comes of the Lord, and there is not anything you may do save attune the body forces to the very vibration of the body itself to the awareness that God is, and is creative in its every purpose." (3042-1)

Mental: For spirit is the life, the mind is the builder, the physical is the result. Constructive, purposeful attitudes are to be cultivated in all who are sick and injured—all who are unhealed. Patience, persistence and consistency are hallmarks of the readings' recommendations for those in search of healing of any kind. Changes in consciousness, release of emotional blocks, and attunement to Spirit (Creative Forces, or God) are the real keys to a lasting "cure," peace and joy.

Physical: "As known by the body itself (reason, for the moment, as to constructive forces, as known from the anatomical structure of the body itself), the body rebuilds itself—*constantly,* through what? The *blood* supply! That lacking or that which is overabundant produces disturbances within the body so that destructive forces may be set up at any time.

"Then, that which will act with the *building* of the body for new blood, *energizing* and *revivifying* same in such a way and manner as indicated, will be the manner to make for constructive forces." (683-3) ". . .if the vibrations are raised sufficiently these [conditions] may be dissipated, and—with the body kept in a *constructive* way and manner—eliminated entirely from the system." (683-3)

III. Suggested Therapeutic Regimen

1. Attitude: Major emphasis needs to be placed on a prayerful, purposeful state of mind. What will the individual do with her life if she does recover? Meditation or biofeedback/relaxation and visualization exercises are particularly valuable in opening one to new awarenesses and attunement to higher ideals and healing forces. Dream study can bring important insights into the healing process. Prayer and the laying on of hands can also be of significant therapeutic benefit.

2. Diet: This should be highly alkaline—rabbit or beef food. Live foods, especially sprouts and wheat grass, should be emphasized. Lots of water is useful for assimilative, eliminative, and general metabolic purposes. Glyco-Thymoline drops by mouth (five to ten drops in water three times daily) may be helpful in alkalinization of the system. Test the saliva with Nitrazine paper—pH should read higher than 7.

Beef juice is recommended as a stimulant/tonic. Cooked asparagus has been suggested from a number of sources as an activator of leucocytes.

Vitamins may be of benefit, particularly ascorbic acid in doses up to 10 grams and more per day. Vitamins A and E may be added. Amygdalin (Vitamin B-15) remains controversial but is not inconsistent with the readings, especially in light of the recommendation to take two or three almonds a day as a cancer preventative. The readings suggest that all vitamins be taken on a cyclic basis so that the body's abilities to extract same from foods and even manufacture its own is not disturbed. Gelatin is indicated to be added to fruits and vegetables to facilitate the absorption of vitamins and minerals.

3. Stimulants: Atomidine is a general glandular stimulant with particular benefit for the lymphatic system, and thyroid and thymus glands. The use of Atomidine alone or in formula will be of value in promoting glandular eliminations, white blood cell function, and general immune responses. Castor oil packs have direct effects on assimilative functions of the small intestine and secondary influences on eliminations, immune capabilities, and nervous system coordination.

4. Ultraviolet light with animated ash: The length and frequency of these treatments varies from patient to patient—from one to five minutes twice weekly to twice daily. Dosage usually was given as one-eighth to one-fourth grain. The violet ray machine can be used as an effective substitute for the ultraviolet. This therapy appears to focus atomic oxygen in the region of the carcinoma (References exist which indicate the anaerobic preferences of tumor cells.) and stimulate white blood cell aggregation and cancer destruction.

5. Local therapy: Massage around the affected breast and axilla with Iodex, Anidex, or cocoa butter stimulates drainage and lymphatic activity.

6. Circulation: Massage, chiropractic or osteopathic manipulation, and hydrotherapy are frequent suggestions to promote vascular function, lymphatic drainage, nervous system coordination, and organic cooperation.

7. Eliminations: Consistent mention is made of the need for proper eliminations in numerous conditions, including cancer, in the readings. Daily eliminations should be maintained by diet (emphasis on fiber, figs, dates, prunes, etc.), castor oil packs, olive oil, vegetable laxatives such as Castoria, Innerclean, syrup of figs, enemas, and colonics.

Robert McNary, M.D.

Edgar Cayce readings referenced:

511-1	5045-1
522-5	5570-1, 2
683-3, 4	5592-1, 2
2457-4	5662-1, 2, 3
3672-1, 2	

BRONCHITIS

I. Physiological Considerations

Bronchitis is an inflammatory condition of the respiratory system brought about by irritant and/or infectious agents. According to the Edgar Cayce readings, in the majority of cases irritants built up within the body are the usual culprit in the etiology of bronchitis as opposed to inhaled irritants, e.g., cigarette smoke, chemical fumes, dust, etc. (which can also cause bronchitis).

The underlying cause was often not to be found in the respiratory system itself but elsewhere. The most recurrent themes throughout the readings were poor elimination, spinal subluxation, and disturbances in the circulatory system. (These, as we see, are the triad mentioned in the readings on "headache.") This is not surprising, for, as indicated in those readings, functional abnormalities which may in turn become structural (pathologic conditions) given enough time may occur in any body organ or tissue as a result of disturbances in these systems in any combination.

The question to be asked now is, "What determines which organs or tissues are affected?" The answer to this is not entirely clear but has to do partly with which of the triad is involved, at what level the involvement is located, the vulnerability of those tissues or organs supplied by that system (i.e., acquired or congenital weakness in such), etc.

Poor elimination results in the accumulation of toxic or irritant material in the alimentary tract, blood, and lymphatics. This implies that the organs of elimination have been unable to keep up with their function and that compensatory changes have been inadequate. Consequently the accumulated toxins produce inflammatory changes in the respiratory system—namely the trachea and bronchi—and in many cases also in the throat, the nasal passages, and the sinuses.

With inflammation, congestive changes occur, further retarding the clearances of waste products in these tissues, thus aggravating the problem. These changes can further impair the nervous impulses controlling circulation (blood, lymphatics) in the respiratory system (overabundance or paucity may result), further compounding the problem.

Subluxation, usually in the third or fourth dorsal centers (but any area of the spine may be involved) causes changes or diversion of nervous impulses (nerve forces) reaching the lungs, bronchi, etc.; this results in circulatory congestion (plethora) in the lungs with attendant inflammatory changes, i.e., bronchitis. This inflammation often extends to the trachea, larynx, nasal passages, and sinuses (lesions in the cervical spine are usually found in addition in these instances). Other organs and tissues in other parts can be affected in a like manner, thus complicating the picture. The digestive system is notably among these. (Note that congestion is associated with toxin build-up.) Case [36] is a good example of multiple organ system involvement.

Qualitative and quantitative changes in the circulatory system have a variety of effects on the body. Overabundant circulation (as in 124-1), apart from causing arterial hypertension, has an adverse effect on the nerve plexuses that regulate blood (and lymph) flow. The result: congestion in various organs, which in the respiratory system produced bronchitis. Anemia, coexisting or resulting from bronchitis, further reduces the functional capacity of the blood.

In a few other cases Cayce mentions other causes and/or coexistent conditions such as superacidity, tendency to cold and congestion, scar tissue in the area of the vagus center causing cold and congestion, "infectious forces," etc. These, in the final analysis, can probably be explained in physical terms through the mechanisms already described.

That our mental/emotional and spiritual attitudes can cause or exacerbate existing illness is illustrated here (pathologic condition produced by a burn [chemical], negative attitude):

In giving the interpretation of the disturbance here, other conditions than the pathological effects produced must be taken into consideration—if there would be real help for this body.

That which is in the physical disturbing is, ever, the result of breaking a law; either pertaining to the physical, mental, or spiritual.

Here we have a misconstruction of some laws pertaining to the physical and mental. Not as of morality alone, but the entity should or must change the general attitude towards conditions about the entity—its hates, its fears; and trust in those promises that have been made.

Who healeth all thy disease? Who supplyeth life itself? Trust, then, in those promises. As has been given, "If ye call, I will hear and will answer." Use the abilities, then, of the body and of the mind, in a service to Him.   3220-1

II. Rationale of Therapy

This may be classified into four main categories:

1. Right attitude (physical, mental, spiritual).

2. Specific treatments for the relief of respiratory symptoms, e.g., nasal congestion, shortness of breath, choking produced by excessive mucous production, etc.

3. Treatment directed at the underlying cause(s), i.e., poor circulation, diversion of nervous activity, circulatory disturbances, superacidity, infections, etc.

4. Preventive measures, such as avoidance of unfavorable conditions, e.g., cold air, irritant fumes (especially smoking), dust, exposure to sudden changes in atmospheric pressure, proper diet, etc.

III. Suggested Therapeutic Regimen

Of the many recommendations for specific and general treatment for bronchitis, certain treatment programs can be selected to suit the patient. One or two of the treatments suggested may be enough to turn the tide in the patient's favor rather than rigidly going through all the available treatments.

1. Respiratory system:

a. *Inhalant* (to combat irritation and stimulate better activity). Composition and quantities varied somewhat from case to case, as well as the order in which the components were to be added. Representative formula:

To four ounces of pure grain alcohol add:

Eucalyptol, 30 minims

Benzosol, 15 minims

Benzoin, 10 minims

Rectified oil of turp, 5 minims

Balsam of fir, or Canadian balsam, 5 minims

Tincture of tolu in solution, 30 minims

Place this solution in glass container twice the volume of the solution, with a glass stopper or cork. Shake well before use. Breathe through the nostril and mouth four to five times per day, several inhalations each time. (See 36-1.) *Note:* 1/60th grain heroin was part of this formula. This can probably be omitted without losing much.

Virtually all the readings recommended some form of inhalant. See reading 5620-1 for another prescription for throat irritation.

A vaporized inhalant was recommended for the pediatric age group (croup, asthma/bronchitis):

Eucalyptol, ½ teaspoon
Compound tincture of benzoin, ½ teaspoon

Put these in one pint boiling water, kept boiling in room.

Onion poultice over throat and chest. Directions: Cook onions, retain juice, mix with finely chopped corn meal (one-half to three-quarters teaspoon). Apply on a very thin cloth or between gauze. Amount about one-half inch thick.

Antiphlogistine poultice. See reading 1346-2.

Ipecac to induce vomiting in case of choking or clogging.

b. *Expectorant* (also beneficial action on digestion and elimination). To four ounces of water add two ounces of strained pure honey (not synthetic). Let come to boil, skim off refuse, when near cool add four ounces pure apple brandy (not apple jack). Then in order named:

Syrup of rhubarb, 1 ounce
Syrup of horehound, 1 ounce
Tincture of stillingia, ½ ounce
Syrup of wild cherry, 1½ ounces
Chloroform, 10 minims

Shake well before use. Dosage: One teaspoonful three times daily. See reading 25-6 for another form of expectorant.

c. *To aid in breathing:*

1) Calcidin in small quantities every five to ten minutes (not to be given with other medicines except during paroxysms of cough).

2) Distilled water, 2 tablespoons
Strained honey, 1 tablespoon

Bring to boil, then skim off refuse; while still warm but not boiling add:

Oil of eucalyptus, 20 minims

Compound tincture of benzoin, 30 minims

Dosage: one-half tablespoon to trickle down throat slowly with saliva.

d. *Chest massage:* Use equal parts mutton suet, turpentine, spirits of camphor, compound tincture of benzoin.

e. *Treatment of associated conditions* that might be aggravating problem, e.g., heart disease, anemia, etc.

f. *Antibiotics when indicated.*

2. Correction of underlying causes:

    a. *Poor elimination*

        1) Colonics (removal of toxins);

        2) Laxatives (Bromo quinine laxative followed by chill tonic, Castoria with syrup of senna, etc.);

        3) Aids to better digestion, assimilation, elimination (Alcaroid tablets, bile salts, Codiron tablets);

        4) Massage;

        5) Osteopathic manipulations;

        6) Electric vibrator for better assimilation/elimination.

    b. *Disturbance in nerve function*

        1) Osteopathic manipulations for lesions in the spine (usually third, fourth dorsal; third, fourth, fifth cervical centers) but lumbar, sacral areas may be involved;

        2) Massage;

        3) Back and neck exercises (sometimes) for subluxations;

        4) Appliances: violet ray (in combination with the ash, sometimes) for correcting nerve imbalance; electric vibrator (relieving pressure on the heart).

    c. *Disturbance in circulation*

        1) Hydrotherapy for coordinating superficial and deep circulation;

        2) Spinal massage—enhances relaxation, circulation/elimination;

        3) Bathing and massaging the feet with hot mustard water followed by a rub (see 1100-7) to improve circulation;

        4) Alophen with 10 grains of aspirin and a good swallow of spirits frumenti is a good stimulant for capillary circulation;

        5) Musterole as a plaster over lower spine draws blood

away from the upper portion, thus relieving congestion.

3. Preventive:

As in #4 under "Rationale of Therapy," an example on dietary advice is found in reading 3220-1, the gist of it being the avoidance of foods hard to digest during acute illness; avoiding starches, warning against mixing cereals and citrus fruits; plenty of beef juice encouraged as well as greens (vegetables, fruits); meats should be fish, fowl, lamb, etc.

4. Others:

For glandular imbalance—Fowler's solution (see 136-66); tonic to create better balance in the body (see 837-1); and for general build-up of the body, Atomidine (see 1100-7).

Hezekiah Chinwah, M.D.

Edgar Cayce readings referenced:

25-6	288-23, 33	1100-7	2309-1	4809-1
36-1	304-39	1346-2	2396-1	4987-2
124-1	379-5, 6	1779-1	2975-1	5436-1
136-6	555-4, 5	1808-1	3220-1	5620-1
265-9 through 15	837-1	1850-3	3332-1	
		1964-1	4111-1	
		2001-1	4252-1	
		2299-5	4731-1	

CATARACTS

I. Physiological Considerations

The major cause of cataracts, as seen in the Cayce readings, is impaired circulation and eliminations leading to accumulations in the sensory system. Other causes less frequently cited include: spinal lesions and subluxations, digestive disturbances, dietary insufficiency, mental attitudes, mechanical injury, and constitutional condition. In one or two instances, no specific cause was given. Even in most of these instances poor circulation and elimination were the final mechanisms that allowed cataracts to form.

For instance, in reading 2193-1 elemental dietary deficiency resulted in anemia, which in turn led to altered circulation and impaired elimination resulting in the formation of cataract deposits in the eyes. The mental strain produced by associated symptoms further led to depletion of the nervous system.

Another variation is seen in reading 3598-1. In this case the cause was digestive disturbance as a result of overactivity of the glandular forces (system) affecting the duodenum. This in turn was caused by pressure on the spine at the level of the fifth, sixth thoracic (dorsal) spinal segment, which affected the hypogastric and pneumogastric centers. The final results were poor assimilations and eliminations.

Improper attitudes can work to bring about physical problems, including cataracts. In reading 3335-1, this was associated with disturbances in assimilation and elimination, resulting in other problems including cataracts. In reading 5451-2 the patient's poor attitude included improper care for his body as reflected in poor dietary habits, which contributed to developing this illness.

In summary, it can be stated that in the great majority of people for whom Cayce gave readings on cataracts, disturbances in circulation and elimination were the final mechanisms through which the disease came about. In a few instances the basis of the problem was of a non-physical nature which set into motion forces that brought about a physical condition.

II. Rationale of Therapy

This may be approached under two broad outlines:

1. Physical causes, the most common underlying problem being circulation/elimination disturbances; others include spinal lesiohs, digestive disturbances, etc. Appropriate therapy is selected on the basis of what is seen as the major underlying problem.

2. Non-physical causes such as attitudes and emotions. Physical problems nearly always overshadow the non-physical and thus the latter may be easily overlooked. In such instances only partial results are obtained when therapy is directed solely to physical causes. The following illustrations will serve to emphasize this point:

Mr. Cayce: So to relieve this condition we would, with the action of mental force, or expression, over the sensory system so control the circulation as to cause the proper elimination, or eliminating channels to be directed to the specific cause. See?
Mr. [3943]: Yes, sir.
Mr. Cayce: And with the assistance of mechanical forces so adjust all of the system as to make the direct action of both mental and spiritual being centered in the condition to be removed. That is by gentle manipulation along the centers that govern the nerves from the cerebrospinal nerve center itself, and the plexus governing the sympathetic or soul forces and their conjunction points with the sensory organism, and we would then direct as it were the energies of the mind and soul forces with the physical attributes in the body to this condition that we wish to remove from this body. Those centers we will find at the cervical region from the 2nd cervical to the 3rd and 4th dorsal. See? **3943-1**

What this passage is pointing out is that we must work on all levels—spiritual, mental and physical—for one is just as important as the others. If the physical body is unable to make use of the channeled spiritual and mental forces, little good is done by using physical applications exclusively. This passage also indicates that the higher forces are channeled through the nervous system.

Another example is to be found in reading 5451-2. This patient was already receiving treatments from other sources and was satisfied with what was being done. Cayce indicated in this instance that as long as he (the patient) felt this way, other treatments would not be advised, for they would be ineffective.

. . .if the body's mind is not to be changed, then wouldn't be best to change the body—for if the body is still convinced within self that that being done is proper, *don't change it!* Let it have its way! For it must learn for itself!
5451-2

III. Suggested Therapeutic Regimen

The following is a summary of the most commonly prescribed treatments. They are aimed at improving the circulation and eliminations and in allowing for better attunement to spiritual forces to provide coordination of the physical, mental and spiritual:

1. *Osteopathy.* Adjustments in the upper cervical and dorsal segments (C1, 2, 3; D1, 2, 3); sometimes in the lower dorsal coordinating with the upper lumbar. Frequency: about twice weekly for five to six weeks with rest periods of two to three weeks. This was by far the most commonly prescribed treatment.

2. *Massage.* With peanut oil (sometimes a combination of oils). Frequency is variable. Again twice weekly would be reasonable, though in one instance it was recommended on a daily basis before retiring. Emphasis to spine, mastoid, temple and chin areas.

3. *Violet ray treatment.* Sometimes recommended only after the first osteopathic series. Would be applied along the spine, head and neck areas for three minutes, then with the double-eye applicator over closed eyes for another one-and-a-half minutes about three times per week.

A Glyco-Thymoline or Epsom salt pack may be used over same areas for 20-30 minutes prior to the violet ray treatments.

    a. Discharge from the eyes may occur with these treatments. This should be wiped off with a non-irritating, antiseptic solution.

    b. Potato poultice may also be used after the violet ray treatment. Wash off with weak eye solution that will remove inflammation drawn by the poultice.

4. *Eliminations.* At least once or twice daily using natural laxatives, e.g., Eno salts, Fletcher's Castoria, bicarbonate of soda with cracker crumbs, etc.; colonics, if necessary.

5. *Diet.* A wholesome diet rich in fruits and vegetables. Seafoods are allowed but no meats or sweets. Raw carrots, lettuce, celery, watercress and the like are beneficial.

6. *Vibratory treatment.* Another way of stimulating blood flow is, first, rub the body with cold water to produce shock, followed by fast vibratory treatment (reading 3943-1). Frequency and duration not specified. Twice weekly treatment is suggested lasting 20-30 minutes.

7. *Spiritual counseling, prayer, and meditation.* These are other modalities available to ensure integration of the triune body, mind and spirit.

Hezekiah Chinwah, M.D.

Edgar Cayce readings referenced:

57-1	2445-1	3566-1
403-2, 3	2638-1	3598-1
1491-1	3168-1	3943-1
1561-7	3288-1, 2	4215-1
2178-1	3335-1	5451-1 through 7
2193-1	3477-1	

COLITIS

I. Physiological Considerations

The cases covered in this review fall into two classifications—acute colitis as found in a one-month-old child and a six-and-a-half-year-old boy; and the other, more common, mucous colitis, often called spastic colitis, more frequent in the adult.

There is a basic etiologic relationship between all cases of colitis, as seen in the readings. They seem to be preceded by a cold or a congestion or what might be called intestinal flu. This acts as a precipitating factor, although occasionally an injury might set the stage for subsequent events. The development of the disease process from that point onward varies to some extent with the individual.

Colitis always occurs in conjunction with lymphatic disturbances. The lacteal ducts throughout the intestinal tract, the lymphatic vessels, the lymph nodes and the Peyer's patches are all involved in a sometimes inflammatory condition. Because of the inflammation in the walls of the intestine, the lymph fluid itself often becomes toxic to the entire body, particularly the liver. Because of the toxic effect on the Peyer's patches and the lacteal ducts that are closely related to the assimilatory process, the food that is ingested no longer can be properly assimilated and made ready to participate in the rebuilding of body tissues.

. . .the disturbances with the physical forces of the body. These have to do with the assimilations in the system. Hence that tenseness as is seen in the system through the *building* or *replenishing* forces, and tendency toward anemic forces in the general system. **3886-1**

The combination of inflammation in the walls of the intestine, the lack of assimilation of needed elements in the Peyer's patch area, the toxins flowing through the lymphatics, and the strains and stresses which are imposed upon the resistances, which should be a portion of the body forces—with all this, the vital energies of the body are consumed, in a sense. As a result the body suffers.

Because of the disorders found in the lymphatics and emunctory centers of the intestinal system, mucus is often formed as a byproduct and the nerve forces throughout this portion of the body become depressed in their energies. Although the statement is never clear in those cases reviewed for this commentary, yet it must be assumed that the body is in a state of excessive acidity when an individual has colitis.

In the young individual afflicted with this condition, the lymph areas become inflamed. With the subsequent disturbance of the assimilation in the lacteal ducts and the Peyer's patches, and usually because of the inflammation present, the liver becomes distressed. This often produces fever, nausea, and a resultant series of lesions in the ganglia and the autonomic nervous system, these not being usually of major significance. Inflammatory centers might then develop in the lymph nodes throughout the body and may create greater disturbances as in [3886].

II. Rationale of Therapy

In approaching therapy, we should remember that the body has a capability of normal function:

Thus, we would administer those activities which would bring a normal reaction through these portions, stimulating them to an activity from the body itself, rather than the body becoming dependent upon supplies that are robbing portions of the system to produce activity in other portions, or the system receiving elements or chemical reactions being supplied without arousing the activity of the system itself for a more normal condition.

1968-3

Since colitis is basically a major disturbance of the lymphatics, then the therapy must be directed at restoring proper function through this portion of the body. This should probably be attempted through the following six measures:

1. Rest,
2. Eliminate the inflammatory process,

3. Balance the acidity-alkalinity by soothing the activity of the lymphatics,

4. Cleanse the lymphatics,

5. Balance the eliminations and the liver functions,

6. Coordinate the nervous system activity.

It is important in achieving the aims just mentioned to be persistent when the individual is an adult and has had the colitis for a period of time. Therapy for the child with an acute colitis would necessarily be directed in a different manner.

III. Suggested Therapeutic Regimen

Children respond rather dramatically, just as they become ill rather precipitously. This was the case with one-month-old [2892], who had acute colitis. He recovered in just a few hours when he was put on a rigid regimen of underfeeding; Glyco-Thymoline packs across the abdomen, put on hot as can be stood and left on until cool—which is 15 to 20 minutes—twice or three times daily; Glyco-Thymoline two drops in water two or three times a day; daily enemas with some Glyco-Thymoline in the enema water or olive oil used first; Castoria one or two drops each hour until movement is obtained every two or three days; and yellow saffron tea sipped in minute quantities during the day, made fresh each day. This combination of substances brought about an immediate response with this infant.

With the six-and-a-half-year-old boy, [3886], the routine of therapy was somewhat different. The enemas and Glyco-Thymoline internally as an antiseptic of an alkaline-reacting nature were used here, as well as underfeeding—in this instance using vegetable and citrus fruit juices and goat's milk. Quiet and rest were insisted upon and beef juice was added to strengthen the body. In addition to the osteopathic manipulations, massage was given daily along the spine with a mixture of equal parts of olive oil, myrrh, and sassafras oil; and a gentle massage over the body with spiritus frumenti (with the alcohol burned off), when fever needed to be controlled.

Chronic mucous colitis or spastic colitis—and I'm sure ulcerative colitis was included occasionally in these—in the older person is approached somewhat differently. The readings sometimes emphasized tuberous vegetables, other times a regular diet and at times a suggestion such as the following:

In the diets, keep away from meats. Only fish or fowl may be taken, and

these never fried. *No fried foods of any kind.* Take rather the body-building and strength-giving foods—especially a great deal of fruits, fruit juices—including citrus fruit juices, of course. Combine a little lemon with the orange juice. Plenty of prunes, prune whip. Plenty of pineapple and the like. All of these would be the principals, though not all of the diet. Refrain from a great deal of pastries. Malted milks and those of such natures may be in the diet. Not too much of candies or sweets, though occasionally milk in chocolate or cocoa or the like may be taken.   **2085-1**

An inch-thick grape poultice—made of crushed grapes and laid on the abdomen for one-and-a-half to four hours until dry—was suggested in many readings apparently for its effect on the lymph centers and the lymph fluid as a cleansing type of preparation. The grapes should preferably be Concord. A wild ginseng fusion is suggested just as frequently. Rest, mild exercise in the open air, alum fusion, massage with camphorated oil to the abdomen and to the spine (especially after the grape poultice is used) are other suggestions. Colonic irrigation is frequently suggested to cleanse the colon and remove toxic products, and osteopathic treatments were recommended to balance the nerve forces and impulses and to remove the lesions which have been formed during the development of the disease process.

Following is a list of various combinations of substances suggested for use in colitis. They are helpful as a reference.

1. First therapy in mucous colitis where there is an excess of lymph activity and a jujunitis (not specified here what function it will perform):

First make a good strong fusion of wild ginseng; not so strong as to be a tincture, to be sure, but: When the wild ginseng is well broken, put an ounce of this in distilled water and boil for at least twenty minutes, until it has produced a good fusion; not using the pulverized ginseng, but broken up; using sufficient water to make two-and-one-half ounces of the fusion. Strain.

Then to the 2½ ounces of the fusion of wild ginseng add, in the order named:

> Tincture of wild ginger, ¼ ounce
> Tincture of valerian, ½ ounce
> Grain alcohol (90 proof), 1 ounce

2846-1

2. After colitis—to rebuild the system:

The greater distresses associated with acute colitis quieted down during the eight days prior to this six-and-a-half-year-old boy's second reading. At that point, it was felt necessary to build up the system more. The following is an extract from his second reading:

Yes, we find the body here, and the conditions show somewhat of the improvements and the reduction of those forces as cause the greater distress. Those that will be more of the general *building,* now, we would add for the system. Those that add iron and the *sodas* to the system, or it may be in a stimul[us] as *this:* These we would add considerably to the stimuli, but would of necessity be given in very small quantities and should be gradually increased until there would be given what would be the division of the whole quantity into thirty pellets. We would take:

> Camphor gum, 20 grains
> Muriated iron, 20 grains
> Sulphate of morphia, ¼ grain

Mix this thoroughly together. Begin with one grain of same, as a stimul[us]—see? Then add those in the food values. These will rest, and those will also *build* the body. Do that.   3886-2

3. Grape poultice for lymphatic disturbances:

Apparently, from readings 5023-1 and 5280-1, grape poultices were used to restore more normal functioning of lymph centers and emunctories throughout the intestinal tract. In the former reading, there was a nerve exhaustion brought on by an injury to the liver area and an amoebic dysentery had developed. Apparently injuries of one sort or another or depression of the lymphatic centers had developed with this excess lymph circulation. In 5280-1 fever from inflammation in the colon had produced disorders of all the lymph centers and emunctories throughout the alimentary canal.

Do apply over the whole abdomen, at least once a week, crushed grapes. These should be used with the hull and the seed. The pack should be at least one inch thick and let this remain on until it has almost dried out from the body heat, which would require four to four-and-one-half hours. Make this pack sufficiently large to cover the whole abdomen. Put the grapes on gauze.
                                                                      5057-1

4. Alum fusion

Prepare this also in a fusion: Put ½ ounce of alum root in 4 ounces of distilled water, and let come to a boil, then strain. Be sure the alum root is crushed. Add to this, ½ ounce of simple syrup and take 1 ounce of grain alcohol or rye whiskey and add. This is only to be taken one teaspoon when there is cramping through the alimentary canal or colon.   5057-1

5. Wild ginseng prescription

To two ounces of distilled water add a tablespoonful of pure honey (not synthetic, but pure honey). Let this come to a boil, skimming off the dross or sediment as it rises to the top. Then add to this ¼ ounce of grain alcohol. Then add, *in the order named:*

> Elixir (or fusion) of wild ginseng, ¼ ounce
> Wild ginger (essence or fusion), ¼ ounce
> Tincture of stillingia, ¼ ounce
> Elixir of lactated pepsin, ¼ ounce

The dose would be half a teaspoonful in half a glass of water twice each day—morning and evening.

This compound taken internally as a stimulant to the activities through the alimentary canal, with the osteopathic corrections given, will gradually make for not only the correcting of the condition but the eliminating of the causes of same; and thus bring about a near normal or equal balance in the functioning of the organs, as well as the glandular forces, and clearing gradually the disturbance wherein the activities through the whole of the alimentary canal may be eliminated and eradicated entirely from the system.
                                                                                    2085-1

6. Fusion of wild ginseng:

Preparation: Put 5 drams of wild ginseng in a pint of distilled water. Let this come to a boil, and boil until, when this is strained, there is only ½ pint. This will be rather strong, but is needed in this particular case.

Then make a fusion of this: Use 2 drams of wild ginger in 4 ounces of distilled water. Let this come to a boil, and boil until there [are] only 2 ounces left when strained.

Add these together and then add 4 ounces essence of lactated pepsin, and 1 ounce of grain alcohol.

This should be taken in the beginning, one teaspoon every four hours for two days. Of course don't arise at night to take this, but if awake during the night take a dose, but not oftener than four hours apart.   5057-1

7. Wild ginseng prescription from 5280-1:

Fusion or essence of wild ginseng, 1 ounce

Essence of wild ginger, ½ ounce
Then add sufficient elixir of lactated pepsin to make 6 ounces.
Directions: Shake and take one teaspoonful twice a day or at about 9:00 a.m. and 3:00 p.m.

8. Pure beef juice:

Beef juice was referred to "as medicine" (5374-1) or "almost as medicine" (1100-10). (See Appendix.) Instructions for taking were explicit:

Take at least a tablespoon during a day, or two tablespoonfuls. But not as spoonfuls; rather sips of same. This, sipped in this manner, will work towards producing the gastric flow through the intestinal system. . .

1100-10

Should we not attempt to awaken the inner forces to God's presence? "For, all healing comes from the one source. And whether there is the application of foods, exercise, medicine, or even the knife, it is to bring the consciousness of the forces within the body that aid in reproducing themselves—the awareness of creative or God forces." (2696-1)

William A. McGarey, M.D.

Edgar Cayce readings referenced:
348-23
2085-1
2846-1
2892-1
3886-1, 2
5023-1
5057-1
5280-1

COLOR BLINDNESS

I. Physiological Considerations

In the single case of color blindness discussed in this Circulating File, the apparent cause is karmic or one that might be called hereditary, since the condition apparently had existed since birth. Other cases are not available for study.

The production of lack of color vision as a physiological series of events is interesting and probably might find many relationships with other conditions of the eye. It begins as nerve energies in the vagus nerve that are deflected from their origin in the second, third and fourth dorsal sympathetic ganglia. (These ganglia have major control over the coordination within the body between the superficial and the deep circulation.) The nerve energies arise here and coordinate through the vagus nerve with the similar areas of control existing in the third, fourth, and fifth cervical ganglia. The latter are the optic centers which control various functions of the eyes. In this series of events then, the nerve energies which should be flowing to the optic centers have been deflected because of disturbances in the upper dorsal area; and the optic centers in turn are deficient in circulatory control energy which might be directed toward the eyes.

Not enough nerve impulse, then, comes from the lower cervical optic centers to care for the replenishing of the eyes and the carrying away of the used forces which are present there. Then, when overactivity comes about (general muscular and visual activity), the primary circulation to the eyes, which is a part of the deep circulation, becomes filled to overflowing with "refused energies." This brings the lachrymals, ducts, and glands of the superficial circulation into action in an attempt to supply the energies needed. Swelling, reddening, and irritation then come to the eyelid, portions of the eyeball, "and to the *character* of that which is *reflected* in the lens and in the iris and in the response to the optic center itself." (820-2)

It would seem—from this series of circumstances among the various consciousnesses of the body—that a specific type of accident to the dorsal area could also conceivably cause color blindness. Other abnormalities in function within the body may or may not be present.

II. Rationale of Therapy

In approaching therapy, we should remember that the body has a capability of *normal* function:

Thus, we would administer those activities which would bring a normal reaction through these portions, stimulating them to an activity from the body itself, rather than the body becoming dependent upon supplies that are robbing portions of the system to produce activity in other portions, or the system receiving elements or chemical reactions being supplied without arousing the activity of the system itself for a more normal condition.

1968-3

The rationale of therapy in this particular condition would be:

1. To correct the condition of abnormality in the dorsal ganglia,

2. To stimulate more activity of those energies coming from the cervical area, and

3. To supply the material with which to rebuild deficient nerve forces.

It would be necessary, of course, to care for the pressures which might exist in the cervical area, and osteopathic care through these courses of therapy would be the primary concern.

III. Suggested Therapeutic Regimen

Therapy should first be directed at correcting osteopathically the pressures which exist in second, third, and fourth dorsal segments. These should be given two or three times a week for a period of three weeks. The cervical vertebrae should not be treated until the dorsal are in perfect alignment as shown by the circulation of the right temple being in balance with the circulation of the left temple. When this is done the cervical should also be treated.

After each osteopathic treatment, the hand violet ray applicator should be used to the cervical and the upper dorsal area but especially to the atlas (the first cervical area). Toward the end of the three-week period, the last treatments should incorporate the wet cell battery, with the gold chloride solution in one grain per ounce of distilled water (use three ounces in the bottle). The positive copper electrode should be placed at the fourth dorsal area, and the nickel plate, carrying the gold chloride, should be placed between the first and second cervicals, which would locate it at the "brain force centers" and the medulla oblongata. Those portions that go to the vagus center on either side of the neck and enter into the arteries and through to the head would be affected. Wet cell therapy should be continued for three weeks.

After this has been completed, rest is recommended for about three weeks. Then the entire series should be repeated and these cycles kept on until the condition is corrected.

Therapy should be aimed at keeping the diet near to alkaline-reacting foods. Green raw vegetables, whole wheat, citrus fruits (never these combined), fruits, berries, and vegetables are all alkaline-reacting foods. Never fried foods, never bananas and never raw apples (unless the raw apples are taken by themselves for three days and then followed with olive oil which will cleanse all toxins from the system). There should be no large quantity of potatoes. Potato peelings are strengthening, carrying those influences and forces that are active in the glands of the system. An 80 percent alkaline/20 percent acid reacting diet is advised.

Should we not attempt to awaken the inner forces to God's presence? "For, all healing comes from the one source. And whether there is the application of foods, exercise, medicine, or even the knife, it is to bring the consciousness of the forces within the body that aid in reproducing themselves—the awareness of creative or God forces." (2696-1)

William A. McGarey, M.D.

Edgar Cayce readings referenced:
820-1, 2, 3

THE COMMON COLD

I. Physiological Considerations

The common cold—also known as coryza, rhinitis, and upper respiratory infection—is an acute infection of the upper respiratory tract by a filterable virus, which is then often followed by invasion of the respiratory tract by pathogenic organisms. It is considered to be highly contagious, although it is usually mild, of short duration, and endemic. The onset is marked by a chilly sensation followed by sneezing, watering of the eyes, nasal discharge, cough, and is often accompanied by a mild fever. Much has been written about this most common of all diseases.

In the Cayce readings much has also been given respecting the common cold, including a complete reading, 902-1, which is included in this File. It is an excellent commentary and worthy of study.

The balance of the body probably plays the most important part in preventing the beginning of a cold. Although Cayce stated that "it is a universal consciousness to the human body" (902-1)—yet a cold develops in the presence of an acid condition within the body and nearly always only when that condition pertains. An alkalizing effect is destructive to the cold germs themselves. The question of acidity-alkalinity is discussed in another Circulating File and seems to be a difficult concept to understand fully. Yet Cayce answered the question whether there were any special precautions to be taken against colds by the simple words, "keep alkalized." (480-45)

Whenever the fine balance of the body in its acid-base relationship is disturbed, then an individual is susceptible to a cold. Any condition—draft, wet feet, change in temperature, or any similar condition—that causes a change in circulation through affecting the body balance, the body temperature or the body equilibrium, can cause a cold if the body is susceptible. Susceptibility comes when there has been extra depletion of the vital energies of the body, which in turn produces a tendency for an excess acidity. Or, psychologically, if an individual becomes aware of a detrimental change in body temperature or environment, this uses energies and makes him thus more susceptible. Loss of sleep; excess emotional turbulence, such as anger, resentment or contention; excess activity leading to extreme tiredness—all these create either a marked depletion of the body's energies or a pouring out of poisons from the glandular system into the lymph circulation, preparing the system so that it blocks the circulation to the eliminating channels, creating again an acidity and a disturbance which predisposes to a cold.

The glands, of course, secrete according to impulse from the emotional system. With anger, these secretions poison the body. "Thus you can take a bad cold from getting mad. You can get a bad cold from blessing out someone else, even if it is your wife." (849-75)

An acid-reacting diet—such as too much of meat and starches—creates a susceptibility to colds within the body. Likewise, incorrect eating does the same thing. Food should be thoroughly masticated. "Bolting food, or swallowing it by the use of liquids produces more colds than *any one* activity of a diet." (808-3)

Overheated rooms, for instance, lessen the oxygen available which weakens the circulation of life-giving forces that destroy any germ. Tiredness, overacidity, or overalkalinity all contribute at times to the production of a cold.

Physiologically we can see that each body is indeed a law unto itself, due to the varying activities of physiological processes which are brought about by the many factors playing a part in each person's body. "Consequently, as we find, this [condition, the cold] is one of the most erratic conditions that may be considered as an ill to the human body." (902-1)

II. Rationale of Therapy

Care of the body externally is certainly one of the obvious factors in prevention. Precautions should be taken as to clothing, drafts, damp feet; one should avoid becoming overtired or too exhausted, and should avoid being in a room that is too hot or too cold. Keeping in the open air often is an excellent preventative, if one does not let the body get too cold.

A normal, alkaline-reacting diet should be kept at all times when one is exposed to colds. This means much in the way of fresh fruits, though citrus fruits and cereals should not be combined at the same meal. Green raw vegetables should be a portion of the diet. The meats should be such as lamb, fowl, fish, or the like. Occasionally the broiled steak or liver would be well. A balance is needed between the starches and proteins with adequate amounts of carbohydrates.

Above all, one should not allow himself the costly luxury of anger, resentment, hate, or argument. He should cultivate instead the quality of forgiveness, teach himself to be tolerant of his brother's mistakes and his own shortcomings, thus developing an equanimity of spirit, which is perhaps the most important prerequisite to a balanced body function.

The body must function as a unit. Thus, care of the body externally and precautions as to diet and emotion must also be combined with specific attention to what might be called therapy as a preventive. Vitamins are substances which stimulate the more normal function of the glands of the body. All vital forces in the body are activities of the glandular system, and these forces are stimulated by specific glandular activity attributed to the functioning of certain portions of the system. Thus vitamins would be helpful when one is exposed to colds. "Vitamins are not as easily overcrowded in the system as most other boosters for a general activity." (902-1) And it would be well to keep the glandular system promoting the normal vital forces within the body at times of stress.

Yet, there is a word of caution about too many vitamins either as a preventive or where infection already exists. "For, that which may be helpful may also be harmful—if misapplied—whether by the conscious activity in a body or by an unconscious activity in the assimilating forces of a system. If this were not true, there would never be an unbalancing of *any* portion of the functioning system; neither would there be the lack of coordination or cooperation with the various organs in their attempt to work together." (902-1)

In addition to the proper use of vitamins as a preventive in keeping the body balanced, the readings suggested that it was necessary to keep the eliminations adequate, both through the intestines and through the kidneys. Thus a cathartic or an enema in the early stages of body unbalancing would be helpful.

For purifying the kidneys, one to three drops of sweet spirits of nitre or 15 drops of onion juice is suggested. Another rather unusual therapy for prevention is the use of a mixture of equal parts of mutton tallow, spirits of camphor, and spirits of turpentine massaged into the feet and ankles and legs of an individual. Why massage the feet for an oncoming cold in the head? Perhaps the same answer could be used here as would be appropriate for the question—why is it when your feet get cold and wet that you may get a cold in the head? The body is indeed a unit.

III. Suggested Therapeutic Regimen

Because of its erratic occurrence in the course of human events and because it meets within each body a separate law of function and activity, the common cold becomes a difficult and puzzling condition to treat successfully. There are, however, certain general rules that have evolved in the readings which might prove helpful.

1. Rest is a primary factor and apparently has no substitute. This is due to the need within the body for a balanced function of the autonomic nervous system. During rest and sleep, balance of the autonomic is, to a great extent, restored. If the body is contracting a cold, something has been stressed through exhaustion, and rest is usually necessary to undo this condition.

2. Much water should be taken during these times. An alkalizer should also be added to the system, such as a teaspoon of baking soda in a glass of water or something similar. The water helps to cleanse the body and eliminate drosses, and the soda tends to produce alkalinity within the body.

3. A diet that is right (as proven over a period of time) for an individual is probably the best at these times. However, it should conform to the dietary suggestions already mentioned. For the acute phase of a cold, a liquid diet generally is best. Little meat should be taken until the recuperative stage, and certainly too much should not be eaten. For [540] Cayce suggested citrus fruit for two days with an occasional teaspoonful of spiritus frumenti in a large glass of lemonade.

4. Vitamins of all kinds are helpful when the body has been weakened to any degree. These supply, through boosting the glands of the body, the vital energies needed for health.

Many things in many ways are beneficial to those who have contracted cold—dependent, to be sure, upon the general constitution of the body, the amount of vitamins stored in the system, and so on. Also the response depends greatly on whether or not there is the opportunity given for rest and

the not eating too much, so that the body may be aroused to gain its equilibrium.

Hence it is necessary that there be given the booster for those portions of the body needing the stimulation; and those elements that produce more of vital energies are the more helpful influences.   **902-1**

5. Weaknesses which are present within the body should be recognized and corrected. This may be due to old injuries, or it may be some factor that has already been understood as being a weak, or susceptible, portion of the body functioning. Constipation is a factor which contributes to many illnesses. Assimilation may have been inadequate for a long time. These various weaknesses must be tended to.

6. Various special therapies were suggested in many instances in the readings. For [585], the reading suggested Sal Hepatica, three doses, two hours apart; to be followed by a half teaspoon of Castoria every hour until the digestive tract was cleared. This same individual was told to treat his fever by bathing his feet in hot water every four hours, and following this, to take a rubdown from the hips to the feet and including the feet with the combination already mentioned (equal parts of mutton tallow, spirits of turpentine, and spirits of camphor).

Such a combination was also suggested at times to be used on the throat and chest, or over the sinuses. Fume baths with rubdowns; steam cabinet treatments; massages; manipulative therapy; nose sprays and gargles with Glyco-Thymoline and Listerine alternated; a variety of cough syrups (see Appendix), such as taking the white of an egg, juice of a lemon, teaspoonful of honey, and two drops of glycerine carefully concocted—all of these are apparently helpful in various circumstances to restore the body to a normal balance.

Perhaps the most interesting specific suggestion Cayce gave followed an injunction to [288] to keep the body alkaline and eliminate the cold. Then he said: "Instead of snuffing, *blow!* Instead of resentments, *love!*" (288-44)

In concluding the commentary, perhaps we should remind ourselves that the body really has a capacity to function normally and we must urge it to do so without sacrificing other functions within the body.

Thus, we would administer those activities which would bring a normal reaction through these portions, stimulating them to an activity from the body itself, rather than the body becoming dependent upon supplies that are

robbing portions of the system to produce activity in other portions, or the system receiving elements or chemical reactions being supplied without arousing the activity of the system itself for a more normal condition.

1968-3

William A. McGarey, M.D.

Edgar Cayce readings referenced:
480-45
540-2
585-5
808-3
902-1
1208-11
IRF pp. 88-93

Causes of Common Cold

Q-1. In case of severe cold such as I have now, when I first take same, what is the first step I should take to correct it?

A-1. What causes it? Then, just as has been indicated here for this body, in the present. This may not be the same the 3rd of February, when you'll take another one if you don't watch out! for that may be from an entirely different cause!   340-32

. . .there has arisen the acute conditions not only from physical reactions but mental conditions that have been as resentments, which have been builded into the mental forces of the body.

These are indicated in the toxic conditions from cold as well as the poisons from gum conditions have settled in joints, as in hips, shoulders, neck and head.   1523-17

In the present the unbalanced condition in the physical of the alkalinity and acidity has caused, and does cause, congested areas in the functioning of the body. These as to their sources have in the main arisen from anger (physical) produced by the activities of environs about the body; thus causing the throwing into the lymph circulation those poisons which reacted upon the general physical body-relationships with the mental and spiritual activities of the body.

For the glands secrete according to impulse from the emotional system. This has been, then, the source of the disturbances in the body.   294-208

Q-6. Is the body getting rid of the poisons discharged into the bloodstream as well as can be expected?

A-6. As indicated, it is getting rid of some, but when there is the ruffling of your disposition when there is any anger, it prepares the system so that it blocks the flow of the circulation to the eliminating channels. Thus you can take a bad cold from getting mad. You can get a bad cold from blessing out someone else, even if it is your wife.   849-75

Q-15. What causes colds? Can you give me a formula or method of preventing them, or curing them?

A-15. Keep the body alkaline! Cold germs do not live in an alkaline system! They do breed in any acid or excess of acids of *any* character left in the system.   1947-4

Prevention of Common Cold

Q-2. What can I do to build resistance against head colds?

A-2. Keep the normal acidity and alkalinity, by occasionally taking the test with litmus paper—both from the urine and from the spittle. Use the blue litmus, see?

When there is the inclination for acidity, use any of the sodas or their derivatives (citrocarbonates) as would make for producing a better balance. Thus we will find the colds will be eliminated.

1100-20

Q-2. What should be done to build resistance against colds?

A-2. Keep the body more alkaline. This may be done by taking food values that are more alkaline in their reaction, and occasionally—say once a week (but do not take it every day)—take a small quantity of plain baking soda; using Glyco-Thymoline as a mouth wash, and occasionally swallow a few drops, for it's an intestinal antiseptic—and there is none better for keeping the eliminations throughout the body, tending toward alkalinity in the alimentary canal—where most disorders arise. 413-4

Q-3. How can she prevent taking "flu"?

A-3. As given. To prevent taking cold is to prevent the body from reaching that point where the blood is acted upon by that bacilli known as cold, or the preventative is to create in the system that which combats cold (which is pure rich blood!) by keeping the system nominally balanced, keeping the metabolism of the body at or near normal. 654-3

Q-17. How can I prevent from having colds all the time?

A-17. It would require volumes to give that which would prevent anyone from having colds! for all those conditions that produce colds would have to be considered; diet, eliminations, drafts, changes of temperature, and everything of the kind. But if a body is sufficiently balanced as to make for resistance, there will be sufficient leukocytes in the blood supply to choke a cold to death immediately! But to keep such a resistance is to keep a body normally balanced, and to be mindful of those things that we have given. For, colds are plasms that find their reaction in the blood supply itself, and *feed* upon the white more than upon the red blood, until they have become some form of the strep nature. Then they work through to the organs in the system, see? They first begin with the lymph, or the water and white blood, and get hold upon the system unless the supply of leukocytes or warriors is present in the system to choke them to death. A cold can't make headway when the warriors are sufficient, or the leukocytes.

386-3

Q-4. How can I overcome susceptibility to infections such as colds, influenza, etc.?

A-4. As we have just indicated, by keeping the body alkaline. Only in acids do colds attack the body.   3248-1

Treatment of Common Cold

[Background: Reading in response to phone call from Mr. [257]'s secretary; Mr. [257] choked up with cold, unable to speak above a whisper.]

Yes, we have the body here. This we have had before.

The use of those properties that have been indicated for such conditions would be well; that is, taking first an eliminant—or about eighteen hundred (1800) drops of the Castoria, but *not* at once. Take it in very small or broken doses. After the first container or bottle has been taken in these proportions, which should be about eight-thirty or nine o'clock this evening, *then* take the Turkish bath; that is, first the sweats, then the salt rum rubs, and then the alcohol rub after the oil rubs, see?

And during the whole period keep more of an alkaline diet. No white bread. Principally use fruit juices, and citrus fruit juices at that! A little coffee without cream may be taken as a stimulant, or a little whiskey and soda later in the evening may be taken.

And the body should feel physically fit by morning.

Afterwards, then, keep the general rubs and the stimulations through especially the lower dorsal and throughout the lumbar area.

[Gladys Davis's note: Each bottle of Fletcher's Castoria contains 900 drops. By "broken doses" the reading means a teaspoonful every hour, or half a teaspoonful every half hour. On 2/2/36 we received a report by Mr. [257]: "I felt miserable, but after taking the day's rest and the bottle of Castoria, and the rubs, I could talk the next morning and was at work all day. . ."]   257-159

Now, we have had these conditions here before, and we find that— with some fresh cold and congestion, combined with reinfection—the conditions have again become exaggerated from that as when last we had this here, and we find, too, that the condition as has been treated in part is as treating the effect rather than treating the cause; or as trying to remove blades of grass and not removing that that grows same—for with the fertile soil, same continues to put forth those hindrances as here. With the continual congestion from conditions in the hypogastric and gastric regions—we find the disturbed circulation, the hindered elimination, continue to cause pressure in the head, neck, throat and the whole of the sensory system.

By the use of antiseptics alone, in congested portions—as in nostrils, ears, throat, eyes—relief will be found from the external secretions as are formed, and prevent the reinfection—for tissue is involved, as is seen, and by applying those elements as given, internally, for the gastric conditions, and by stimulating with the massage of the equal portions of myrrh and of the olive oil in the centers as are seen from the solar plexus to the base of brain— stimulation to those centers—will enable the body to throw off these conditions through their normal channel, and thus reach the base or cause of these conditions.

Rest necessary—as is rest for the digestive system in the manner given, for to cause this center (the gastrics) to again become in that condition of throwing refuse in the upper circulation, rather than eliminating same through the dross channel, is as but adding fuel to the flame—and in the manner as *outlined* should this be handled, see?

Ready for questions.

Q-1. What antiseptic should be used for the eyes, nose, ears, etc.?

A-1. That in throat, eyes and the nose, use that of the Glyco-Thymoline and Listerine, alternately. One as an alkaline, the other as an acid—gargling with these; bathing with the weak solution, or snuffing or spraying nostrils, as to clear this portion of the head.

Use the massage and rub at least twice each day.

As soon as the physical conditions permit we would change to the warmer clime—such as Cuba, or Bahamas. These would be well, see? for six to eight weeks.

Q-3. In what proportion should the Glyco-Thymoline and Listerine be used?

A-3. In the throat and nostrils as gargle or spray, in normal quantity. That for the eyes would be weakened very materially, of course—but when used in throat and nostrils, little will be required for eyes, see? 137-95

Prepare this compound in two solutions, you see, that is, melt the mutton tallow and this would be a separate solution, until the others are added. Do not attempt to mix the tallow in its original state, but melt it. Then—while it is not too hot, but before it congeals—add an equal amount of each of the other ingredients; first the turpentine, then the camphor.   2175-2

Keep up the gentle rubs each evening. . .Liquefy the mutton tallow, then add the same quantity of the turpentine, and *then* the same quantity of camphor, see? Stir these together.   2051-3

Massage the glands on the throat and upper portion of the chest, in the hollow of the throat and neck, on the glands of the side, with an equal combination of mutton tallow (melted), spirits of turpentine and spirits of camphor; and in the evening put two thicknesses of flannel around same.

This should within twenty-four to forty-eight hours, as we find, reduce the conditions [for this body].

With the diet, of course, take those things that are more of the liquid nature.

Have good eliminations, preferably with either the Castoria or syrup of figs, or any compound that is of senna base.

Do these, as we find, for the immediate; and have a good, general, thorough osteopathic treatment to relax the body thoroughly afterwards.   1100-29

Q-1. Should anything further be done to eliminate present cold? What produces these poisons?

A-1. As has been indicated; the colonic and the eliminations set up; *keeping* the alkalinity—though don't overdo this, see?

Instead of snuffing, *blow!* Instead of resentments, *love!*   288-44

CONSTIPATION

I. Physiological Considerations

Constipation—inadequate, difficult, or infrequent evacuation of the fecal content of the bowels—probably causes greater disturbance of function and more symptoms of dis-ease in the human being than any other single condition.

Most commonly, constipation has its origin in an acidity created in the assimilating system of the body. We call this acidity "stomach trouble." Implied in the readings—though not explicitly described—is the concept that stress, tension, arguments, disagreements, anger, and other negative manifestations of the adrenal gland bring the acidity into being in the stomach/duodenal area.

The Peyer's patches provide for the body the alkaline forces necessary in the acid-base balance that must be maintained. (See Acidity-Alkalinity Circulating File.) With excess acid present in the stomach, lymphatic function decreases and creates an inactivity in the liver. A relative lack of enzyme production with a subsequent decrease in proper assimilation follows. This in turn cuts down markedly on the rebuilding forces available for producing normal eliminations. Then some foods which are at times acceptable to the body become as poisons and the system becomes overloaded with "used forces"—those end products of metabolism and the substances produced by improper metabolism and intestinal wastes that begin to be reabsorbed through the lower intestinal walls. After this occurs, a condition which might be described as an intestinal indigestion comes into being which causes a packing of fecal material in the large bowel. The system, reabsorbing waste into the bloodstream, reinforces the beginning factors which brought the constipation into being.

Certainly it must be recognized that constipation occurs as a result of various types of diseases, but the development as described above is probably the most common. Associated with constipation nearly always and sometimes acting as a cause of constipation are varying pressures and subluxations of the cervical, dorsal, and lumbar segments. Improper diet, such as an acid-reacting one, kept up as a regular practice, is also a major factor. The consequences of constipation are consistently underrated, possibly because they are not understood. When toxins are reabsorbed into the circulation, the liver progressively loses its ability to excrete as well as to secrete. The kidneys usually respond to this relative liver shutdown by becoming overtaxed in their function of eliminating substances from the body. Symptoms of dysuria appear, associated with inflammation of the kidney, bladder, and the tubes associated with the renal system. The skin and lungs—two other organs of elimination—are called upon to exercise their functions more vigorously in order to keep the body in a good general balance. Thus halitosis or various skin disturbances may occur.

In case [550], the accumulation of toxins produced a general nervousness with bad dreams—an incoordination of the cerebrospinal and the autonomic nervous sytems. What caused all this? "This same restlessness as was produced in the nerve system, which carries, as it were, its message of those conditions awry in the system to the brain. This, then, produces restlessness, and the tendency for the body to have hallucinations or visions that would harm physically the body." (550-1) From the disturbance of the incoordination comes also the inability to rest well, a constant waking during the night, and a tiredness when rest should have brought about resuscitation. These symptoms arise because the recuperative processes malfunction due to the toxins throughout the system. The eyes might become inflamed, the hands become cold on occasion, and skin eruptions appear. Headaches are a common symptom, nausea at times, and a heaviness in the feet. Also a dryness of the mouth; sometimes a swelling of the feet; and the color and circulation are reported as "bad."

In looking at the various types of incoordination produced, it becomes evident that disease syndromes can be built upon the simple condition that we know as constipation. It becomes important, then, to regard the elimination system with a great deal of respect.

There should be a warning to *all* bodies as to such conditions; for would the assimilations and the eliminations be kept nearer *normal* in the human

family, the days might be extended to whatever period as was so desired; for the system is *builded* by the assimilations of that it takes within, and is able to bring resuscitation so long as the eliminations do not hinder.   311-4

II. Therapeutic Considerations

Constipation that has progressed beyond a single episode must be given due respect when therapy is being considered. A wide variety of treatments, certainly, is available. However, for constipation that has progressed to the point where it becomes a problem for the individual, there seems to emerge a pattern of three basic therapies.

1. Diet: Unless a condition of alkalosis is present, the diet should be a highly alkaline-reacting one with many leafy green vegetables. Starches and protein should not be combined, such as bread with beans or high protein vegetables, and white potatoes with bread. Cereals and juice (citrus) combinations should be avoided. *Important:* The diet should be kept to consistently and for a long period of time.

2. Osteopathic treatments were advised for [926], who was to have three treatments a week for five weeks, then two a week for perhaps 10 weeks, then rest 10 days—then another series of six to eight treatments. Sometimes a longer series would be needed, depending to a great extent on the chronicity of the constipation. (Relaxation or manipulation should be used at all times with the exception of one adjustment of specific nature every three to five treatments.)

3. Cleansing of the intestines includes colonics, which are very helpful and frequently necessary; enemas; various types of eliminants, such as Fletcher's Castoria, olive oil, Agarol, and cleansing diets. These may all be necessary at one time or another to keep the bowels cleansed. Castor oil packs may occasionally be needed or abdominal massage. Massage with olive oil should follow the course of the stomach to the duodenum, past the Peyer's patches to the jejunum and ileum, and then across to the caecum, up over the ascending, transverse and descending colon, for as long as the body will absorb the olive oil.

Most often treatment for constipation will be in conjunction with treatment for other conditions, so this must be kept in mind when the above suggestions are utilized. (See Appendix.)

An Elimination Program for a Torpid Liver

After each meal for two or three days, take about a quarter teaspoonful of the Alcaroid.

After the third day that this has been taken, leave it off, and take two Zilatone tablets at bedtime—on the day after the Alcaroid has been left off, you see; drinking plenty of water!

Let this go then for two or three weeks, then do this again.

But to keep the eliminations each day that there is not the evacuation through the alimentary canal, the high enemas—salt and soda enemas. Preferably take these yourself, using a fountain syringe. Not necessary that the water be hot. Do *not* have the water warmer than the temperature of the body, but use this each day when there is not a natural evacuation from the alimentary canal.   1269-1

Constipation—Acute Infection

In case [25], Cayce suggests that an eliminant be given that is of the lactic nature rather than of the acid nature. In this case the teenage boy had tonsillitis which was causing pains in the joints and a toxic condition.

Hence it would be necessary that, not too much excitement to the secreting organ but, sufficient and rather the lactic nature than of the acid; that is, these properties taken to produce elimination shall be lactics and of the saline nature rather than of an acid nature. That is, such as these would be well for the body to take regularly for some time after this was done:

Plain phosphate of soda, half a teaspoonful in half a glass of water, and add five to six drops of oil, or syrup of sarsaparilla.   25-2

This boy was advised to have his tonsils removed and to clean out the intestinal tract.

The following extract helps us to understand the balance of mind and body that is needed, for emotions *do* have an effect upon our physical beings:

Do not become overanxious—for, to be sure, the mental is the builder; and overanxiousness may bring about barriers to proper reactions throughout the system; whether as related to the circulatory forces or the assimilations or eliminations of the body.

But these influences kept in a body—normal eliminations, near to normal assimilations—without accident—it, the body, reproduces itself in every phase of its experience. The natural balance is an eighty percent alkaline to a twenty percent acid reaction. This means *reaction* in the system, and these should be kept.

Keep these physically, mentally, with a spiritual basis of *constructiveness*

for the mental attitudes. For grudges, animosities, hates, overanxieties are a part of the mental and become conditions reactory in the physical forces.
816-8

William A. McGarey, M.D.

Edgar Cayce readings referenced:
311-4
550-1
816-8
926-1
1069-4
1713-17
2553-3
5080-1
5116-1

CYSTITIS

I. Physiological Considerations

Cystitis, or inflammation of the bladder, is brought about by a number of conditions which act in such a way as to disturb the circulation through the kidney and bladder area, resulting in congestion, stasis, and at times outright infection of the tissues. Cystitis is more often a reaction of the bladder to a diseased state occurring elsewhere in the body than a distinct disease in itself. A single cause or a number of factors acting together may bring about one or more of the symptoms of burning and frequency of urination, spasm of the bladder and bladder neck, a sensation of heaviness in the bladder area, difficulty in emptying the bladder and in retention of urine. Pus, blood, or protein may or may not be present in the urine.

The bladder, an organ assisting the kidneys in the elimination of waste products, is sensitive to the many imbalances that may occur in the eliminative systems of the body. It may react to burdens placed upon the liver in its efforts to rid the body of toxic products through the kidneys; or it, as well as the urethra, may become irritated in a more direct manner from the passage of certain poisons and waste products being eliminated from the hepatic circulation by the kidneys. Too high a concentration of either acid or alkaline substances passing through the bladder and urethra are frequently mentioned as causes of irritation.

A survey of the readings reveals that most cases of cystitis are associated with disease states in other parts of the body which act in such a way as to disturb the hepatic circulation. In very few cases was cystitis the only, or even the major, condition for which a reading was given.

The hepatic or portal circulation is that part of the venous circulation that flows from the organs of digestion through the liver before returning to the heart via the inferior vena cava. The kidneys also comprise a part of the hepatic circulation.

As an organ (for the more perfect understanding of the body, for this may be disputed by some), the liver and kidneys form the hepatic circulation. The blood supply of the whole body goes through the liver twice, even to once through the heart. 1140-2

Disturbances in the hepatic circulation may be brought about by a rather wide variety of causes, due not only to the many and varied functions of the liver but also to the rather close coordination between the liver and kidneys.

Then there is that circulation called the hepatic, as indicated, wherein there is the *coordinant* reaction between the liver *and* the kidneys. The liver is an excretory as well as a secretive organ. The kidneys are *secretive* and take *from* the system, also from the liver and from the general circulation of the whole abdominal area, poisons that are not eliminated through other ways and manners.

When toxic forces arise in the body from the inflammation through the abdominal area, or through the uterus itself, combined with the disturbances through lack of proper eliminations in the alimentary canal, *then* we have a sparse activity of the bladder or of the kidneys through the bladder. Then this produces in the body an irritation, owing to the great excess of acidity, that produces a burning even through the clitoris and the mouth of the uterus and in the portions of the body.

This is not an indication that the kidneys are involved but that the activity of the whole hepatic circulation and the organs or eliminations through these portions of the system become involved in same. 1140-2

The causes of disturbances to the hepatic circulation as given in the readings are too numerous and too diverse in nature to be included as a comprehensive part of this discussion. They include such imbalances to the system as infection and congestion in the liver and gall duct areas (815-1, 882-2 and 1446-1), a torpid liver (19-1 and 3050-1), cirrhosis (2729-2), prolapsed descending colon (69-3), improper colon eliminations combined with uterine inflammation (1140-2), disturbances in the red cell element of the blood (2729-2, 3050-1 and 3822-1), cerebrospinal lesions (2462-1 and 3822-1), adhesions causing a thinning in the lacteal duct areas of the jejunum (2050-1), and emotional disturbances (2402-1).

We have at times the condition with the lower portion of the hepatic circulation; when the kidneys are affected, not other than sympathetically, in their attempt to aid in the elimination of these toxic forces that are created in the body. A burning through the urethra, with the evacuation of the bladder, occurs at times.

These are from a form of acidity. . .   2462-1

The liver torpid in its activity, as is the stress at times and overactivity of the kidneys and the hepatic circulation—pressure on bladder at times— painful when passing of urine at times, or burning. This an overacid reaction, and the effects of the disturbance as is seen in that portion of system as given.

19-1

In the following case, overalkalinity is found to be the cause:

There has been a gradual increasing in the lack of activity of the liver and gall duct area, with the accumulation not of stones but of gravel in the gall duct itself. This tends to produce activities that prevent a normal elimination and the normal flow of the gastric juices that keep certain elements out of the system by the poor assimilation; making then rather a complex reaction. For there have been those quantities of foods and of medicinal properties that have caused an excess alkalinity. Thus the reaction existing between the circulation in liver and kidneys is gradually, through this alkalinity, causing irritation to the bladder and the tubes through which the urine passes.

5009-1

In general the bladder, when it becomes inflamed, may be regarded more often as the victim of disease rather than the source.

II. Rationale of Therapy

Since most cases of cystitis in the readings result from some disturbance to the hepatic circulation, the rationale of therapy will center mostly around efforts to improve the hepatic circulation and coordinate the function of the organ systems, and the specific relief of bladder inflammation and discomfort.

Whenever a diseased condition occurring elsewhere in the body is found to be disturbing the hepatic circulation or otherwise contributing to bladder inflammation, treatment is directed toward relieving the cause. This would indicate that a thorough physical examination at the beginning of the undertaking is usually essential to the overall treatment and ultimate cure.

Efforts are made to eliminate any irritating or toxic elements present in the system. Good bowel habits should be established and maintained in all cases. Adequate removal of the accumulated toxic refuse from the lower bowel makes a thorough cleansing by enemas or colonics necessary in many instances. Ample fluid intake is essential in aiding the kidneys in their elimination of toxic waste products.

The diet should be kept on the alkaline side to correct the acid tendencies which more often accompany disturbances in hepatic circulation. At least six to eight glasses of water are prescribed in the daily diet as well as a plentiful supply of fresh fruits and vegetables. Caution is given against the use of white bread, starchy foods, and too much fried foods and sweets, all of which contribute toward an over-acidity in the system. Carbonated beverages should not be taken in any quantity except as prescribed.

Osteopathic adjustments help to stimulate the blood and lymph circulation in the disturbed areas to assist in the more efficient removal of accumulated waste products. This is one of the first steps necessary in assisting the body in its repair of the damaged tissues and restoration of balance to the system. Various physical therapies and local applications of counterirritants are used in some instances to aid in stimulating circulation. Hydrotherapy and cabinet baths are, when indicated, usually prescribed in close conjunction with thorough cleansing of the colon so as to coordinate the elimination of wastes from the system more completely.

Watermelon seed tea, which contains a preferred form of nitre, is often used to help purify and clear the activity of the kidneys.

Q-1. What is the condition of the kidneys?
A-1. As just indicated, this is an incoordination between the eliminating systems. Thus the necessity of that character or quality of nitre as may be obtained from watermelon seed tea. 2434-2

In general throughout the readings it is advised that very little carbonated beverages be taken; however, a little Coca-Cola syrup is advised in those instances where there tends to be an acidity in the urine. This acts in much the same way as watermelon seed tea.

Afterward—that is, for that day, or for that evening—use a little of the watermelon seed tea; this will help to purify. Or if desirable drink Coca-Cola—a little Coca-Cola; this will act almost in the same way and manner in

purifying or clearing the ducts through the kidneys, and thus reduce the general forces and influence there.   **540-11**

Local therapy consists of using an antiseptic solution such as Glyco-Thymoline for feminine douching and for general application over the pubic area in the form of hot packs. Atomidine when prescribed as a douche solution (1140-2), included in the Circulating File on cystitis, is stated to act in such a manner as to work directly upon the hepatic circulation, acting not only as a cleansing solution for inflammatory conditions but aiding in the functioning of all the reproductive glands that become irritated or inflamed.

A combination of laudanum and aconite can be applied to the skin locally for relief of pain. Laudanum is a tincture of opium. Aconite is described in *Dorland's Medical Dictionary* as a poisonous drug whose systemic use has been largely abandoned. It is a cardiac and respiratory sedative, analgesic, diaphoretic, and diuretic. Its active principle is aconitine.

III. Suggested Therapeutic Regimen

Since the underlying causes of cystitis are often complex and involve imbalances in other parts of the body, no system of treatment should be undertaken in those cases of chronic or recurrent cystitis until there has first been a complete physical examination. Specific treatment of the underlying disease will of course depend on the diagnosis made.

More general therapy consists of improving the eliminations and balancing the diet, using nitre in the form of watermelon seed tea, stimulating the circulation, and further coordinating the activities of the various organs through osteopathic adjustments and physical therapy, and using medicinal douches and/or local applications for the relief of pain and irritation. (These will be taken up and elaborated on separately.)

Good bowel eliminations are essential to successful therapy. One of the milder laxatives such as senna is often prescribed. Senna acts with the digestive forces to produce the proper condition within the blood that is to be carried through the hepatic circulation. (3972-1) Certain foods such as figs, dates, raisins, prunes, pieplant [rhubarb], and stewed fruits are also advised for their laxative qualities. A particular combination is prescribed in reading 2050-1.

Then follow the regular diets that aid in eliminations. Use such as figs; or a combination of figs and dates would be an excellent diet to be taken often. Prepare same in this manner:

> 1 cup black or Assyrian figs, chopped, cut or ground very fine;
> 1 cup dates, chopped very fine;
> ½ cup yellow corn meal (*not* too finely ground).

Cook this combination in 2 or 3 cups of water until the consistency of mush. Such a dish as part of the diet often will be as an aid to better eliminations, as well as carrying those properties that will aid in building better conditions throughout the alimentary canal.   2050-1

Harsher laxative compounds are sometimes suggested.

First we would begin with a series of cleansing properties, prepared in this manner. Prepare at least six (6) capsules, with this amount in each capsule:

> Podophyllin, ¼ grain
> Leptandrin, 1 grain
> Sanguinaria, 1 grain

These would be taken one each evening, until all six are taken.

During this period take little besides liquids or semi-liquids in the diet. And do drink at least six to eight glasses of water each day.   3050-1

Podophyllin, of course, is a contact irritant. Leptandrin acts directly with the functioning of the lower intestinal tract. (3972-1) In the same reading sanguinaria is stated to produce the condition necessary to cause the flow of blood through the lower portion of the body.

If a more thorough cleansing of the lower bowel is indicated, then professionally administered enemas or colonics are used.

Then we would use the enemas, rather the colon enemas; not too often, but so that the body may be cleansed from toxic forces that naturally arise from this inactivity through the system. Do not use such large quantities of water, but use a saline solution that—through these *manners* of application—will add an element that *will* form *with* the natural secretions of the body, as *well* as the oils. Not those that would make for a collecting of influences through the alimentary canal (as those that carry the paraffin in same), but rather small quantities of olive oil; that would be not only a food for the intestinal system but would—in such minute quantities—be assimilated without causing disturbing factors.

In using the colonics, combine the solutions in this manner: To each quart of tepid water that would be used, use a level tablespoonful of salt and half a tablespoonful of baking soda; this well dissolved before it is used. 1140-2

At times an antiseptic solution such as Lavoris or Glyco-Thymoline is used in the enema or colonic solution with a tablespoonful to a gallon or gallon and a half of water.

The matter of diet relates primarily to the acid-alkaline balance of the system. In most cases of cystitis—and especially where there is a disturbance of the hepatic circulation—the system has a tendency to be overly acidic. Hence, the diet is generally alkaline in nature.

As to the diets—these are very well if kept in a balance of at least eighty percent alkaline-producing to twenty percent of the acid-producing. This would then indicate not great quantities of sugars or of sweets, though honey may be taken. But beware of cakes or icing or great quantities of sugar or candy. Honey, especially with the honeycomb, may be taken as the sweets. Not a great quantity ever, of course, of fried foods. Not great quantities ever of white bread, but rather use rye or whole wheat or the like—these are the more preferable.   540-11

As to the diet—after the period of the cleansing of the alimentary canal, and making for the activity of the liver, the spleen, the kidneys, as to their general activity—there should not be a great deal of meat. Never any hog meat, except occasionally a little crisp bacon may be taken. Fish, fowl and lamb should be the meats, and these not every day—and never fried.

Leafy vegetables are preferable to the tuberous or bulbous nature. A raw salad should be one meal each day, or at least part of same. Include raw carrots, lettuce, celery, watercress, and especially beet tops. These may all be taken raw, if properly prepared. For this particular body, these would be better in bulk than just taking the juices of same; though for some bodies the juices would be better.

As for breads—only cornbread, using the yellow meal, with egg, and whole wheat bread. These are preferable.   3050-1

A method for obtaining a rough idea of the acidity or alkalinity of the system is given in one of the readings.

A general activity for a body in much of a normal condition is to keep the acidity and the alkalinity in a proper balance. The best manner to indicate this is to test the alkalinity or acidity of the body through the salivary glands or through the salivary gland membranes, or by taking the litmus paper in the mouth. This also may be indicated through the urine.

Whenever there is disturbance with this, if it is in the glands themselves, then take citrocarbonate—that is, if it is indicated in the salivary glands that there is an acidity, then take a small quantity of citrocarbonate. If the acidity is indicated through the kidneys, or from the urine itself, then drink a little of the carbonated waters, as would be indicated with Coca-Cola—but that which is *bottled* is the better; *or* use a little of the watermelon seed tea. Either of these would tend to make for a balance. **540-11**

Osteopathic adjustments, at the discretion of professional judgment, tend to be given in the areas of the ninth dorsal, which leads to the solar plexus, and to the lumbar and sacral segments of the spine which innervate the pelvic area. Lesions of the spine most often affecting the hepatic circulation are found in the lower dorsal area.

Stimulation of circulation to promote better coordination throughout the system is further aided by physical therapy. This includes hydrotherapy treatments and peanut oil massage (see 2462-1). Where cystitis was in part due to improper oxidation of the blood as manifested by excessive tiredness and weakness, a program of physical therapy was advised.

After these properties have reacted upon the system, begin with hydrotherapy treatments. When giving the first two or three, watch the pulsations—or the heart's activity. Each treatment should include a mild cabinet sweat, first beginning with dry heat. Then add to this the fumes from witch hazel, by using a teaspoonful of witch hazel in the open boiler or croup cup of boiling water in the cabinet, inside the cabinet with the lights, you see, though the lights would be turned off after the water begins to boil—and after the body has been slightly heated from sitting in the cabinet. Use a teaspoonful of the witch hazel to four ounces of water. These should be taken every week until ten or twelve are taken.

Follow each fume bath with a hot and then cold shower. Sitz baths would also be well for the body. This will aid in alleviating the tendencies in the rectal area for those disturbances there, as well as through the lower lumbar area.

These should be followed by a thorough rubdown with a combination of three parts olive oil and one part oil of pine needles, thoroughly mixed. Massage this thoroughly into the spine, especially across the area of the diaphragm and the liver, close over the spleen and the abdominal area.
3050-1

In reading 882-2 massage—using a compound of equal parts heated mutton suet, spirits of turpentine, spirits of camphor and compound tincture of benzoin as a counterirritant—is applied to the lower dorsal and lumbar spine and across the abdomen, followed by application of a heated salt pack to the area. A hot salt pack is preferred to a heating pad as a source of local heat and is said to help carry those properties through the pores that would enable the body to overcome congestion in the area. The same is indicated in the following reading:

Q-1. What causes and what can be done for burning in the bladder?
A-1. The improper circulation. Apply Glyco-Thymoline packs over the pubic area. . .
Use three to four thicknesses of cotton cloth saturated with the Glyco-Thymoline for the packs. Place salt heat over same; not an electric pad, but salt heated in a sack or bag and laid over the Glyco-Thymoline pack. These will ease and relieve these tensions.   **3469-1**

For relief of pain it was frequently advised that the area be painted with a combination of three parts laudanum to one part aconite, then followed with the application of a hot salt pack.

When there are acute pains across the bladder, then we would apply hot packs of heavy salt. First paint the area, though, with a combination of three parts laudanum to one part aconite, which as we find would give relief. Then apply the heavy salt, heated and put in a sack or bag, of course. These we find will relieve and bring the better conditions for this body. 1446-1

Glyco-Thymoline douches, using a teaspoonful of Glyco-Thymoline to a quart of body temperature water, are recommended for occasional use as well as taking five drops of Glyco-Thymoline in a glass of water one to three times a week to help relieve the irritation of the bladder. (3469-1) In cases of vaginal or pelvic inflammation an Atomidine douch is indicated.

Also we would find it well to use the Atomidine douches, for the irritation through the pelvic organs. These should be body-temperature. Do not have the water cooler than body-temperature, nor very much higher. Test same, not by hand but by thermometer. That means ninety-eight and a half to one hundred or a hundred and one, not above that. The proportions would be a teaspoonful of the commercial strength Atomidine to half a gallon of water. Give these at least every other day, but if there is *acute* disturbances they may be taken oftener.   1446-1

Frederick D. Lansford, Jr., M.D.

Edgar Cayce readings referenced:
19-1
69-3
540-9, 10, 11
815-1
817-1
882-2
1140-2
1446-2, 3, 4
2050-1
2402-1
2434-2
2462-1
2729-2
3050-1
3469-1
3822-1
3972-1
5009-1

DIABETES

I. Physiological Considerations

The primary physiological consideration in the condition known as diabetes mellitus seems to be a malfunction in the pancreas gland with ramifications that extend through its coordination with the liver. At times there seems to be a stimulation in the functioning of the gland as a whole, at other times a sluggishness. There is a tendency in the pancreas, in both of these conditions, to create too much sugar and to handle the carbohydrates in such a way that they also form an excess of sugar.

In the causation of diabetes is a disturbance of certain cerebrospinal centers which are associated with the sixth, seventh, eighth, and ninth dorsal sympathetic ganglia. These "pressures in specific centers" of the nervous system give an impulse to the liver and pancreas primarily and apparently also to the spleen. This impulse may be one of stimulation because of the pressure or it may be one of creating a sluggishness. The type of injury or muscular spasm or degree of incoordination of the nervous system itself probably mediates what type of impulse will be sent out from the centers.

In nearly every case the disturbance in the autonomic ganglia brings about the greater imbalance through the pancreas and the circulation and the coordination between the liver and the pancreas. This, in essence, causes the condition of glycosuria and what we commonly know as diabetes. Then these conditions of excess sugar in the blood bring about other strains and incoordinations in the system, creating other difficulties within the body.

We find also that the assimilations of the body can become disturbed and create an incoordination between the assimilations and the eliminations. In one particular case, such an incoordination created a lower bowel stasis with improper eliminations, which in turn created a strain to the liver and caused the circulation, especially in the left lobe of the liver, to be sluggish. (953-1) The liver then became principally excretory in its function rather than secretory as it should be. This malfunction of the liver caused the Peyer's patches and other local lymphatic vessels and centers to cease production of substances which recreated blood elements, in this case probably the lymphocytes. Thus the circulation lacked new blood, which taxed the cerebrospinal centers in the autonomic nervous system. This created unusual nerve impulses to the pancreas and the liver, and gradually the condition of sugar in the bloodstream.

This impulse of an aberrant nature coming from the sixth, seventh, eighth, or ninth dorsal ganglia might be considered as reacting on the hepatic circulation or causing a tendency for imbalance or sluggish or "cold" circulation in the liver and pancreatic area. It would sometimes undoubtedly aggravate the pancreas. It can be seen that these would create varying types of manifestations associated with the diabetic. This is nearly always the physiology.

A dysfunction of the pancreatic-liver circulation might create an excess in the kidney function with a subsequent strain on the heart because of the accumulation of body metabolites. Likewise, improper assimilation might be brought into being with reflexes to the nerve supply, to the prostate, or to the heart and lungs and sometimes to the locomotor nerve centers of the system, causing difficulties in all or parts of these areas.

The excessive pancreatic activity in some instances would produce obesity. The starch and sugars prevent the normal functioning of the liver and sometimes create an excessive kidney function with a subsequent heaviness in the bloodstream and an increase in the red blood cells with a decrease in the white. Some consequences of this condition might be anticipated as a result of the system trying to adjust itself. This would make for a type of normalcy but it would be apart from the true normal functioning of the body and would probably create a depression of nervous and mental function and unusual emotional responses to some degree.

II. Rationale of Therapy

In approaching therapy, we should remember that the body has a capability of *normal* function:

Thus, we would administer those activities which would bring a normal

reaction through these portions, stimulating them to an activity from the body itself, rather than the body becoming dependent upon supplies that are robbing portions of the system to produce activity in other portions, or the system receiving elements or chemical reactions being supplied without arousing the activity of the system itself for a more normal condition.

1968-3

The therapy for diabetes mellitus should be directed at correcting the basic physiological malfunctions. Again, it is important to remember that this should be done gradually, not changing other therapies abruptly, especially where insulin has been used. Attention should be paid to correcting the sugar-forming condition within the pancreas and this should be done in conjunction with correcting the causation. A diet should be adhered to which would help restore the normalcy of the pancreas and the liver. Any attendant conditions such as gastro-intestinal imbalance and an incoordination between the cerebrospinal and the autonomic nervous systems should likewise be cared for.

In this manner, the original cause would be corrected and should remain corrected. The pancreas itself would be gradually restored to normal and the other conditions which pre-exist the change in the pancreas and those which come as a result of the pancreatic malfunction would gradually normalize.

III. Suggested Therapeutic Regimen

Undoubtedly, diabetes exists without the definite subluxations of the vertebrae which have been named. In these cases, however, abnormal autonomic impulses still appear to be coming to the pancreas. Thus it would be advisable in all cases of diabetes, since we cannot always appraise the need for this type of therapy, to institute a course of osteopathic manipulations and adjustments. Specific adjustments of these particular vertebrae should be made as well as general adjustments. They should be given in series, six to eight at a time, perhaps with a rest, and then another six to eight. They should coordinate the fourth lumbar with the third cervical in conjunction with the dorsal vertebrae that are being treated. It is important to remember that a pressure might be alleviated, but correct flow of nerve impulses cannot come about consistently unless the balance is maintained over a period of time. This is why more than one treatment is necessary.

Diet is highly important. From 3086-1, we see that the diet has more to do with the reactions obtained than almost any other application. Jerusalem artichokes are suggested in every case of diabetes. These provide a type of insulin material for the body which helps restore normal function of the pancreas. These should be taken in varying amounts of perhaps three a week or, if the case is more severe, one a day for five to six days a week. They should be cooked—one artichoke about the size of a hen's egg—in Patapar paper, prepared with the juices and eaten in that manner. If they are taken five or six days a week they should be used raw one day and cooked the next. From reading 1878-1, "for taking the artichoke—especially this Jerusalem variety—is using insulin but in a manner that is *not* habit-forming, and is much more preferable—if it is governed properly—with the rest of the diet."

The Jerusalem artichoke or *Helianthus tuberosis,* also called the gerasole, is unique in that it stores its carbohydrates as inulin or inulides (which yield levulose on hydrolysis) rather than as starch (which yields glucose). The levulose is not as harmful to the body in diabetes as is glucose. Medical opinion has been divided on its use. For sake of reference, it is noted that insulin is a protein hormone, inulin is a plant-derived fructose polysaccharide, while glucokinin is a hormone-like substance obtained from plants which will produce hypoglycemia in animals and will act on depancreatized dogs in a manner similar to insulin. Some plants contain glucokinin, but apparently this has not been demonstrated yet in this type of artichoke.

Otherwise, in the diet, it should be advised that one eat no red meats, not too much sweets, not too much meats, less starch, no white sugar, no white bread. Pastries, pies, etc., should be markedly decreased. Coffee or tea should not be taken more than once daily. Fish or fowl should be eaten in small amounts; there should be much of leafy vegetables in the diet, but very little of the pod variety; no vegetables grown below ground with the exception of oyster plant, carrots, or beets occasionally (and the beet should be taken with the beet top). No fried foods should be eaten.

After osteopathic adjustments have been started, then Atomidine could be begun in small amounts—for instance, one drop twice a day, increasing one drop daily for the next eight days until five drops are being taken twice daily. Then, decrease one drop per day until the original dosage is reached. Rest a week or two. Then repeat this regimen three or four times. Atomidine cleanses the glands and the glandular forces of the body.

The balance of the assimilation and elimination should be established through one of several prescriptions. There are two prescriptions in reading 674-1 whose purpose is "to keep the eliminations, and is as an active force producing with the liver and the hepatic circulation an increasing of the lymph without disturbing the activities of the spleen and pancreas secretions." The following prescription should be used to create a balance in the assimilation and to rejuvenate the excretory function of the emunctories (lacteals, Peyer's patches, and excretory ducts and organs).

To one gallon rain water or distilled water add eight (8) ounces of clary flower (garden sage). Reduce by simmering, not boiling, to one quart. Dissolve four (4) ounces of beet sugar in just enough hot water to dissolve it. Then add—while warm—to other solution. Dissolve fifteen (15) gr. ambergris in one (1) oz. of grain alcohol and add to solution. Then add: grain alcohol, four (4) ounces; oil of juniper, fifty (50) minims, balsam of tolu cut with alcohol, three (3) drams.   674-1

Directions: One dessertspoonful three times a day. (953-1; see also 730-1 and 767-1.)

Other medications should not be taken with the exception of insulin, which may already be a part of the routine. This should be slowly decreased in dosage until not used at all. Caution should be made here that blood and urine determinations guide the gradual discontinuance of the insulin.

Vitamins should rarely be used. From case [5345], we see that "when there is applied those elements even in the forms of vitamins alone they are against the activities of the liver, the spleen, especially the pancreas as related to conditions."

Should we not attempt to awaken the inner forces to God's presence? "For, all healing comes from the one source. And whether there is the application of foods, exercise, medicine, or even the knife, it is to bring the consciousness of the forces within the body that aid in reproducing themselves—the awareness of creative or God forces." (2696-1)

William A. McGarey, M.D.

Edgar Cayce readings referenced:

584-1, 6, 8	951-4	3086-1
674-1	953-1, 8, 9	3386-2
730-1	1603-2	5341-1
767-1	1878-1	5345-1
834-1	2578-1	

DIVERTICULITIS

I. Physiological Considerations

Diverticuli are pouchlike out-pocketings consisting of the mucosa and serosal layers, i.e., the inner and the outer layers respectively of the bowel walls, and are more common on the left side of the colon. These are said to protrude through the muscularis, i.e., the middle layer of the bowel wall in areas of weakness (points of penetration of nutrient vessels). The mechanism by which this happens is not well understood, but it is postulated that this is due to increased intraluminal pressure as a result of narrow caliber of the colon stemming from lack of bulk in Western diet.

Symptoms usually do not occur until complications arise, such as inflammation and abscess formation in and around the pouches (i.e., diverticulitis). Further complications as a result of this include perforation, bleeding and fistula formation (i.e., unnatural channels between various organs and tissues). Spasticity of the colon (alternating bouts of diarrhea and constipation) may exist with diverticular disease. For a more detailed discussion, the reader is referred to the textbooks on gastroenterology.

Turning now to the Cayce readings on diverticulitis, one finds that in case [805] the underlying problem is traced back to lesions (adhesions) formed at the time of abdominal surgery (appendectomy). Toxins accumulated in the blood from this area, causing irritation of the bowel wall with excessive mucus production which hardened into "strings" and "threads" as well as sloughing of tissue from the mucosa, tending to make for more accumulation and irritation.

This led to an increased temperature, pain, and pulsation in the colon. The irritation and increased pressure resulted in strain on the whole nervous system, and abnormal autonomic discharge further leading to impairment in colon function.

Although no definite mention was made in this reading of diverticuli formation, it can be readily seen how increase in pressure and disorganized peristaltic activity can lead to saclike herniations through areas of weakness in the abdominal wall.

Widespread signs and symptoms may be associated with autonomic nervous system dysfunction, the more common ones being pain, heaviness and burning sensation in the lower limbs as a result of altered circulation and tiredness.

Case [3079] may serve as another example of how this disease might develop. Here the problem was poor eliminations leading to toxic accumulations, which in turn produced deposits around the ligaments, cartilages and segments of the lower spine, resulting in stiffness in the spine. The autonomic nervous system could thus become involved at this level with dysynergy in the activity of the colon.

Also there was seen a deficiency in certain elements in the hemoglobin of the blood "that is a creative and active force from digestive forces through the liver itself." The meaning behind this last phrase is not entirely clear to me; but it seems to indicate that the missing component arises from the diet and is processed in the liver before being incorporated into the hemoglobin. This deficiency presumably contributed to toxic accumulations and poor eliminations. These abnormalities may then act on the colon and the autonomic nervous system through the mechanisms already discussed.

It can be seen from the foregoing that there are several factors involved in the genesis of diverticular disease of the colon, some of which remain to be further elucidated.

II. Rationale of Therapy

1. *Good dietary habits:* A well-balanced diet should act as a deterrent, especially in people who may have predisposing factors, e.g., poor eliminations, prior surgery, etc. Those who have established disease may benefit from bulk-forming diet (high fiber).

2. *Good eliminations:* This raises the necessity of redefining what is considered normal eliminations. It is true that there is great individual variation, but considering the increasing amounts of undesirable additives or deficiencies in processed foods, a more stringent criterion should be established. In my opinion, evacuation of the bowel daily or at least every other day would be most desirable.

3. *Physical therapy:* The modalities most commonly recommended include castor oil packs, colonic enemas, osteopathic manipulations, and violet ray therapy. These collectively alleviate distressing symptoms and aid in bringing the body back to balance.

4. *Medicinal:* Thyroid replacement and/or Atomidine was recommended for underactive thyroid which might aggravate or cause constipation.

III. Suggested Therapeutic Regimen

1. *Castor oil packs:* These may be used for three to four hours at a time daily for acute symptoms, then one-and-a-half to two hours at a time three days a week (same days and times if possible) after improvement is noted. Olive oil, one-half teaspoon every two to three hours initially for one to two days, may be helpful. For subacute or chronic cases, one to two tablespoons of olive oil after the third day of castor oil pack (i.e., once a week) may be used. [*Note:* It was recommended that the affected area of the abdomen be painted first with a mixture of three parts tincture of laudanum (opium) to one part aconite before application of the castor oil pack to this area. This "focuses" the desired effect to the affected area. This prescription is no longer available; but if it does become available in the future, its use is strongly recommended.]

2. *Colonic enemas:* These should be gentle and would be most beneficial after the third day of castor oil packs. The recommended frequency would be one or two treatments per week initially for two to three weeks, then one monthly for the next two to three months.

3. *Gentle or mild laxatives* as necessary to keep the bowels open, e.g., Fletcher's Castoria, Sulflax, Serutan, etc.

4. *Osteopathy:* Manipulations once or twice per week for three to four weeks with two-week rest periods before repeating for three or more series.

5. *Total body massage* with emphasis along the spine, using a combination of equal parts of peanut and olive oils. This again should be once or twice a week, if possible, for a five- to six-week period. This may be repeated as often as necessary.

6. *Correct underactive thyroid* by using thyroid hormones (dosage dependent on severity) and/or Atomidine.

Suggested program of Atomidine:

One drop daily for seven days, rest five days
Two drops daily for seven days, rest five days

Three drops daily for seven days, rest five days
(Repeat this cycle two or three times.)

7. *Diet:* An alkaline-reacting diet is recommended. During acute attacks, food intake should be limited to liquids and semisolids for the first 10 to 14 days. Drink plenty of juices, at least four ounces per day from the following: watercress juice, carrot and lettuce juice, beet juice, celery and lettuce juice, apple juice from fresh apples, grape juice from fresh grapes (may alternate among these). Seafoods are also recommended two or three times a week.

8. *The ultraviolet ray* may also be used, placed 38-40 inches from the body for one-and-a-half to three minutes at a time, three to four times a week for one to two weeks.

9. Have adequate *rest.*

The treatments outlined here aid in the purification of the body. In some cases, after initiation of these treatments, the condition may appear to worsen. This may be attributed to the liberation of "dross" which has accumulated in the system. With patience, persistence, and consistency, improvement usually occurs.

Hezekiah Chinwah, M.D.

Edgar Cayce readings referenced:
805-1
3079-1, 2, 3
3499-1
3616-1, 2

EMPHYSEMA

I. Physiological Considerations

Emphysema is classified as an obstructive lung disease which is probably best defined in pathological terms as a replacement of normal lung tissue by coarse air spaces of variable size.[1] Clinically, the patient with emphysema experiences increasing exertion because of shortness of breath and he has difficulty in exhaling. This produces a gradually increasing barrel-type chest as accessory muscles of the chest are called into play. Other problems arise sequentially.

Historically, there has been a close relationship between chronic bronchitis, asthma, and emphysema, and some theories hold that the mucus produced in chronic bronchitis predisposes to obstruction and thus loss of normal tissue in the lung distal to the obstruction. This mechanism is unlikely since destructive emphysema occurs infrequently in patients with allergic bronchial asthma. In addition, emphysema often occurs without any evidence of predisposing bronchitis. In destructive pulmonary emphysema, there are often areas of normal lung tissue as well as areas of destruction of the lung tissue. This and other factors add to the confusion that exists in differentiating between chronic bronchitis and pulmonary emphysema, and some observers believe that true differentiation can occur only with pathological examination.

As the destructive process begins in pulmonary emphysema, the normal tissue loses its elasticity and its normal structure, the circulation to those areas becomes severely diminished, and increased resistance to air flow is brought about by a narrowing of the bronchial lumen by mucus and swelling of the mucosa, and also by the unequal ventilation of various portions of the lung. Progression of the disease brings further destruction of lung tissue and the findings and symptoms which are typically found in this disease.

In the Cayce readings only one case is suggestive of emphysema, and this is not a clear diagnosis from the material available. This 31-year-old man, [5642], had epilepsy as a result of a World War I shell explosion, which caused a fracture of the skull. He also apparently had emphysema, or the beginning stages of this condition.

It is inferred here that the autonomic nerve supply to the lungs was too "relaxed," but other physiological inferences are difficult to come by. Work done by Nakayama, Overholt, Phillips and others[2] during the past 20 years seems to bear some relationship to Cayce's comment regarding the nerve supply. In more than 10,000 cases of asthma and emphysema, these men removed one carotid body, which is a nerve ganglion situated at the bifurcation of the common carotid artery. This carotid body, Phillips felt, is sort of a relay station in the autonomic nervous system from the mid-brain to the bronchial tree, and by removing it he felt he was interrupting the spastic element to the bronchial tree.

Throughout the body, a balance is achieved in the functioning of an organ through the influences of the antagonistic sympathetic and parasympathetic nervous systems, which are part of the autonomic nervous system. If, indeed, the lung is under the control of nervous impulses, then either excessive spastic impulses from the parasympathetic or a weakening (relaxation) to an excessive degree of the sympathetic would bring about a process within the lung tissue which could conceivably be the beginning of emphysema. There is no doubt that hormonal influences also play a significant role in the maintenance of a normal function within the lung tissue. The readings do not discuss this.

It is an obvious fact that early cases of emphysema can be treated more successfully than far-advanced ones, in the event a reasonable therapeutic program can be achieved. The further advanced the disease is, the more the deterioration of function and tissue. Secondary problems would arise as the emphysematous process progresses.

II. Rationale of Therapy

In approaching therapy, we should remember that the body has a capability of *normal* function:

Thus, we would administer those activities which would bring a normal reaction through these portions, stimulating them to an activity from the

body itself, rather than the body becoming dependent upon supplies that are robbing portions of the system to produce activity in other portions, or the system receiving elements or chemical reactions being supplied without arousing the activity of the system itself for a more normal condition.

1968-3

It should be kept in mind that most people with asthma develop emphysema. Thus it would be helpful to consider the objectives already developed relative to therapy in asthma. The following is an extract from the asthma commentary:

> Asthma, when viewed as a condition which has its origin and basis in the nervous system, should then be approached in therapy with the objective in mind to remove the stimulatory factors in the nervous system and to correct those adjunctive, correlated and resultant imbalances that may prevent a return to normal function.
>
> Since pressures are present in the dorsal and sometimes the cervical ganglia, these should be relieved osteopathically and treatments should be continued long enough to allow continuance of normal nerve function. The eliminations should be restored to normal, and assimilation should be balanced with the elimination. The deep and superficial circulation which is often disturbed should be restored to a balance of coordination. The glands of the body should be brought to a balance, and the resistance of the body should be stimulated through improvement of assimilation and function of the Peyer's patch area of the intestines.[3]

In [5642], the apparent purpose of therapy is to bring about a diet which will supply easily digested food so that the assimilative needs of the body will be met, but not overloaded. The nervous system and the lymphatics are treated with massage, and substances are added to the body which improve the breathing capacity and utilization of substances taken in through the lungs. The bowels are kept active so that eliminations might be balanced with the assimilation, and later on an inhalant is used which, like the first prescription given, improves the lung functioning. Finally, the capacity of the body to assimilate and utilize food substances needs to be increased.

The rationale for therapy in both asthma and emphysema is based on the concept that the autonomic system as a whole must be balanced in its relationship to the lungs. Once this is achieved and the circulation to the lungs is improved, then the lung tissue can conceivably begin rebuilding. It would seem reasonable to assume that the readings recommend bringing the body from a homeostasis of disease to a balance consistent with normal health.

III. Suggested Therapeutic Regimen

It becomes quite obvious that far-advanced emphysema cannot be treated as was [5642], who had no evidence of a progressed condition. However, it is interesting to look at the various phases of therapy suggested here, perhaps as a basis or as a springboard for further therapy in the chronic emphysematous patient.

This man's first course of therapy was a diet, easy to digest, with predigested foods and liquids, and a caution not to overload the stomach at any time; and medication for a period of 12 to 14 days—a capsule taken every other day each containing the following:

> Eucalyptol, 1 minim
> Canadian balsam, ½ minim
> Rectified oil of turpentine, 1 minim
> Benzosol, 1 minim
> Heroin, 1/60th grain
> (This makes three capsules at a time.)

During this two-week period, a massage was suggested over the entire back and spine with an equal mixture of olive oil and tincture of myrrh, as much as would be absorbed. The oils should be mixed at the time of use. The olive oil should be heated and then the myrrh added. At least half an ounce should be applied every night.

A second course of therapy followed this and came from a subsequent reading:

1. A vegetarian diet was suggested since meat was not considered to be good for the body in its present condition.

2. Enemas were suggested for constipation rather than cathartics at any time.

3. The olive oil and myrrh mixture was to be used as a massage every two or three days.

4. An inhalant was to be prepared and used twice a day. This was to be placed in a jar at least twice the capacity of the ingredients. To four ounces of grain alcohol was added the following in order:

Eucalyptol, 20 minims
Rectified creosote, 3 minims
Balsam of fir, 5 minims
Compound tincture of benzoin, 5 minims
Rectified oil of turpentine, 5 minims
Tolu in solution, 30 minims
(To be inhaled only after shaking.)

5. A substance was suggested to be taken 20 or 30 minutes before meals and at bedtime in doses of one teaspoonful, which would provide what Cayce said would be an "active force" for the stomach and the digestive system. It is prepared as follows:

Take a half gallon of distilled water. Add eight ounces of wild cherry bark and reduce by simmering, not boiling, to one quart. Add four ounces sugar. Reduce again to 1½ pints, then add:

Sarsaparilla comp., ½ ounce
Tincture or essence of yellow dock root, ¼ ounce
10% potassium iodide solution, ¼ ounce
Elixir of celerena: essence of celery, ½ ounce
Tincture of capsici, 3 minims
(Shaken before using.)

Massages were often used interchangeably with osteopathic manipulations. Rest from massages might be advisable after a period of two to three months on such therapy, and then, after two or three weeks, a series of osteopathic manipulations. It would be advisable to continue the inhalant for a long period of time while particular attention is paid to the assimilative process and the eliminations.

For weakness, beef juice was often suggested (although it is not found in this particular reading).

Particularly where asthma has been present, it would be consistent in the readings to advise Atomidine in series. This could be given one drop in a half glass of water, on first arising in the morning, daily for five days. Then rest two days, then repeat over a period of two to three months. Then a rest from the drops should be taken and the cycle started again.

An important concept from the Cayce readings says that any therapy should be given for a period of time, then a rest should be taken by the body. It is well to remember also that patience, consistency, and perseverance or persistence are necessary elements for the patient and the doctor to observe and use as the body is being rebuilt and brought back to a normal balance.

Keep up what we have given. Be a little patient, but know that there is being brought about those conditions that will correct the disturbances *in* this body, and that the body's strength—the body-physical and the body-mental—*is* gaining. Set before self, mentally, that the body would attain. Make it *high,* and keep the mental *lifted* in that direction; for to heal the physical alone, and to have the mental still distorted—would only be the return of the conditions when *activities* would be renewed physically. But make the body physically fit, that the body-mental may act through same— and *make* the efforts to bring about that as *is desired,* in a mental *and* physical body—but make it high! Don't be satisfied with less!   5545-2

William A. McGarey, M.D.

References:
1. Cecil-Loeb: *Textbook of Medicine,* 12th ed., P.B. Beeson & W. McDermott (ed.), Philadelphia: W.B. Saunders Co., 1967, Vol. 1, 502-507.
2. Nakayama, Komei: "The Surgical Significance of the Carotid Body in Relation to Bronchial Asthma," *J. Thorac. Surgery,* 39: 374-389 (No. 4), 1963.
Overholt, R.H.: "Resection of Carotid Body (Cervical Glomectomy) for Asthma," *JAMA,* 180: 91-94 (No. 10), 1962.
Phillips, J.R.: "Removal of the Carotid Body for Asthma and Emphysema," *S Med J,* 57: 1278-1281 (Nov.), 1964.
Read, C.T.: "Glomectomy: A Survey," *Annals of Thor Surg I:* 590-606 (No. 5), 1965.
3. "Commentary on Asthma," based on readings 5642-1, 2, 3.

EPILEPSY

In the Edgar Cayce readings a total of 95 cases have been indexed to date as some form of epilepsy. For the purposes of this study these 95 cases were divided into three groups. Classification was complicated in most cases by inadequate medical history and lack of description of the symptoms of the disease. Questions asked in the readings as well as the correspondence for each case were found useful for this purpose. In some readings epilepsy was mentioned by name as the basis of the condition, but in most cases a description of the causes and treatments was the chief consideration. Group I contains the 46 cases in which the diagnosis was most certain. These readings named the condition as epilepsy, a medical history was supplied in the correspondence, or some ideas relating to a description of the convulsions or seizures could be ascertained. Group II contains 33 cases in which the diagnosis was less certain because no description was given other than that the patient had some type of convulsions, seizures, fainting spells, black-outs, or falling-out spells. Group III contains 16 cases in which the diagnosis did not seem to be epilepsy as ascertained from the correspondence or readings or both. In many cases in Group III the diagnosis was able to be established as something else. Therefore, for the purposes of this study, the 79 cases in Groups I and II formed the basic data which were analyzed.

Because of the incompleteness of the follow-up information and the inexactness with which the treatments were followed in the cases where such information was available, the adequacy of the treatments can only be ascertained by biological experiments to test the mechanism suggested and by extensive and well-controlled clinical trials of the treatments suggested.

I. Physiological Considerations

In the 79 cases of Groups I and II (see "Case Breakdown by

Groups" at end), two interrelated types of lesions predominated as the basic cause of the conditions: lacteal duct lesions and spinal lesions. Lacteal duct pathology was described in about half (39) of the cases. This ratio is the same in both Group I (23 out of 46 cases) and in Group II (16 out of 33 cases). Mechanical, circulatory, or neurological lesions located by reference to a spinal segment are specifically mentioned in 31 cases (19 from Group I and 12 from Group II). The incidence of these two classes of lesions would have been higher if a lesion were assumed to be present because of the type of treatment recommended. For example, specific manipulation was indicated in 51 cases, and castor oil packs were suggested in cases where lacteal duct lesions had not been specifically described. A relationship seemed to be indicated by means of nerve reflex action via the autonomic nervous system between the lacteal duct area and certain spinal segments.

An initial lesion was described in the lacteal duct area in 23 cases; and an original injury was located by reference to a spinal segment in 23 other cases. That the readings assumed there was a definite relationship between the two types of lesions was shown from the fact that in 37 of the 39 cases in which lacteal duct pathology was mentioned, the presence of a lesion in a spinal segment or segments was either directly described or indirectly indicated because of specific treatments consisting of manipulations and massage on and around the spinal column. Therefore, it can be assumed that in almost half the cases these two types of lesions were considered as occurring together.

The most common cause given for the lacteal duct lesion (when a specific cause was described) was reflex action from an initial injury to a spinal segment, particularly in the sacral-coccygeal region. Direct trauma to the right upper quadrant of the abdomen or in the region of the umbilicus during or after birth was also repeatedly described (e.g., cases [3801] and [5732]. Post-natal infection in the umbilical area was also given as a cause for [2441]. In case [2019], prolonged fasting in the past produced some sort of injury to the umbilical and lacteal autonomic plexuses so that a tautness was produced in the lacteal ducts periodically. A sudden drop in a fever without sufficient water in or activity of the alimentary canal was described as the cause in [2153].

The basic lesion in the lacteal duct area was an interference in the flow of chyle. This seemed to be in some cases caused by an actual constriction or narrowing of the lacteal vessels by adhesions or thickening, and in other cases by some type of spasm. It is hard to understand anatomically how the lacteal ducts themselves could constrict since they have no smooth muscle. A spasm of the smooth muscle in the walls of the jejunum and ileum could conceivably cause such a blockage of the flow of chyle in the lacteal ducts. According to the readings, this basic lacteal duct lesion had far-reaching effects in the body by reflex action via the autonomic nervous system. Interference with elimination through proper functioning of the large and small bowels was repeatedly stressed (e.g., case [1980]). There was an interference and decrease in the hepatic circulation (see [4091], [5642], [567]). In case [1025], an interference with oxidation in the body was mentioned. This could conceivably come about as a slowing of metabolic reactions by almost complete stoppage of fat absorption. Also in [1025] a disturbance to the liver and pancreatic secretions was described. All these conditions described a malfunctioning of the digestive system. Also by autonomic reflex, lesions in spinal segments were set up—most commonly in the sacro-coccygeal region, ninth and tenth dorsals, and first, second and third cervicals.

The lesions in the spinal segments and the lacteal duct lesion produced what was described as an incoordination between the cerebrospinal nervous system and the autonomic nervous system. From the data above, it can be implied that there was a type of reciprocal action between lesions in the spinal segments and the lacteal duct lesion. Where the lacteal lesion was produced first, these lesions in the spinal segments developed by reflex action and vice versa.

The endocrine glands were involved in 21 cases—also by reflex via the autonomic nervous system—with the adrenals and gonads affected and triggering a response in the pineal and pituitary glands. The mechanism of this reaction was not given in detail. No specific hormonal relationships were described. It was indicated, however, that one way to influence the pineal and pituitary glands was via nerve reflex in the autonomic nervous system which would affect centers in the medulla oblongata. The readings suggested that these glands have reciprocal relationships with the brain, particularly the autonomic centers. Thus, the basic incoordination between the cerebrospinal and the autonomic nervous systems was caused by reflex action from the lacteal duct and spinal segment lesions via the nervous system and the glands. The end result of these disturbances was an overflow of neuronal discharge via the central nervous system in the case of grand mal seizure or the temporary loss of consciousness in a petit mal seizure.

Such an explanation is a somewhat general and rather incomplete description with many statements which have not been verified by present medical knowledge. The readings were more concerned with treatment than cause and usually gave only as much theory as was necessary to understand and carry out the treatments. The theory presented above was pieced together from various readings.

As indicated, the lesions—or adhesions and lesions—in the lacteal ducts are the basic cause for the disturbance in the nervous system. And these arise from the inability of the assimilating system to function with the sympathetic nervous system in its reaction to the nerve reflexes or impulses. For these conditions, as we find, exist:

When there is an expression or activity from the sympathetic nervous system, or the sensory system that responds through the sympathetic nerve system, we find there is movement or impulse to and from the brain centers themselves. Then with a lesion or adhesion the impulse is cut off—or deflected. For, as indicated, we have a lesion in the lacteal duct area, from an injury there in times back; this is the right side, just below the liver area.

Hence we have first an intestinal disturbance through the activity of the assimilating system, producing at times disturbances to the liver; at others producing to the pancrean secretions, at others to the activities through the peristaltic movement; not only in the lower intestinal tract but to those activities through the jejunum itself.

Then this coordinating or connection with the solar plexus nerve centers, making for an incoordination with the cerebrospinal nerve system, produces at the base of the brain—or through the medulla oblongata—an incoordinant reaction. . .

Q-7. Do you find any condition existing in the brain, or is it reflex?

A-7. As we find, and as indicated, the accumulations that have been there are rather reflex—and are produced by the condition in the lacteal duct area.

Q-8. Of what nature was the injury, that caused or brought about this condition in the lacteal area?

A-8. This was a pressure, or a lick [a blow].   1025-2

These as we find are hidden, in a nature, and the causes arise from an injury received some years ago, in the coccyx area, and then a contributory cause later in the area above the lumbar axis.

These caused a slowing of the circulation through the areas of the lacteal ducts, thus producing a *cold* area there, that has produced a partial adherence of tissue.

With the activity of the lymph through the area, we find that periodically, when there is the lack of proper eliminations through the alimentary canal, there occurs a reflex to the coordination between sympathetic and cerebrospinal system area; that takes the governing of the impulse, as it were, to the brain reactions; *or* a form of spasmodic reaction that might be called epileptic in its nature.

If this is allowed to remain, or if there are the attempts to allay by or through the applications ordinarily in such cases, we will not only continue this reaction but cause greater destructive forces in the areas along the impulses to the sympathetic and cerebrospinal centers in lumbar and coccyx area; thus increasing and making more severe the attacks that occur from this deflection of impulse. . .

Q-2. *What was the nature of the original accident?*
A-2. Striking the end of the spine—on banister.   1980-1

As has been indicated—and should be noted by the masseur or osteo-path—the lesions that cause attacks are in the lacteal duct and those areas about the assimilating system and the upper portion of the jejunum and caecum.

There are *no* brain lesions, but there is that which at times hinders the coordination between the impulses of the body and the normal physical reactions—or that break between the cerebrospinal and the sympathetic or vegetative nerve system, that coordinates from the lacteal duct through the adrenals and their reaction to the pineal; causing the spasmodic reaction in the medulla oblongata, or that balance at the base of the brain. . .

There are, to be sure, lacteal ducts. There are the strings or ducts all through the upper portion of the alimentary canal, or jejunum; but the larger patch or area is that lying just below the lower end of the duodenum, and where same *empties* into the jejunum, see? *This* patch is not only an *internal* activity, but an *external,* that makes for the production of assimilation.

The adhesions in these ducts here were produced by an excess temperature, which the body suffered at some period when there was too *sudden* dropping of the temperature (which they may check and find to be correct), and *not* sufficient water, or manipulations, or activity, through the alimentary canal.

This has gradually caused the disturbances to the general breaking of coordination in the nerve systems, and brings about—for this body—the *source* of the attacks.   2153-4

As was indicated above, in only about half the cases was lacteal duct pathology described. Of the remaining cases brain damage was described as the cause in seven cases. In others, the pathological description was complicated by the existence of another disease present along with epilepsy. For example, case [3521] had both epilepsy and multiple sclerosis. Other cases combined epilepsy with mental retardation. It might be assumed that lacteal duct pathology (although not specifically described) and related mechanism led to the production of convulsions in some of the remaining cases because of the similarity in the treatments suggested.

Although the Edgar Cayce readings gave as the etiologic factors a lacteal duct lesion in association with a spinal segment lesion in slightly less than half the cases (37), these were the largest group of cases with a consistent mechanism and type of treatment. For example, in 29 of these cases castor oil packs were recommended and in 22 of these same cases incoordination between the autonomic and cerebrospinal nervous systems was specifically mentioned as a definite factor. If it is taken as a presupposition that this type of pathology and the mechanism of pathologic physiology described above is the etiology in some types of epileptic conditions, an explanation could be suggested for a portion of the 50% of all cases of epilepsy which are now termed idiopathic.

It is interesting to note the diagnostic sign which was given in six of the cases where lacteal duct lesion was described—a cold spot on the skin of the right upper quadrant. This sign was usually only present at the time of the seizure. Another possible diagnostic sign noted in the correspondence of case [561], which resulted in a complete cure of the condition, was an occasional feeling of pressure or a "stitch" in the right side. Trouble with eliminations also seemed to be present fairly consistently.

II. Discussion of Treatment

Treatments aim at the elimination of the basic causes and restoration of the normal functioning of the body. All the treatments were somewhat interrelated in their actions and effects. In order to break up the lesions and adhesions in the lacteal duct area, a combination of hot castor oil packs, massage, olive oil taken internally, and spinal manipulations was employed. In addition, proper elimination and diet also were supposed to have their effect upon the lacteal area. Hot castor oil packs were usually given in a three-day series and were kept on for from one to three hours over the entire right abdomen, both anterior and posterior from the right costal margin to the crest of the ileum and covering the area of the caecum and umbilicus. These hot packs were said to start the breakup of the lacteal lesions and adhesions. The heat alone would certainly tend to increase the circulation of the area. It was also implied that the castor oil itself would have a beneficial effect by absorption through the skin. In many cases a period of abdominal massage and kneading of the right side of the abdomen was instructed immediately after the removal of the packs, to help in the breakup of the lesions and adhesions. This massage was recommended with either peanut oil or a mixture of olive oil and myrrh, and sometimes with a combination of all three.

The olive oil, given internally (usually two tablespoonfuls), was to be taken at bedtime on the last day of the series of packs. As a fat it would be absorbed through the lacteal ducts and might help to increase the flow through them.

Osteopathic massage and manipulation on and around the spine followed the series of castor oil packs. The relationship mentioned above between spinal and lacteal lesions is significant here. The manipulative treatment was supposed not only to correct any mechanical abnormalities in spinal segments, but also to stimulate the autonomic nervous system to help overcome the imbalance between it and the cerebrospinal nervous sytem. The effect upon the lacteal duct area was to aid in the elimination of the lesions and/or adhesions by an increase in circulation and a relief of nervous tension or spasm induced via the autonomic nerve plexuses in the abdomen. The hot packs seem to be an essential preliminary step, so that the manipulations would have their maximum effect on the lesions and adhesions in the lacteal duct regions. Elimination of the lesions would in turn have a reciprocal effect upon the spinal segment lesion and vice versa.

It is necessary that there be sufficient of the castor oil packs taken to relax the lacteal duct area, the caecum and the central portion about the umbilicus center.

Also in giving the adjustments necessary from the 9th dorsal to the lumbar axis, or 4th lumbar, there must be the massage—or the kneading, gently, of the whole right portion of the abdomen, specifically. And then there must be the relaxing of those centers also in the coccyx area.   1025-2

Have sufficient periods of the castor oil packs. To be sure, they are disagreeable, but they will break up lesions as no other administrations will. The best time to take these is the evening, to be sure. These should be given in series; applied for an hour each evening for two or three evenings *before* each osteopathic adjustment is to be made, see?. . .

Keep these up until this coldness *and* the lesion in the right side is removed—which is just a hand's breadth below the point of the rib, or over that area of the ducts. . .

The idea of the treatments, of course, is to correct those subluxations, or tendencies, which exist; deep in some areas, superficial in others, along that area given; but mostly to eradicate—causing the system to assimilate—the tautness, coldness and the lesions in the right side of the body, in the areas indicated.   2153-4

Stimulation of the autonomic nervous system by manipulation would also affect the functioning of the glands which in turn would have an effect upon the brain by the mechanism that the readings suggested.

The problem of inadequate elimination was addressed from a number of different angles. The olive oil, a natural laxative, also acts as lubrication in the intestines. Other laxatives were sometimes suggested, such as Fletcher's Castoria, or Innerclean. Colonics were recommended for those who seemed to have a particularly difficult problem with elimination. Manipulations would presumably also help here. Proper functioning of the alimentary canal was aided by a diet designed to include food as easily digestible as possible. This in turn would aid eliminations. The diet was low-fat in nature, definitely prohibiting fried foods, pork, fat meats, and sweet milk. Alkaline-forming foods and vegetables were recommended, but most tuberous vegetables were excluded. Acid-producing foods such as meats, sugars, starches, and condiments were discouraged.

A boiled concentrate which was prepared in a definitely prescribed manner from the passion flower was recommended to replace the use of sedatives. Although the readings occasionally approved the temporary continuance of sedatives such as dilantin or pheno-barbital, the ultimate goal of successful treatment was the elimination of the need for such drugs which act as poisons in the system. The passion flower fusion was described as a non-habit-forming herbal compound and not a sedative itself. It was supposed to have a calming action on the nervous system and to aid the eliminations, as well as to help retard muscular contractions.

Exercise in the open was recommended both for a means of helpful outlet of physical energy and as a means of securing physical relaxation of the body during rest.

To be sure, the body should take as much physical exercise—and in the open—as is practical each day, not to be overstrenuous. Calisthenics, or *anything* which has to do with the general movements of the body in the open, is well. Walking is one of the *best* of exercises; walking, swimming, *anything* that has the calisthenics; tennis, handball, badminton; *any* of those activities for the body.   2153-4

The readings stressed the importance of a balanced program of treatment, with equal stress on all phases. The importance of completeness, continuity, and consistency was emphasized. In most cases, treatment had to be continued for a considerable period of time, at least six months.

III. Recommendations

1. The medical literature for the last 50 years should be reviewed to determine if there is any experimental work which throws any light on or gives any evidence for the mechanisms suggested in the readings. For example, the action of the chemical ingredients of castor oil; the action of castor oil on adhesions; or any instances of gastrointestinal pathology, particularly in the lacteal duct area, which have caused convulsions.

2. The suggestions for the mechanisms involved in the lacteal duct type of epilepsy referred to in the readings would furnish leads for experimental research. For example, the passion flower fusion compound could be analyzed and its chemical compounds checked for pharmacologic activity.

3. Pathologists could be alerted to the possibility of gastrointestinal pathological conditions of epilepsy. Port-mortem examinations of known epileptics could include a special concentration on examination of the gross and histological specimens from the lacteal duct area in the jejunum and ileum as well as from the mesenteries to these regions of the small intestine.

4. A controlled clinical trial of the most frequent and consistent types of treatment could be undertaken on a selected group of epileptics at the same time and place under the supervision of qualified physicians. The number of patients in such a study should be

large enough to make the results statistically valid. Both the patients receiving the Cayce treatment and the control group should be divided according to the type of epilepsy (grand mal, petit mal, or psychomotor) to determine the effectiveness on each type. The 79 cases in Groups I and II were not able to be adequately separated into types because of the meagerness of the case history data available.

With the presupposition that there is an intestinal type of epilepsy with a lacteal duct etiological factor, the treatment could be expected to be effective only in such cases where such pathology is present. Obviously, the most satisfactory trial would be on a group of epileptics of this type. At present, the only guides which can be used to separate this type of case are the cold spot described above, discomfort in the right abdominal region, or disturbances in eliminations from the digestive tract. If such a selected group could not be found and the treatments were tried on a general group of epileptics with no apparent brain damage, it should be remembered that in no more than 50 percent of the cases (Groups I and II) were lacteal duct lesions described as an important etiological factor.

With the possibility of such a clinical trial in mind, the following treatment outline has been prepared. The suggestions given below occurred repeatedly and fairly consistently in the readings. All patients in such a trial should have a complete medical workup for epilepsy, including an electroencephalogram. Definite brain pathology would presumably rule out the possibility that a type of intestinal pathology was the cause of the convulsions and that the treatment could be expected to be effective.

In general, treatment involves the application of castor oil packs for three-day periods in conjunction with daily massages of the right abdominal and spinal area. The osteopathic manipulations are to follow the three-day series of packs on the fourth day. During the first six weeks of treatment, osteopathic manipulations are to be given twice weekly, each following a three-day series of packs. The packs, massages, and manipulations follow a cyclical schedule with three weeks of treatment followed by one week of rest, etc. Starting with the third three-week treatment period (i.e., the eighth week), only one osteopathic treatment is to be given each week, following one three-day series of packs. In addition to these treatments, the passion flower fusion is given, but only after the packs and manipulations have been started.

The above mentioned basic treatment should be supported and

given in conjunction with strict attention to diet, exercise, daily regularity and full eliminations from the digestive tract. The complete treatment should be carried through. The greater part will be done by the patient but, at the time of the manipulations, progress can be checked and persistence in all phases of treatment encouraged. A detailed daily written report of treatments administered and diet followed should be kept and turned in by each patient. Six months is suggested as the minimum period of treatment.

IV. Treatment Outline

1. *Hot castor oil packs:* One to one-and-a-half hours daily for each three-day series. The pack should be applied preferably in the evening, so that the patient can go to sleep immediately after the pack and associated massages have been finished. (See Appendix.)

2. *Massage of the abdomen and spine:* After the packs have been removed and the area sponged off with soda solution, the right abdominal area should have a thorough massage with deep kneading movements. This massage should last for at least 15 minutes and be given with the fingers dipped into a solution made of equal portions of olive and oil and tincture of myrrh. (This oil solution should be prepared by heating the olive oil and then adding the tincture of myrrh.) After the abdominal massage, a 15-minute massage of the spine and the back muscles along the side of the spine should be given from the base of the brain to the tip of the spine with same oil solution.

3. *Olive oil:* Two tablespoonfuls by mouth at bedtime after each three-day series of packs (i.e., on the evening of the third day).

4. *Osteopathic manipulation:* Twice weekly for the first six weeks of treatment and once weekly thereafter (except during the one-week "rest" periods every fourth week). This osteopathic treatment should be both general and specific. In addition to general massage and manipulation of the spine, special attention should be paid to the sacro-coccygeal area and the first three cervicals, as well as the ninth to the eleventh dorsal segments. The coccyx and the sacro-coccygeal junction should receive special attention. An osteopathic massage should be given to the abdominal areas from the liver to the caecum and include the umbilical area. Each manipulative treatment should be preceded by the three-day series of packs.

5. *Passion flower fusion:* One teaspoonful four times daily, one-half hour before meals and one-half hour before retiring. This

treatment should be started during the fourth week of therapy—i.e., at the start of the first one-week rest period. This compound is intended to reduce the amount of sedative needed to control the epilepsy. Sedatives which the patient is already taking should be decreased gradually in accordance with the following schedule: At the time of the second one-week rest period, decrease total dosage by one-third. At the time of the third one-week rest period, decrease another one-third; and by the time of the fourth one-week rest period, discontinue sedatives entirely so that the patient is taking only the passion flower fusion in the above dose. (See Appendix.)

Note: Reduction of sedatives must be undertaken in accord with the individual patient's response and only upon the recommendation of the supervising physician. The goal should be complete freedom from sedatives by the end of the six-month treatment period.

6. *Diet:* The diet should generally contain foods of a non-constipating and easily digestible nature. Overeating should be avoided.

a. Sugars and starches: Use honey for sweetening. Cut down on starches. Avoid sugars and condiments.

b. Fruits: All in abundance except raw apples, bananas, large prunes, plums, cranberries.

c. Vegetables: Especially stress raw, green vegetable salads. Leafy vegetables in abundance rather than tuberous vegetables (except carrots, beets, and oyster plant). Avoid potatoes, turnips, legumes, and rhubarb. Eat Jerusalem artichokes one or two times per week, and okra frequently.

d. Cereal products: Whole wheat, cracked wheat, or pumpernickel bread. Dry cereals, whole wheat or steel-cut oats (not rolled oats) as cooked cereals, but not at the same meal with citrus fruits. No nuts, except filberts and almonds in moderation. Ovaltine as a beverage, rather than coffee or tea.

e. Meats: Seafoods in abundance but never fried. Fish, fowl, lamb, calves' liver (broiled, never fried), no rare meat, no beef except beef juice regularly, no fat meats, no pork except crisp breakfast bacon occasionally. Use gelatin frequently—e.g., in fruit and vegetable salads.

f. Dairy products: Eggs, but only the yolk. Cheese only in moderation. Avoid sweet milk (use Bulgarian buttermilk, dry skimmed milk, or soybean milk).

g. Miscellaneous: No carbonated beverages. No alcoholic drinks. No smoking unless already an addict, then decrease to a minimum.

7. *Eliminations:* The natural functioning of the digestive tract should be kept regular. The two tablespoonfuls of olive oil after each three-day series of castor oil packs will aid in this, but other laxatives may be required. Petrolagar, Fletcher's Castoria, or Innerclean are other possibilities. If the eliminations do not seem to be adequate, even with the use of the laxatives suggested, a colonic irrigation should be given one to two times per month. In cases with a special problem, eat nothing but raw apples (in spite of prohibition of apples in the usual diet above) for three days followed by a half cup of olive oil as a cleansing for the entire digestive tract.

In summary the treatment follows a cyclical pattern with a rest period every fourth week. A schedule based on the plan of treatment given above is as follows:

First three weeks: Castor oil packs plus massages each evening— Sunday, Monday, Tuesday. Olive oil at bedtime following the treatment on Tuesday. Manipulative treatment on Wednesday. Repeat series of packs plus massages each evening on Wednesday, Thursday, Friday. Olive oil following the treatment at bedtime Friday. Manipulative treatment on Saturday. This same schedule is followed each week.

Fourth week: None of the above treatments but start passion flower fusion by mouth and continue four times daily throughout the remaining periods of treatment.

Fifth, sixth and seventh weeks: Same as first three weeks.

Eighth week: Rest from all treatment except passion flower fusion, diet, and control of eliminations.

Ninth, tenth and eleventh weeks: Each week *one* three-day series of castor oil packs and massages, plus the olive oil as before, followed by a manipulative treatment on the fourth day.

Twelfth week: Rest as during the eighth week. Repeat patterns of weeks nine through twelve for the remainder of the six-month treatment period.

V. Conclusion

This report has been a preliminary step in the study of the treatment given for epilepsy in the Edgar Cayce readings. No conclusions can be drawn as to the worth of the treatments without further research. Suggestions for such research have been presented.

Walter N. Pahnke, M.D.

Case Breakdown by Groups

Group I (46 cases): 34, 80, 161, 251, 543, 561, 567, 571, 663, 693, 814, 885, 1001, 1025, 1527, 1625, 1683, 1699, 1784, 1836, 1916, 1980, 1994, 2019, 2149, 2153, 2292, 3057, 3082, 3156, 3210, 3302, 3426, 3438, 3569, 3606, 3688, 3790, 4678, 5232, 5234, 5379, 5386, 5562, 5642, 5736.

Group II (33 cases): 22, 54, 179, 395, 521, 769, 1495, 1653, 2155, 2286, 2441, 2991, 3133, 3217, 3362, 3428, 3465, 3521, 3565, 3568, 3603, 3690, 3788, 3801, 3891, 4091, 4677, 4798, 5033, 5094, 5128, 5333, 5732.

Group III (16 cases): 146, 241, 436, 758, 1198, 1289, 1465, 3071, 3905, 3918, 3995, 4080, 4503, 4844, 5204, 5391.

The Most Common Types of Etiology and Treatment

Classified According to Frequency of Occurrence in the
79 Cases of Groups I and II

Items Specifically Mentioned in Readings	Group I	Group II	Total
Etiology:			
1. Lacteal duct pathology	23	16	39
2. Cold spot present	6	2	8
3. Spinal segment lesions			
(a) All types	19	12	31
(b) Coccyx	14	9	23
4. Incoordination between cerebro-spinal and autonomic nervous systems	22	13	35
5. Glands	13	8	21
6. Brain scar	5	2	7
Treatment:			
1. Castor oil packs	23	14	37
2. Osteopathic manipulations	34	17	51
3. Massage	24	19	43
4. Abdominal massage	14	9	23
5. Passion flower fusion	17	11	28
6. Diet	27	13	40
7. Eliminations			
(a) Laxatives	14	13	27
(b) Colonics	6	6	12
8. Exercise	9	2	11

FLU: Respiratory

I. Physiological Considerations

According to medical texts, influenza, or "flu" is usually an upper respiratory infection caused by viruses of the myxovirus group and related to the larger paramyxoviruses which include mumps, measles, parainfluenza, etc. There are three distinct antigenic types of influenza virus, designated A, B, and C, infection with one type conferring no immunity against the other two.

Influenza B occurs sporadically or in localized outbreaks. Type C causes a very mild disease which is rarely detected. And type A is responsible for major epidemics which tend to recur in cycles of two to four years in the winter months.

Although the upper respiratory tract is the usual site of infection, this can extend farther downwards leading to bronchitis or pneumonia. This can be complicated further by a superimposed bacterial infection, a serious complication indeed. Blood-borne infection occasionally does occur as well as involvement of other organs and tissues, leading to a wide variety of effects and symptoms.

In the readings given by Edgar Cayce on "flu" and "flu aftereffects," the principal sites of involvement were the respiratory and gastro-intestinal systems, occasionally with blood-borne infection. Complications by superinfection were very rare. A distinction is made between the cold and flu germs:

Q-2. Will the "flu" vaccine taken prevent reattacks?

A-2. With the proper care this will prevent; though the conditions that arise from cold or congestion will ever be apparent without sufficient of that in the system to combat with that germ or bacilli known as cold (and is *not* "flu" germ!). *One* may be combated with certain elements in the blood, while the other would be only to create others that would affect other

portions of the body. With proper care, though, the "flu" would be outlawed, or the body would be immune to the effect of "flu" proper.   654-3

Apparently the necessary elements in the blood to combat the cold germ are sufficient and proper function of hemoglobin and also enough of the white strep in the blood. (Perhaps by "strep," Cayce means white blood cells, the defense system of the body.)

While in a few instances the readings merely gave the diagnosis of flu, in many other instances, they say the underlying causes are cold and congestion, poor eliminations, deficiencies in the blood supply (humoral and/or cellular) with lack of resistance to infectious agents, poor diet, or any combination of these. Some of the causes of cold and congestion are overacidity (perhaps through dietary indiscretion) and mechanical pressure on the cerebrospinal system, presumably causing circulatory disturbances.

What seems to emerge from this is that a variety of stimuli—all originating from inharmonies between the spiritual, mental and physical forces, acting through the circulatory system as a final common pathway—does predispose one to acquiring "flu," the severity and extent of which depends on the class of flu organism and the associated or underlying conditions of the person thus infected.

Reading 274-12 makes a brief mention of astrological influences, while 845-2 gives some insight into how extensive complications can arise from "flu." These complications often occur years after the initial attack, particularly in the cases of gastrointestinal flu (which are found in the Circulating File, "Flu: Aftereffects").

II. Rationale of Therapy

Therapy may be broken down into two general areas: treating the underlying problem, such as poor eliminations, poor diet, circulatory disturbances, etc.; and treating distressing symptoms. With correction of the underlying problem, all symptoms will eventually disappear, but this may take some time.

Proper elimination is brought about through colonics and laxatives. Equally important is the improvement of circulation through massages and osteopathic manipulations so that the other organs of elimination can function better. Hydrotherapy may be utilized in severe circulatory disturbances, as this helps to balance the superficial and deep circulations.

An alkaline environment is detrimental to the "flu" organism, hence alkalizing agents and an alkaline-reacting diet are helpful.

III. Suggested Therapeutic Regimen

The following is not meant to be an exhaustive list of the therapeutic modalities prescribed by Cayce, but only a guideline— what one might consider a reasonable approach with the average patient.

1. An inhalant. Two to three inhalations taken through the mouth and nostrils three to four times daily, as described in reading 304-15.

The mono-ichthyolate spray (preserved with a weak solution of alcohol to counteract irritation in the nasal passages and throat). (274-11)

A throat purifier (expectorant) and alkalizer prepared thus: To the white of one fresh, beaten egg, add the juice of one lemon very slowly and stir; then a tablespoon of strained honey added drop by drop and beaten into same; then glycerine—two minims (not more than two drops). *Dosage:* One tablespoonful twice daily until condition clears. Dosage was as frequent as every two to three hours in one instance. (274-11)

For lower respiratory involvement, additional measures are necessary, and these might include chest massage, onion poultice, ultraviolet ray treatment, Calcidin to relieve congestion and improve breathing, antibiotics, etc. (See File on bronchitis.)

2. Establish good eliminations by use of laxatives, such as Fletcher's Castoria, taken two teaspoonfuls every two hours until good bowel evacuation ensues. The properties in this product are claimed to help lessen the activity of the infectious forces. (274-11) Eno Salts may be used as an alternative. (464-18)

Colonics once or twice a week may be resorted to if satisfactory results are not obtained with laxatives.

3. Diet is very important. An alkaline-reacting diet is recommended.

Some alkalizers: Alka-Seltzer, rectified bicarbonate with cracker crumbs (348-6), etc.

4. Others: spinal massages, osteopathic adjustments. These may be necessary in more severe conditions to improve circulation and elimination and to relieve pressure along the spinal centers.

Occasionally one sees a case of respiratory and intestinal "flu" combined. The File on flu or flu aftereffects should be consulted.

Hezekiah Chinwah, M.D.

Edgar Cayce readings referenced:

143-3, 4	348-6	755-3
274-11, 12	464-18, 19, 30	845-2
286-2	538-43, 62, 63	1010-8
304-4, 15, 16, 17	654-3, 4	1861-3
341-46	710-2	

FLU: Aftereffects

I. Physiological Considerations

Some clarification in terminology is necessary to avoid confusion in discussing this topic. The medical texts tell us that the influenza virus is not one of the viruses that causes gastroenteritis, although gastrointestinal symptoms such as nausea, anorexia, constipation sometimes do occur with this infection. The main features that are lacking for the diagnosis of gastroenteritis are abdominal cramps, vomiting, and especially diarrhea. The enteroviruses (Coxsackie, Echo, rheovirus) are the agents usually responsible, but unfortunately the term "intestinal flu" has been in common use for all viral gastroenteritis.

Whether this common usage was adopted in the Cayce readings is a moot point, but the following observations would lead me to believe otherwise. In one reading (654-3) Cayce made a distinction between the flu and cold germ; and in another reading (341-46) he indicated that the infection was caused by a variant of the flu germ.

The mechanism involved in the production of the symptoms and signs due to intestinal flu are as follows: Infection results in inflammation and congestion in the intestinal tract, which leads to improper assimilation/elimination. (Involvement of the lacteals leads to impaired production of the digestive juices.) Toxic accumulations occur. This together with the congestion results in pressure on the ganglia, leading to abnormal sympathetic (autonomic) discharge. A vicious cycle sets in, producing more inflammation, congestion, poor elimination, etc., which ultimately might lead to multiple organ system dysfunction, which could in time become an organic condition. The mechanism and the complexity of the interactions can be better appreciated by the diagram pictured on next page:

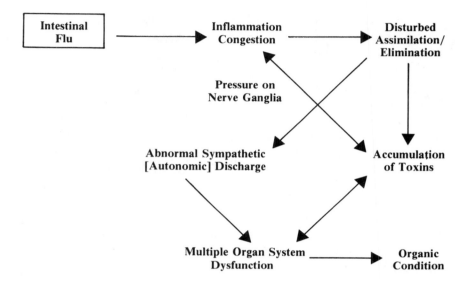

Overt symptoms and signs manifest themselves sometimes years after the initial attack.

The effect on the gastrointestinal tract is as depicted in the diagram. In addition, involvement of Peyer's patches leads to diminished resistance and impaired ability to rebuild. Other effects that were described included collapse of the stomach with near autodigestion; and collapse, prolapse, and impaction in the colon.

The liver and kidneys become involved through abnormal sympathetic (autonomic) discharge and irritation from accumulated toxins. This leads to impaired circulation in these organs with attendant metabolic changes. This further enhances toxic accumulations. Similar changes may extend to the spleen, pancreas, heart, lungs, pelvic organs (which in the female may lead to menstrual problems and infertility), etc. The glandular system, not infrequently, is thrown out of balance as a result of this.

The effect on the nervous system is mediated through abnormal sympathetic (autonomic) discharge, this producing muscular tension and pressure on the cerebrospinal system. This is how lesions are produced in the spine. Less frequently the infection may produce inflammatory reaction directly around the nerves. Central nervous system signs and symptoms may occur, including impaired mental functioning and a variety of abnormal sensations (incoordination).

In the cardiovascular system, circulatory changes may lead to high blood pressure; irregular heart action may result from increased pressure and irritation (from congestion) on the cardiac plexus. With persistence of these stimuli, organic heart disease may be the outcome. The inflammatory process is usually reflected by an elevation in the white blood cells when an adequate defense response occurs, and sometimes in anemia with the result that there is diminished vitality, resistance, and ability to rebuild damaged tissues.

The emotional response to the illness may be an additional stress to the system, the magnitude of which is dependent on the state of consciousness (spiritual maturity) of the individual. In other words, the way one reacts to an illness is very important regarding its outcome. If proper use is made of such experiences, just as in all other experiences in our daily lives, this brings us closer to the real purpose of our existence, i.e., spiritual alignment with divine will. The following passage illustrates this:

These are then conditions to be met and to be overcome; not only effects but the basic causes of same.

As we find, this will require then some patience, some persistence, some periods of the body taking not only precautions but being very persistent, very consistent with itself and with its activities. But if these are done, consistently, persistently, we may bring back to the body quite a different outlook upon life. And we will arouse those emotions not only to be good but to be good for something; and this the body has almost lost sight of.

Being merely good for self's own satisfaction doesn't satisfy a very great deal in the last analysis of the purposes of an individual experience in associations with others. But to become a channel through which hopefulness, helpfulness, patience, long-suffering, endurance, loveliness in its expressions to others, makes for life and its experience and its expressions and its outlook upon life more and more worthwhile. Something to hope for! It's not all just to live nor yet all *just* to die. For as the tree grows (and when it passeth or falleth), so it lies, and it has not changed that it has lived or experienced. For only that an individual soul is able to give out does the individual have. And ye cannot create a surrounding or an environment for self or others of that ye do not express or experience within, not only the own mind but the own body itself.

These hindrances have come, then, for a purposefulness—if they are to be used as stepping-stones to understand self and self's relation within a creative world—yea, a really beautiful world, if the beauties will be sought and not the sordid darkness of disappointments or failures or ill health. For if you

continue to look for ill health or sordidness or disappointments or darkness, how has the law been given? "As ye seek, so ye find—as ye sow, so ye reap." If you are looking for these, ye cannot find happiness or contentment or harmony or peace, either in body or mind; neither can ye give out other than discontent to others in thine own self of self-expression.

First then begin with this ideal and this idea; that the corrections can be made, will be made, "*If* I will only choose to have same that the usefulness of this experience may be worthwhile, not so much for self but spent for others; that I may indeed have love and hope and faith in my own experience."

1303-1

II. Rationale of Therapy

This may be subdivided into the following categories:

1. Specific measures directed against the infective organism,

2. Alleviation of distressing symptoms,

3. Treatments directed at the underlying problem(s) and/or associated conditions, such as overacidity from dietary indiscretion, poor eliminations, circulatory disturbances, mental/emotional attitudes, etc.

Usually, each of the therapeutic modalities encompasses more than one or all of these categories.

III. Suggested Therapeutic Regimen

All cases of intestinal flu do not progress to involvement of multiple organ systems, but sometimes such extensive complications do occur. With this in mind, one can tailor the therapy to suit the patient. The following may be considered a reasonable approach to the average patient.

1. Enhancement of bowel elimination and destruction of the infecting organism.

    a. Bicarbonate of soda (rectified bicarbonate, not baking soda) one-third teaspoon and fine cracker crumbs one tablespoon; this to be eaten. Wait at least 20 minutes, then take drinks of water with a pinch of elm. (This produces an alkaline reaction and is lethal to the flu germ.) If the temperature is elevated, yellow saffron tea should be taken instead of the elm which otherwise would be belched out or become rancid. This should be continued every three to four hours until good bowel movements ensue. For more difficult cases, other laxatives may be used, for example Fletcher's Castoria, Fleet's Phospho

Soda, etc. Only non-irritating laxatives should be used.

b. Colonics or enemas were recommended in practically all the readings. One every week to 10 days for two to three treatments seems a reasonable number. Sometimes it was recommended as often as twice a week in more severe and complicated cases.

c. The combination of elixir of lactated pepsin, 12 drops, plus milk of bismuth, one teaspoon, added to a half glass of water and taken daily for three weeks is helpful in clearing intestinal scales. (3455-1)

2. Alleviation of symptoms.

a. When digestive disturbances are present, dietary aids were prescribed, e.g., Alcaroid tablets with meals, one or two tablets, or Glyco-Thymoline taken internally, a few drops once a week (both are alkalinizing agents).

b. Grape poultice over the stomach area for excessive gas. (See 2320-2.)

c. Castor oil packs for three days followed by two table-spoons of olive oil. This done for a three- to five-week period was prescribed in one instance.

3. Treatment directed at underlying causes and/or associated condition(s).

a. A prescription to improve the circulation and lymph flow:

To two ounces of strained honey add two ounces of distilled water, letting it come almost to a boil. Then to this solution add:

Fluid extract or essence of wild ginseng (not tame but wild ginseng), ½ ounce

Tincture or essence of Indian turnip, 20 minims

Tincture of stillingia, ¼ ounce

Lactated pepsin, essence of, ½ ounce

Essence of wild ginger, ¼ ounce

Shake well before use; one-half teaspoon before each meal three times daily. (913-1)

b. *Dietary:* An alkaline-reacting diet was recommended, elimination of heavy starches such as potatoes, rice, white bread, etc., and red meat was advised. Blood-building diet is also beneficial, especially if anemia was present. Pure beef juice is good for this. Red wine with black or pumpernickel bread taken some afternoons helps to absorb poison from the system. (1044-1)

c. Atomidine was recommended for glandular imbalance.

4. Other measures.

a. Spinal massages, osteopathic manipulations were recommended frequently. The frequency of treatments varied greatly. A reasonable approach might be one treatment each at weekly intervals for four to five treatments.

Cabinet sweats followed by rubdown and massages were recommended less frequently, again the frequency of treatments varied greatly (ranging from three treatments 12 days apart to three a week for a two-week period). This cleanses the circulation.

b. Zilatone stimulates liver activity. Dosage: Two tablets one-and-a-half hours after dinner for three days. This may be followed by Fleet's Phospho Soda the morning after the third dose.

c. Appliances.

1) Violet ray applied front and back with the bulb applicator for eight to ten minutes in the evening before retiring—this usually when the condition has started to improve.

2) The wet cell and/or diathermy may also be used for coordination of nerve activity.

3) The radio-active appliance is also beneficial for balancing the superficial and deep circulations. Sometimes Atomidine was recommended in its use. (See 4175-1.)

The therapy outline has been arranged in such a way that one might start off using one or two of the treatments under each category simultaneously. For more difficult or complicated cases, one might then proceed down the line under each category, adding on in a stepwise fashion. Other measures may be reserved for last.

Hezekiah Chinwah, M.D.

Edgar Cayce readings referenced:

Volume I:			
913-1	1700-2	2726-1	4178-1
989-1	1724-1, 2	3025-1	4250-1
1023-1	2313-1	3033-1	4283-1 through 5
1044-1, 2	2320-1	3455-1	4374-1
1303-1	2334-1	3622-1	5376-1
1358-1		3644-1	5399-1
1400-1	*Volume II:*	4149-1	5604-1
1561-22	2580-1	4175-1	5737-1

FRACTURES AND SPRAINS

Care of fractures is obviously an orthopedic problem. The primary consideration in such care is preservation of life. With this assumed, proper reduction of the fractured bone then becomes paramount to healing. If such reduction is not performed, changes might come about within the part of the body affected which would be irreversible. For a naturopathic doctor who applied for a reading (4457-1) Cayce saw conditions that would "necessitate an operation before the body could be *entirely* relieved and brought back to a normal condition. . ." This was a skull fracture, apparently depressed and causing pressure on the brain. This man was advised to have surgery at Johns Hopkins Hospital, another one of Cayce's specific recommendations.

In another case, [1715], the care and reduction of a fractured arm was "improper," and it was reported that the hand and the finger were becoming stiff and there was sensory loss to the little finger. In his comments, Cayce did not see a full healing of the conditions likely to come about, apparently because of interruption of the nerve supply to tendons and muscles of the extremity.

Assuming, however, that the reduction of a fracture is proper and other factors are equal, healing comes about as a manifestation of the spirit acting within the body itself, in a manner that demands the proper balance between the physical body and the mental body. Case [564] was urged "then, give self the *opportunity* to function normally, mentally, physically, spiritually. The *spirit* will act, irrespective of what a body does with its physical or mental body—and it may make a very warped thing if you keep it under cover or expose it too much!" (564-1)

The healing comes through hormones that "coagulate" those electrical energies from food and from the red blood cells, etc., into form or into tissue that is the rebuilding of the fracture. This rebuilding, which in medical terminology is called callus formation, needs to be balanced in its effects on the rest of the system by means of the nerve centers in the sympathetic ganglia and the cerebrospinal nervous system so that the body as a whole may remain adjusted, in harmony, and in coordination with itself. Also the products of rebuilding, which become "refused" or rejected or used energies—waste products or end products of metabolism—must also be eliminated properly from the system. Elimination becomes a very important factor, as does the balancing of the sympathetic ganglia through adjustments and manipulations.

When the body is not properly balanced to bring about normal healing or when improper reduction of fractures brings problems in healing, the healing forces within the body can be assisted in bringing conditions as a whole back toward normal. A stiffening was coming about in the knee ligaments after a fracture of the patella in a 40-year-old man. (438-5) Cayce suggested massages to supply calcium, acids, and oils that "will prevent accumulations of water—or prevent the tendons becoming so taut as not to allow movement in the knee and the kneecap." On one day he suggested using olive oil and tincture of myrrh, equal parts, while on alternate days salt soaked with pure apple vinegar was to be used. The salt and vinegar combination was perhaps the most common massage or pack recommended in care of fractures or sprains.

The normal healing of a fracture is stimulated and aided with massage in case [3823] on the arm and brachial area of the shoulder with the same salt-and-vinegar combination, twice a day. This was for fracture of an arm and was used after the splints were removed.

Ligamentous sprain becomes a problem often, both acute and chronic. The "loosening" of the tendons to prevent further disturbance in these areas has already been described above in case [438]. For sprained ligaments about the knee, for ankle sprain, for torn ligaments—for all these conditions, table salt moistened with pure apple vinegar or a solution of pure apple vinegar saturated with table salt or a pack of salt soaked with vinegar seems to be a beneficial, corrective, rebuilding application. Other suggestions to speed up the healing process appeared in the readings. An oil for massage can be made up by taking four ounces of peanut oil, then adding in order: two ounces of oil of pine needles, one ounce of oil of sassafras root, and one tablespoon of melted lanolin. This was suggested to alternate with salt-vinegar rubs in restoring a fractured knee back to health.

Almost a specific for backache, sprains, aching in joints, swellings, bruises, etc., would be: To one ounce of olive oil, add:

 Russian white oil, 2 ounces
 Witch hazel, ½ ounce
 Tincture of benzoin, ½ ounce
 Oil of sassafras, 20 minims
 Coal oil (kerosene), 6 ounces

"It'll be necessary to shake this together, for it will tend to separate; but a small quantity massaged in the cerebrospinal system or over sprains, joints, swellings, bruises will *take out* the inflammation or pain!" (326-5)

The violet ray hand applicator was suggested for use in [1715], in which case there had been improper reduction of the arm. About every third day the violet ray was to be applied to the brachial plexus area of the neck, and about once a week or once in two weeks gently over the entire arm. This was used in addition to the massage once a day with a combination of one tablespoon each of olive oil, tincture of myrrh, and sassafras oil made up fresh for each treatment. (The olive oil is to be heated first, and then the others added in turn.) This treatment brought the condition of near immobilization of the hand back to full normalcy.

Much then can be done to assist in healing of fracture or restoration of sprained muscles and tendons to normal.

Do these as we have indicated, in a consistent and persistent manner; and we will find we will bring the normal conditions for this body. Not as rote, but knowing that within self must be found that which may be awakened to the *building* of that necessary for the body, mentally and physically and spiritually, to carry *its* part in this experience. For the application of any influence must have that which is of the divine awakening of the activative forces in every atom, every cell of a living body. 726-1

William A. McGarey, M.D.

Edgar Cayce readings referenced:
564-1
1715-2
4457-1

Readings Extracts on Fractures and Sprains

Male, age 70, strained kneecap from fall

The ligaments about the knee we would massage well with almost a saturated solution of pure apple vinegar and common table salt, preferably the very heavy salt [rather] than that carrying too much of chalk or ingredients to prevent the sticking. We rather prefer the baser or common salt for this purpose. . .   304-3

Male, age 70, fractured foot

The condition. . .in the [right] foot. . .where the injury both to the flesh in the bruising of muscular tissue and also the fracture to the bony portion, and the crushing of soft portion in toe proper, this we find giving a great deal of trouble. . .be careful of infection. . .[For] the stimulant necessary to make the circulation. . .take small quantity of strychnine, under the directions, however, of a physician. . .with the temperature as will come from these conditions. Bathe well in solution that will disinfect the condition, using bichloride of mercury in as warm water as can be applied to the afflicted parts. Dress then with. . .Unguentine, a combination of oil and of sedative, and of a cleansing of the bruised portions. . .

Be well that the portion where the end of the bone has been mis-shapen, and out of alignment, be corrected properly.   304-6

Female, 20's, lumbar sacral injury, ankle sprain

Also the adjustments by the manipulations, osteopathically given, of the conditions in spine and lower limbs, applying, whenever the pain is severe in the lumbar and sacral region, and in any portion of limb (for it changes), those properties of saturated solution of salt and apple vinegar, heated as hot as body can bear.   49-1

Female, 60's, strained back

[This would be a very good specific for backache, sprains, joints, swellings, bruises, etc.]:

To one ounce of olive oil, add:

        Russian white oil, 2 ounces

        Witch hazel, ½ ounce

        Tincture of benzoin, ½ ounce

        Oil of sassafras, 20 minims

        Coal oil (kerosene), 6 ounces

It'll be necessary to shake this together, for it will tend to separate; but a small quantity massaged in the cerebrospinal system or over sprains, joints, swellings, [and] bruises will *take out* the inflammation or pain.   326-5

Female, age 59, arm in cast for fracture
   . . .we would use those foods that carry in a soluble manner that which may be absorbed and become replenishing or rebuilding for the blood; or the calciums, irons, glutens that make for the urea. . . [Sample daily menu followed.]
   When there is the removal of those braces, or that which holds same in place (and, as we find, this is knitting—and very well done), we would massage the arm with salt and vinegar. This will be most helpful; also—when knitting—that the shoulder and the brachial center be massaged with same. Do this once or twice a day; it will relieve, and the absorption through this manner would be well.
                                                3823-2

Male, age 40, fractured kneecap
   To prevent the recurrence in the muscular forces about the knee and the limb of the stiffening, so as to pull the ligaments loose again, we would massage the whole of the limb each day, as follows:
   One day we would use equal parts of olive oil and tincture of myrrh for the massaging.
   The next day we would use the salt (plain sodium chloride; not that carrying other properties, but this well powdered) and *pure* apple vinegar.
   Use one one day, the other the next. Continue in this manner, and we find that these ingredients will supply calcium, acids and oils that will prevent accumulations of water—or prevent the tendons becoming so taut as to not allow movement in the knee and the kneecap.   438-5

Female, age 24, torn ligament in knee
   The specific disturbances that we find from the injury in the left limb or knee—where there is a strained ligament, between the upper and lower portion (and this in the right side of same under kneecap)— it would be better *not* to have operative measures, but to apply— daily—in the afternoon or when ready to retire—wet heat; that is,

heavy towels wrung out of hot water, as hot as body can well stand. Apply these once or twice and then thoroughly massage the knee, especially around the cap and on the inside and under side, with *salt* that has been well saturated with pure apple vinegar.

Do this for several days, and we should find—with the precautions—this disturbance being removed.

In the second and third day it may bring some excruciating pain, but it will disappear as *dry heat* is applied—as from the infrared light.

But continue with this and we will save a great deal of trouble later.

Of course, do not apply the infrared unless there is excruciating pain from the massage of the salt and the vinegar—and this should be well dampened with the vinegar, to be sure. This would be in the evening, you see—that is, the infrared—following the massage; but only if there is excruciating pain. 1771-4

Female, age 77

In the area of the knee, where ligaments have been torn, use about twice a week this combination: Moisten table salt (preferably iodized salt) with pure apple vinegar, not having it too liquid, but that it may be gently massaged into the kneecap, the end of the ligaments. While this will hurt a few times at first, if this is kept up each day for quite a while, we will get better results here. 3336-1

Male, age 67

When there is excruciating pain, we would paint the areas with a combination of three parts laudanum to one part aconite; then apply the heavy salt pack (coarse, heavy salt, you see) saturated with pure apple vinegar. This, heated and applied will relieve any tension or strain, and the reaction of the sedatives and also the healing forces, as well as the rubs given as indicated, will continue to keep improvements. Put the salt in a sack or bag, see? Then saturate with vinegar. 2051-3

HEADACHES

I. *Physiological Considerations*

From the viewpoint of the readings, the mental forces (attitudes), the nervous system, the digestive system and the circulatory system are all closely interrelated in the pathogenesis of headaches, i.e., the cause of the headache was most often not in the head itself but elsewhere.

The mental and spiritual forces are said to govern the circulation to a great extent. In case [171], these forces, and consequently the circulation, were in fairly good order. The cause of the headache was traced back to production of toxins in the colon in combination with deficiencies in the important secretions from Peyer's patches leading to pressure in the nerve plexus opposite the pneumogastric center, which in turn reflexly transmitted this pressure to the brain as headache.

The deleterious effects of the toxins were not limited to this; imbalances in sympathetic discharge also occurred, as well as over-stimulation of the sensory organs through the areas of connection of the sympathetic nerve plexuses, the pneumogastric center, and the sensory nerves producing a variety of sensory defects which might include visual, speech, hearing, smelling abnormalities.

The abnormal conditions in the nervous system can, through the pneumogastric center, react in turn on the intestinal tract (and on other systems as will be seen from other readings), causing pain, nausea, vomiting, etc. Thus, if the condition has been there long enough, virtually all organ systems of the body can be affected. Excessive mental strain can initiate the process in at least three ways; either through the digestive or circulatory systems, or both.

In reading 263-16, lack of storage of resistance in the body in the form of vitamins A and D was the cause; this leading to disturbances in the nerve forces, which together with changes in the general activity of eliminations produced stress in the glandular system in an attempt to compensate for these changes. Vitamin B_1 was also deficient. This finally led to pressure on the cerebrospinal and sympathetic systems, resulting in headache and other symptoms.

Overtaxation of the nervous system can produce lesions in the spine which can result in muscular contractions leading to headaches, fatigue, vertigo, etc., as was illustrated in case [294]. Mechanical injury to the spine can result in headaches through the mechanisms already described (case [1387]). Here the effect was mediated through the circulatory system, resulting in congestion and toxins which could not be properly cleared. In the case of too much stress on the nervous system, it is not necessary for lesions to be produced in the spine, for the stress can be transmitted to the circulatory and digestive systems, resulting in headaches. In anyone who has a predisposing condition— as already described in the early parts of this writing—sudden changes in atmospheric pressure apparently can cause congestive changes, overacidity, which can bring on a headache.

In conclusion, any stimulus that can react adversely on the nervous, circulatory or digestive system can result in headaches. Through the very close relationship that exists between these systems, isolated abnormalities of these systems are seldom seen.

II. Rationale of Therapy

From the material in the readings, it seems logical that there would be four areas of therapy that could be instituted in every patient to bring about resolution of the headache problem. The four areas deal with underlying causes such as:
1. Subluxations,
2. Mental or emotional stresses,
3. Intestinal abnormalities or malfunctions, and
4. Circulatory problems or acid-base imbalances.

Perhaps it could be better stated that from these four areas of therapy, one or two could be drawn that would lead toward correction of the headache.

Removal of underlying causes should be accomplished, such as spinal adjustments to correct subluxations and removal or attenuation of stimuli that tend to overtax the nervous system (mental, emotional stress); correction of anatomic abnormality in the intestinal tract (e.g., corrections of the positions of the stomach through osteopathic adjustments, stomach brace, etc.); elimination of toxins from the intestinal tract and correcting overacidity in the system; proper diet (easily assimilated foods); correction of circulatory disturbances through osteopathic adjustments to improve flow; through diet building up the proper blood elements in the right quantities; development of higher spiritual ideals.

III. Suggested Therapeutic Regimen

1. For the prevention of making and absorbing toxins and for better assimilation and elimination and the relief of pressure on the pneumogastric center, the following was recommended:

> Tincture of valerian, 4 ounces
> Iodide of potassium, 2 grains
> Bromide of potassium, 4 grains
> Elixir of celerena, 4 ounces
> Tincture of capsici, 5 minims

in sufficient syrup to make 12 ounces to be taken one teaspoonful four times a day. (171-1)

2. The violet ray over the whole portion of the body from the sacral to the seventh dorsal, especially about the lower lumbar and the solar plexus center both along the spine and over the abdomen, along the right side especially. Total treatment not more than three minutes. This should be done in the evenings before retiring. Total number of treatments not specified. (171-1)

3. When the cause was seen as lack of storage or resistance in the body leading to disturbances in the nerve forces, eliminations, glandular system, etc.:

a. Spinal massage with peanut oil every other day and once a week with combination of peanut oil and oil of pine needles. This to be done in the evening.

b. Wet cell appliance alternating with gold and camphor. (Special instructions—see reading 263-16.)

c. Diet—well balanced (see 263-16).

d. Being helpful and nice to others; being with other people.

e. Other—with return of headaches, quiet environment was recommended, covering the eyes with cold cloth, bathing the temples with camphor and tincture or oil of lobelia, massage of the sacral and lumbar area.

4. When anemia was coexistent, a blood-building diet which

included beef, iron and wine was recommended (Wyeth's Beef, Liver & Wine). (1387-2)

5. When overacidity of the stomach was present, Alcaroid or Codiron tablets were recommended, the Codiron with meals for the duration of the spinal adjustments. (Intestinal antiseptics—Lavoris, Glyco-Thymoline.) (2290-2)

6. Others: Electric vibrator; colonics; castor oil packs; fume baths; olive oil by mouth; milk of bismuth mixed with elixir of lactated pepsin for better digestion; hydrotherapy (witch hazel), three to ten treatments followed by shower, massage, four to five short wave treatments to area of brachial center.

From the foregoing a reasonable therapeutic program might consist of 1, 3(a), 3(c), as initial therapy with the addition of colonics, ultraviolet ray, etc., as further therapy is needed.

Hezekiah Chinwah, M.D.

Edgar Cayce readings referenced:
171-1
263-16
294-3, 4
1387-2
2290-2

HEMOPHILIA

Hemophilia is described in *Dorland's Medical Dictionary* as "hereditary hypoprothrombinemia characterized by the delayed clotting of the blood and consequent difficulty in checking hemorrhage. It is inherited by males through the mother as a sex-linked character." From the 1966 edition of Best and Taylor's *The Physiological Basis of Medical Practice,* it is understood that there are two types which are called Factor VIII and Factor IX. Both involve genetically determined transmission to the male from the female. Cecil-Loeb's *Textbook of Medicine* (twelfth edition) describes a true hemophilia (a lack of the clotting factor), also a vascular hemophilia, and a vascular pseudohemophilia. In these latter two, the vessel walls are involved in the hemorrhage process.

For description of these conditions the reader is invited to study at least these two sources of information. It is interesting to note that not all hemophilia is transferred by genetic mechanisms. Thirty percent of all hemophiliacs are mutants or those who develop hemophilia without any family history of such. Looking at this fact in a rather objective manner, one would be influenced to think that so-called "mutation" activity could as easily correct the condition of hemophilia as, in the case of those 30%, bring it into being. This should be kept in mind in the discussion which follows.

I. Physiological Considerations

Hemophilia is seen in the readings to be a condition which is correctable. It is a deficiency due to improper assimilation in the elements which are necessary to build the vital energies in the glands and their functions in the body, which in turn would bring about proper coagulation of the blood and the ability of the body to build the walls of the blood vessels properly. (See reading 2832-1.)

Coagulation, as is described elsewhere in the readings, is the process whereby hormones create, in a real sense, structure out of energies which are supplied in the bloodstream. The structure, of course, would be proper rebuilding or generation of blood cells and walls of the blood vessels in the circulatory system. From the area of the Peyer's patches are taken into the system those substances which are then incorporated into lymphocytes and thus carried to various glandular tissues throughout the body, giving those glands the proper structure themselves, that they may in turn produce hormones and rebuild, regenerate, and keep in a vital condition other cellular structures throughout the body. Vitamins, iodine, and apparently globulins of various types interdependently take part in this whole procedure. The blood vessels and the blood cells are apparently under a single control.

Physiologically, then, we should look at the hemophiliac as one whose chromosomal genetic defect gives certain qualities to the organism which prevents it from assimilating certain specific substances necessary for the proper functioning of the blood and circulatory system. This same lack of assimilation might well be developed during a lifetime by the creation of a change in the genetic makeup of the individual.

In the same manner in which characteristics of growth are found as electrical imprints, so to speak, on DNA molecules, the defects causing hemophilia are imprinted or might be removed by a process involving delicate electrical energies or metabolic processes.

Aside from the rather general information found at the beginning of case [2832], the readings do not indicate specifically what glands are involved and the specific nerve areas. However, the wet cell appliance was suggested for consistent use in this case—the purpose being to affect, in a constructive manner, the lacteal duct center, the largest Peyer's patch. This would indicate that the vibratory energy necessary to change the genetic makeup itself would be needed in this very important area which in a sense controls all assimilation and which relates specifically to the autonomic ganglia and the coordination between the cerebrospinal and the autonomic nervous systems. This lymphatic area also has an indirect relationship to those centers of the control which exist within the ganglia and which control the circulation itself.

This single case [2832] and also reading 2769-1, which seem to indicate a tendency toward hemophilia, pose the possibility of a very interesting explanation for the physiological events involved here. Also suggested is a possibility not only of correction but of a method by which this disease may be aborted or prevented.

II. Therapy in Hemophilia

In approaching therapy, we should remember that the body has a capability of *normal* function:

Thus, we would administer those activities which would bring a normal reaction through these portions, stimulating them to an activity from the body itself, rather than the body becoming dependent upon supplies that are robbing portions of the system to produce activity in other portions, or the system receiving elements or chemical reactions being supplied without arousing the activity of the system itself for a more normal condition.

1968-3

Therapy suggested for a child of 10 months, [2832], is rather simplified, consisting only of dietary addition of blood pudding and the daily use of the wet cell appliance. Gold, camphor, and Atomidine were suggested as elements to be carried in the wet cell to be used on alternate days. (Details of this can be seen in the reading itself.) It is to be assumed that, had the parents of this child followed the instructions, further readings would have been obtained. It would have been interesting to see what would have been suggested after this. However, it is implied in the reading that following these two suggestions would bring about a return to normal in the child. Prevention of hemophilia is suggested as a possibility in case [2769]. Here the same general factors seem to be present—improper assimilation and involvement of the autonomic nervous system, produced by improper reactions of glandular tissue (again these not being specified). In bringing this particular body to a normal condition the following statement is of interest:

We find that these may be met easily by the consistent application of that as may aid in improving the activities of the glandular forces. Not by the adding or attempting to make the chemical reactions, though this is what becomes necessary; but there is in each body, as in this body, those necessary influences to produce body-sustenance and body-rebuilding—if the activities of the glands and organs are made to coordinate.   2769-1

These suggestions can be read in their entirety but involve basically fume baths, massage with oils of various types, osteopathic treatments in series, and certain dietary adjustments.

III. Summary

In summary, hemophilia was not, in the readings' estimation, a disease that carried with it the dire outlook seen in medicine today. Rather, it is a simple case of a deep-seated defect in the assimilations of the body which is correctable if proper steps are taken. The body may be restored to normal as a result of patience, persistence, consistency, and proper application of vibratory force that influences the very genetic centers of electrical function.

Do these, as we have indicated, in a consistent and persistent manner; and we will find we will bring the normal conditions for this body. Not as rote, but knowing that within self must be found that which may be awakened to the *building* of that necessary for the body, mentally and physically and spiritually, to carry *its* part in this experience. For the application of any influence must have that which is of the divine awakening of the activative forces in every atom, every cell of a living body.   726-1

William A. McGarey, M.D.

Edgar Cayce readings referenced:
2769-1
2832-1

HEMORRHOIDS

I. Physiological Considerations

Hemorrhoids, more commonly called "piles," are defined in medical literature as varicose dilatations of veins of the superior or inferior hemorrhoidal plexus. (*Dorland's Medical Dictionary,* 24th ed.)

Hemorrhoids are sac-like developments filled with lymph and blood vessels, and always located in conjunction with the two rings of sphincter muscle tissue that guard the opening of the rectum to the outside. The sacs often extrude out of the anus. Sometimes hemorrhoids are located higher in the canal and stay inside. They often bleed, especially when the lining of the anal orifice is irritated and thinned. And they sometimes bleed into the sac and cause a thrombosed hemorrhoid, this being the most troublesome.

Itching and bleeding are the two most significant symptoms, although often there is also pain associated with the condition.

In reviewing some 104 readings given for 65 different individuals, one finds a consistent story: There is always an underlying disturbance of function in the physiological balance. The most common disturbances are:

1. Excess acidity in the body (superacidity);

2. Disturbance of the hepatic circulation and related autonomic nervous system imbalances;

3. Nervousness, worry, emotions, anxiety, irritation—those things that we usually term "stresses";

4. Constipation, which usually has its own set of predisposing factors.

In one instance, [98] was on her feet too much, helping to bring on the condition in this 34-year-old woman; but there were other factors involved. An osteopathic "lesion," circular in type, had laid the foundation. The lesion was in the sixth and seventh dorsal sympathetic center, reflexed to the fifth and ninth. As the reading described it, "The blood supply does not carry the eliminations properly; neither does that assimilated build properly, and the functioning of the organs—as has been hindered—is the cause of same. Namely, the pancreas and the spleen, with the liver and hepatic circulation." (98-1) These in turn produced other sympathetic problems and irritations in various parts of the body, including the rectal area.

It seems as if the entire body is involved in the development of a hemorrhoid. When eliminations are decreased, the assimilation of foodstuffs into the body is lessened, the lack of nutrient elements creates glandular deficiences, anxieties, and often an increased acidity. The lymph is suppressed, irritations arise; incoordinations develop between parts of the nervous system and the deep and superficial circulation; the hepatic circulation and the balance between the eliminatory channels are all upset.

Throughout this happening, the homeostasis of the body is so magnificent that all an individual might notice is a greater anxiety, perhaps loss of sleep to a degree, a slight weight gain and the beginning of hemorrhoids. But the change is all very real, destructive in nature, and promising more destructive things to come unless there is a turnabout. The following extract tells the story in Cayce's words:

In the activity of the liver, as coordinant with the hepatic circulation as these are a part of the excretory as well as the secretive forces of the system—this as a gland or an organ gradually becomes involved the more often there arises this unbalanced condition.

With the superacidity produced, the reaction to the lower portion of the hepatic circulation is to cause a lack of the lymph circulation through the alimentary canal as related to *eliminating* channels of the system.

Thus, as has arisen, when there arises this disturbance, its reaction through the system is to affect the activity of the glandular system as related to the kidneys in *their* elimination.

Hence an excess of acidity has at times caused the folds of the sphincter centers, and the lower portion of the alimentary canal, to become involved in the disturbance because of the very lack of the lymph and the elimination through the proper channels of the excess drosses in the system.

Then, as has been indicated again and again for the body: There are the needs for the hydrotherapy treatments occasionally; that is, those that stimulate the superficial circulation and that make for a better coordinant

activity between the superficial and deeper circulation, by stimulating the whole of the glandular force as related to the eliminations through not only the alimentary canal but the better respiratory reaction, the better perspiratory reaction, the better stimulation for the emunctory and gland forces of the superficial or the skin itself. All of these become necessary as a part of the activity.   **257-199**

Cayce described to a 38-year-old man (555-7) the manner in which an excess of acidity in the system creates these distresses, by "producing a strain by the activity at the time in the muscular forces of the lower portion of the intestinal tract; this forming folds in the lower sphincter muscular forces, segregation of the blood supplies, and producing the form of a blood tumor." A thrombosed hemorrhoid!

Although it is difficult to ferret out the information dealing with the mechanism of anxiety-generated problems of physiology, the readings are explicit about the fact that "anxiety has caused and does cause those disturbances at times." (257-172) Anger, frustration, or stresses of that nature do create greater acidity in the system, and thus more opportunity for the process already described.

In pregnancy, pressure to the lower bowel and rectum may apparently cause hemorrhoids. It is questionable, however, whether the pressure of the child's head is the only factor. There may be other predisposing causes not readily discernable.

Perhaps it is safe to say that life stresses, a constant acid-reacting diet, and constipation are the three most common problems bringing on the condition.

II. Rationale of Therapy

In gaining an understanding of an approach to successful treatment of hemorrhoids, one must be aware that the general condition of the whole person must be taken into consideration. In two instances of the 65 individuals, surgery was advised. (2701-1 and 5327-1) Both were women past 60 years of age and afflicted with numerous problems. They needed immediate relief from the severe hemorrhoids and would benefit from surgery. The other 63 were all given indications that, if a therapy program were followed as suggested, permanent cure would be the result, or at least a condition "nearer normal."

Q-2. Will Tim [a compound recommended in the readings] cure or dry up these hemorrhoids without any other action?

A-2. Consistently used, it will not only remove the cause but remove hemorrhoids. 257-200

As we find, while conditions are good in many respects, there is still much that might be desired in the body building resistances, and for a better coordination of the assimilating system.

However, with the assimilating system made to coordinate with the blood supply, the nerve energy, and the activity of the liver as related to spleen, pancreas and kidneys, we would have a much nearer normal condition.

1102-6

Q-7. Any further questions for the relief or cure of this body?
A-7. These as have been given, if met properly, would bring near normal conditions. As to how to meet these, this has not been given or asked for. In meeting these, there is necessity of more consistency with the mental and physical activities of this body. In the diet, in the nominal activities, keep the body near equalized in elimination and assimilation. This will be accomplished more by consistency than any definite outline, other than *knowing* that it is necessary to keep these conditions nominal for the body. Do that. 654-3

Among these 65 patients (from 19 years of age, a young man, to a woman 76), the age grouping was well distributed. Each decade was represented. There is obviously much more likelihood of generalized troubles of the body in the older age group than in those in their 20s or 30s. But in every individual afflicted with hemorrhoids, there are those specific localized symptoms of itching, local irritation, frequent protrusion of the sac and sometimes bleeding. And, as described in these readings given, there must be underlying disorders bringing the specific problem into focus—such as constipation, improper diet, "superacidity," life stresses, incoordination of the nervous systems, lower intestinal acidity, and hepatic circulation imbalances as well as an incoordination between the deep and superficial circulation.

Obviously, use of Tim only in all instances will not bring removal of both the cause and the hemorrhoid, as Cayce indicated might happen for 257-200. But consistency is a part of that promise and needs to be a part of *all* therapy programs that are planned for relief of this problem. This is a spiritual quality, related closely to patience, wherein one possesses his soul. Thus its importance.

Most individuals are interested primarily in the relief of symptoms and unfortunately do not follow through on clearing up the systemic malfunctions that brought the symptoms into being. Cayce was not unaware of that in his information, and gave much material on caring for those irritations, the itching, the protrusion and the bleeding. In the course of doing this, however, he chose treatments that were more far-reaching and thus more helpful than many that might be used.

Tim is a product which was originally described in the readings specifically for the relief of hemorrhoids. There were numerous variations in its composition as Cayce described its formulation over the years. It was suggested more often than any other one therapy for treatment of hemorrhoids and was to be used both externally and injected with a bulb syringe (or such) into the anus and into contact with the rectal and anal mucosa.

One of the early descriptions of the formulation of Tim was for [294]. It probably derived its name from some of its original contents: T-tobacco, I-iodine, M-mentholatum.

To the oil as would be found from ¼ pound of butterfat (fresh) add:
    1 dram pulverized tobacco or snuff, with
    2 minims mentholatum, or oil of same, with
    1 drop or minim of tincture iodine.
This to be used as salve or lotion for such conditions or abrasions, internal or external. Apply that to the body. We will bring better relief and relations to the whole physical body, with the action of the physical when in the subconscious or subnormal condition.   **294-24**

Two other suggestions of interest came from reading 953-9:

    Butter rendered, 4 ounces
    Mentholatum, 3 minims
    Pulverized tobacco, 6 grains
    White castile soap, 2 grains
And 4709-5:
    Butterfat, 3 ounces
    Berton's snuff, 15 grains
    Spirits camphor, 1 minim
    Eucalyptol, 2 minims

This the proportion in the preparation of Tim:
As we find, there are other properties much preferable in the use of same than the old formula. Here's the better formula:
To 1 ounce of oil of butterfat, add:

Tincture of benzoin, 10 minims
Atomidine, or atomic iodine, 5 minims
  (or iodine, though atomic iodine is that with the poison
  out—but plain iodine is not as expensive as the
  Atomidine)
Powdered tobacco or snuff, preferably the snuff—the powdered,
  3 drams
Stir well together. Preferable that this never be put in tin, but rather in the
porcelain or glass; and should be in an ounce or ounce and a quarter
hexagon-shaped jar, preferably. The directions would be to apply as an
ointment to affected portions once or twice each day. Rest as much as
possible *after* application, with the feet elevated above the head. It'll cure it!
                                                              1800-20

This preparation (1800-20) is more of an ointment, with more of the
snuff or tobacco in it, and is probably meant only as an external
application. It lacks the mentholatum, present in earlier formula-
tions. It is not easy to determine which of the suggested formulas is
best to use consistently.

Cayce suggested for some of his questioners an ointment or
suppository called Pazo. It is still on the market and has as active
ingredients: a combination of benzocaine and ephedrine sulphate,
zinc oxide, and camphor in an emollient base. Other currently
available products include Rectal Medicone (benzocaine,
oxyquinoline sulphate, zinc oxide, menthol, balsam of Peru and
cocoa butter); Calmol 4 (Norwegian cod liver oil, zinc oxide, bismuth
subgallate, balsam of Peru and cocoa butter); Nurses Brand
suppositories and ointment (benzocaine, zinc oxide, bismuth
subgallate, para-cholormeta-xylenol and balsam of Peru); and
Preparation H (live yeast cell derivative, 2000 units skin respiratory
factor per ounce of suppository, shark liver oil and phenylmercuric
nitrate); among others.

It is interesting to look at the composition of these various
substances and see how similar they are. All of them lack the butterfat
and the pulverized tobacco found in Tim, but Pazo is probably the
closest to the Tim formulation. These substances no doubt work as a
soothing agent as well as an astringent, making the folds of the tissues
retract and become more normal.

Cayce suggested also quite frequently another substance which
always was to be inserted or injected into the anal orifice, a
combination of glycerin, carbolic acid, and Nujol or Usoline (Russian

white oil). The three substances were always the same although in differing quantities at different times. The action of this formulation was not the same as Tim. It was described best for a 50-year-old woman who had just experienced bleeding and asked the question as to why:

The conditions that formed in the lymph pocket, thus allowing for the emptying of same. Thus the character of enema indicated is not only to act as a healing influence and to prevent the folds reforming, but is to allay the disturbance and prevent the tissue that has broken from becoming scar tissue and again causing disturbance.   404-8

In giving instructions regarding the compounding of this substance, Cayce was specific in insisting that the glycerine and carbolic acid be *very* thoroughly mixed before being combined with the Nujol. Here are some of the differences from several readings in compounding the substance:

Glycerine	1 ounce	1	1	1	1	1	1
Carbolic acid	7 drops	2	3	5	2	4	2
Nujol (or Usoline)	16 ounces	1	3	4	4	4	2

The most frequent combination was one ounce of glycerin, two drops of carbolic acid and two ounces of Nujol. It was suggested nine times in the readings. This was to be injected with a bulb syringe, forcefully enough to go above the first and second sphincter muscles; usually about one to one-and-a-half ounces at a time, and about once a week up to once a month. "Use this in syringe that may *force* same, as a pump, you see; with the body reclining upon the knee and the elbow, or knee and shoulders." (404-8)

Another direct therapy described in the readings is a specific exercise. Cayce told a 19-year-old young man what he might expect from using this exercise: "This done several times each day, very slowly, will gradually lift the sphincter muscle and thus remedy the hemorrhoid condition." (3678-1)

Directions were somewhat complicated. To put together several suggestions, it would go something like this: First, wear as few clothes as possible. Then, while standing erect, slowly rise on your toes, inhaling through your nose, and at the same time, bring your arms slowly upwards till the hands are high above your head, your palms toward the front. Then, while exhaling through your mouth, slowly bend forward, keeping your hands still above your head, finally touching them to the floor, while still on tip toe. Then, again flat on both feet. Then still keeping your hands in the same position above your head, inhale again through your nose as you rise once more on your toes till you have again become upright. Then repeat the bending as described. Do this five or six times, very slowly, both morning and evening, more often if desired. But continue the frequency chosen consistently until the condition has cleared up and the underlying causes have been eradicated. Otherwise, the same forces that brought hemorrhoids into being the first time will cause them to recur.

For very painful acute hemorrhoids, ice can be used directly on the protruding part. Cold, then hot packs are also useful. In our own experience, castor oil packs can be very soothing and help the swelling to subside.

The underlying causes, however, are to be dealt with in other ways. Incoordination between the nervous systems (cerebrospinal and autonomic) becomes most acute in these conditions in the lumbo-sacral area, but sometimes involves the whole spine. Since it is the sacral parasympathetic outflow that controls the lower bowel, it is then this area that deserves the most attention.

Osteopathy plays an important role in correcting the body. In reading 654-3, Cayce told a woman: "Use Tim ointment as has been given for such conditions. This applied, with the proper manipulation in the lumbar and sacral region, will *permanently* relieve this body of such conditions."

Exercises, however, do much of this; and another woman who had failed to do her exercises needed the osteopathic or chiropractic corrections afterward. (288-47)

A 35-year-old woman, [98], was advised to have osteopathic treatments to the dorsal region—once a week only. Every other treatment, however, "should be a full gentle massage, manipulating all of the centers throughout the cerebrospinal system; not neglecting the sacral and coccyx." (98-1) One osteopath was directed to treat the third, fourth, and ninth dorsal areas especially concerning liver activity. (416-14) Another direction was to have treatments after the glycerin-carbolic acid combination was used and salt heat was applied across the lower back—then colonics in three days. And then, the manipulations. (462-14)

The violet ray was to be used for 15 minutes along both sides of the entire spine in one instance, immediately after the osteopath had finished. In reading 106-12, manipulations were suggested to "relax the body from the centers that radiate through this portion of the body, or specifically from the seventh and eighth dorsal to the fourth lumbar."

So it can be seen that more general malfunctions of the body need attention. Hot Epsom salt packs or hot castor oil packs were recommended to be used across the lumbar and sacral areas to relieve tension and aid when manipulations were given. In one instance (288-47), gentle rubs were suggested to be given across the small of the back with mutton tallow, spirits of turpentine and spirits of camphor—equal parts—with a hot pack placed over the back afterwards. And in another instance, diathermy was to be applied "giving low heat between cerebrospinal and sympathetic systems." (337-23)

Diet is always important in keeping the body balanced. Here it is advised to keep down the acidity which is often very high. An alkaline-reacting diet then is most important. Less sugars, less starch; fish, fowl, or lamb, but no red meats. Little coffee or tea—rather Ovaltine or cocoa for most individuals. Whole wheat bread is OK but cut out beer especially, and liquors. No fried foods. Condiments or pickles or the like hinder the flow of lymph through the lower portions of the abdominal area; with hemorrhoids, it is in that area that lymph is absent and acidity is highest. Fresh green vegetables help the eliminations, which in turn aid in the assimilation of substances which build and replenish the physical body. In specific questions asked by [257] both raw and canned tomatoes were said to be well for the body.

Olive oil in small amounts was suggested several times as food for the body and helpful to the intestinal tract. Although not in this particular set of readings, it is present elsewhere that garlic is highly beneficial to the intestines.

For better eliminations, colonics were frequently suggested, as well as ordinary enemas. Glyco-Thymoline added to the water was often seen to be beneficial. Eno salts were suggested as alternatives to the colonics. Two selections describe interesting information about this particular laxative:

Q-9. Is it good for the system to soften the stool with a salt which I am now using? Carlsbad Salts?

A-9. The use of the Eno salts would be preferable. Here is the variation: Eno is a vegetable or fruit salts, while Carlsbad is a mineral—and hence [the

Eno is] active more upon the upper portion of the duodenum and through the upper portion of the jejunum in creating a great quantity of the lymph circulation.

And read or study that which we have indicated, as to what takes place with the lymph in the activities of assimilation. The fruit salts would be the better, and occasionally an oil.   257-200

Q-6. What is a good laxative for this body?
A-6. Eno salts is the best laxative for this body, for this is of the fruit nature and not mineral—that would cause disturbance or hardening activities through the conditions in the stomach, as well as through those activities in the liver and the kidneys. This also should be taken in just small doses, almost every day, for periods of a week at a time—and will be most beneficial.   462-13

It would seem that the fruit laxative increases the flow of lymph in the walls of the upper intestines where assimilation takes place; whereas a mineral laxative would make assimilation more difficult through a "hardening" process. Improper assimilation of nutrients affects not only the organs involved but the entire body, and in this instance is a hindrance to the process of overcoming the hemorrhoids.

To correct hemorrhoids in the early stages, simply treat the local condition with an application and follow through with the stretching exercise. But when significant body malfunction has brought about the condition, the underlying causes must also be attended to, or the hemorrhoids will not be resolved.

III. Suggested Therapeutic Regimen
Therapy for hemorrhoids should be directed first at the local condition, then at the underlying causes. A simplified program of therapy is the procedure Cayce followed most often, with many variations, of course. The following regimen might be termed a basic approach, with deviations made according to the needs of the particular individual, and in line with the material already presented in the earlier part of this commentary.

Local Treatment
1. Use Tim (preferably) or Pazo or a similar substance after each bowel movement. It can be used directly on the hemorrhoid or

injected with a bulb syringe into the anal orifice, or both. When used with bulb syringe, one to two teaspoonfuls may be inserted into the area above the sphincters. Preparations other than Tim are now available with applicators for use internally. This should be used consistently, then, until the hemorrhoid is gone and the body returned to normal.

2. For acute, very painful, hemorrhoids, ice can be applied directly; or cold, then hot, sitz baths; or castor oil packs directly to the hemorrhoid.

3. The glycerin-carbolic acid-Nujol mixture is helpful in preventing scar tissue and in alleviating irritation, so is very useful for rectal bleeding; this best used once a week until all signs of bleeding or irritation have disappeared.

4. The exercise—stretching on tiptoe and bending forward—should be done in every case of hemorrhoids five or six times, very slowly, morning and evening, and should be continued until all evidence of this trouble can no longer be found, and until the causative factors have at least been addressed.

General Care

1. Diet. An alkaline-reacting diet, including green vegetables, fruits, vegetable and fruit juices, fish, fowl and lamb. Avoid too much starch, fats, fried foods, pork and beef, spices and condiments, beer and liquor. These are the basic rules. Studying diet books helps to develop a new way of eating and thinking about foods.

2. Manipulative treatments by osteopath or chiropractor—with special attention to the lumbo-sacral-coccygeal area. The rest of the spine may also need attention—this to be according to the need of the specific body and the capabilities of the physician. Abnormal relationships between the cerebrospinal and the autonomic nervous system need to be corrected.

3. Correction of constipation, either through colonics, given regularly, by having manipulations, or by using laxatives, such as Eno salts, which were mentioned specifically in these readings. It has been my experience also that several drops of castor oil on the tongue at bedtime provides for better regularity of the bowels.

4. Packs across the low back—hot Epsom salts or hot castor oil—used either at home or prior to manipulative treatments would be helpful as long as the hemorrhoids persist. They—as well as the diet, the manipulations and the rest—aid in correcting the high acidity and

lack of normalcy in the rectal area. Soaking a flannel pack in a strong solution of Epsom salts (two cups to a quart of water) or castor oil; then applying hot over the lumbo-sacral area. Then, placing plastic over the pack and a heating pad over that will continue the heat for the next hour or hour and a half. These packs can be applied twice a week, if used at home.

5. A general exercise program should be adopted (walking is the best, according to the readings), and then continued as a regular part of one's life.

6. Stresses are usually the result of one's rebellion against what one has chosen to meet in this lifetime. Thus rebellion is really against oneself. There are many ways to work at the level of the mind and the emotions. Cayce always suggested the fruits of the spirit in one's life as a way of facing oneself: gentleness, kindness, forgiveness, long-suffering, understanding and the like. Study Group work (Search for God Groups) is one way of strengthening one's approach in this manner. Ideals must be set at some point in life, and this is always a choice. The mind builds either obstructions or a way of success: and it is ours to choose.

Perhaps the best way to end a commentary on a problem so close to the manner in which we eliminate the drosses in our bodily life is to quote Edgar Cayce's spiritual injunctions to two of these people who suffered from hemorrhoids:

Q-12. Any other advice?
A-12. Keep the mental and spiritual attitudes in constructive ways of thought; for, the mind is the builder.   462-13

Keep the purpose right—creative ever; judging no one, but keeping self in that attunement to Creative Forces.   2823-2

William A. McGarey, M.D.

Edgar Cayce readings referenced:

91-1, 2, 3	288-46, 47, 53
98-1, 2	294-24
106-1, 2, 11, 12, 13, 14	304-20
109-2	325-50
137-50	327-4
147-34 through 37	337-23
257-172, 184, 193, 197, 198, 199, 200	404-7, 8

408-3
416-14, 16, 18
457-9, 14
460-6
462-13 through 17
480-45
540-2
555-6 through 11
563-4, 5
573-7
636-10
654-3 through 7
678-2
761-1
935-2
953-9
954-3
984-2
1102-6
1223-7, 8
1230-1
1278-1
1334-1
1540-1
1665-1
1713-22, 23

1800-20
2056-3
2130-1
2157-2
2280-1
2323-2
2457-6
2701-1
2711-2
2811-1
3039-1
3190-4
3356-2
3489-1
3678-1
3754-1
3818-6
3896-1
4202-1
4709-5
4769-3
5060-1
5087-1
5226-1
5327-1
5609-1

HERPES ZOSTER

I. Physiological Considerations

Shingles (herpes zoster) and chicken pox (varicella) are caused by the same infectious agent, a virus. In shingles the virus attacks the spinal or cranial nerves and has a characteristic distribution (unilateral) reflecting the segments innervated by the involved nerves.

The thoracic section is most commonly involved, followed by the cervical, lumbar, sacral and the ophthalmic division of the trigeminal nerve (i.e., the fifth cranial nerve).

In young, otherwise healthy individuals the skin lesions go through the various stages and heal within two to three weeks, though pain may persist another week or two. In the majority of people over 60 years of age, the illness is usually more protracted, the pain lasting two to three months after the lesions have healed.

According to the readings given on this condition, poor eliminations are invariably at the root of the problem, this being initiated by a variety of mechanisms. Thus in reading 106-4, hyperacidity "is produced by the overtaxation of the body with those properties that create an unbalance [imbalance] in the hydrochloric portion of the system. . ." which in turn affects the circulation (capillaries, emunctories or lymphatics), the gastrointestinal tract, the kidneys, liver, etc., with resulting poor eliminations. Irritation is set up in the skin which leads to the rash (the virus presumably is able to set in and cause problems under these conditions).

Other causes of poor eliminations cited in these readings were:
1. Poor diet (527-3),
2. Respiratory flu causing congestion in the colon (338-9),
3. General debilitation (1944-1),
4. Spinal lesions (3139-1),
5. Malfunction in the hepatic circulation (322-4).

Nowhere in these readings was specific mention made of a primary infectious etiology for herpes zoster, so it would seem that the basic pathology is disturbed eliminations through a variety of mechanisms which set up toxic irritants in the capillary-lymphatic circulation, thus laying the foundation for the eruption of skin lesions.

The readings make no mention of invasion of the nerves and skin by the virus, so at what point this occurs is left at present to speculation.

II. Rationale of Therapy

This would have to be directed toward enhancing eliminations through proper diet (which is alkaline reacting); laxatives and colonic irrigation; and alleviating pain through local applications.

III. Suggested Therapeutic Regimen

1. *Local therapy* for alleviating pain:

   a. Ice packs over lesions or hot packs with soda salt, whichever provides more relief.

   b. Oil of sassafras, 1 dram

   Tincture of laudanum, ½ ounce

   Spirits of camphor, 1 ounce

   Glycerine, 1 ounce

   Distilled water, 6 ounces

   Shake well and dab with cotton to affected areas twice daily. Follow this immediately by dusting with a combination of balsam of Peru, dusting powder of stearate of zinc, and chalk.

2. *Diet:* An alkaline, easily digestible diet should be followed, keeping away from all acid-producing food during this period. Examples: all fruits except apples, citrus fruit juices, cooked vegetables and their juices, vitamin B_1 in addition to vitamins from food sources. Avoid sweets, alcohol, meat of any nature. Avoid citrus-cereal combinations.

3. *Eliminations:*

   a. To stimulate circulation and blood purification, gold chloride, 10 grains in 20 ounces of distilled water, at five drops daily. (106-5)

   For a resistant condition:

   Extract of cascara sagrada, ½ ounce

   Syrup of rhubarb, 2 ounces

   Podophyllum, ½ grain

   Simple syrup, 2 ounces

Shake well before use. Take one teaspoon every three hours until good bowel movement ensues, then take enough to maintain movement twice daily (322-5); or Rochelle salts alone, or a combination of Epsom salts, cream of tartar and sulphur in equal amounts thoroughly mixed. (Note: Avoid getting the feet wet while using this, as this makes the system more susceptible to colds.) One-half teaspoon two to three times daily until eliminations begin. (322-4)

b. Watermelon seed tea to stimulate eliminations through kidney lymphatics: one-half ounce tea to 20 ounces water steeped or simmered for five minutes, strain and use as beverage (106-4); or sweet spirits of nitre, three to five drops two to three times daily to improve eliminations through kidneys and bladder. (322-4)

c. Colonics (irrigation) as frequently as necessary to eliminate mucus from the stools, otherwise once or twice weekly for several weeks (two to four weeks).

4. *Other:*

a. Manipulations, generally the dorsal and cervical spine, sometimes coordinating with the lumbar; from two to six adjustments over several weeks.

Massages once or twice a week for three to four weeks. A combination of peanut oil and witch hazel in equal parts might be used.

b. The wet cell used in a manner similar to the radio-active appliance was recommended in one case (1994-1) in which there was general debilitation.

Directions: Connect leads in a diagonal fashion to the limbs as with the impedance device (i.e., positive lead to right wrist and negative lead to left ankle) and alternate with the other two limbs; i.e., one does not need to make a complete cycle going from one limb to the next. No solutions need be connected with the cell. However, the feet should be immersed in a small quantity of water at body temperature in a glass container and the hands in a weak solution of copper sulphate (1 dram to 1 pint of water), also in a glass container. The duration of treatment should be 20-25 minutes on a daily basis.

If used with the other therapies Cayce suggested for this particular case, the lesions could heal within 10 days.

c. The head and neck exercise is helpful in improving circulation to the head area when a cranial nerve is involved.

Finally Cayce had this to say to [338] who asked for spiritual advice:

Much has been given this body as respecting the mental and spiritual attitude, and that the attitude is reflected more in that in which the individual entity meets its problems with itself as well as with others. If there are the worries and aggravations, these worries and aggravations will reflect in the functioning of the organs of the central nerve and blood supply as well as in the sympathetic. Then know in whom ye believe and know He is able to keep that ye may commit unto Him against any experience.   338-9

Hezekiah Chinwah, M.D.

Edgar Cayce readings referenced:
106-4
322-4
338-9
527-3
1944-1
3139-1
3185-1

HYDROCEPHALUS

I. Physiological Considerations

The physiology of the development of hydrocephalus in the human being is considerably different in the Cayce readings from that concept held rather consistently today in the field of medicine. In the readings, there is seen an incoordination between the patches of emunctory or lymphatic tissue which act as the centers of coordination between the cerebrospinal and the autonomic nervous systems. The patches are located in the sympathetic ganglia, the dorsal root ganglia, or the spinal cord. The larger patches, which have the most significant roles in this function, are found in the coccygeal area; in the sixth, seventh and ninth dorsal areas; and in the cervical first, second and third.

Lack of coordination of this particular type apparently produces an excess of lymph fluid from impulses in the coccygeal area of the spinal cord. Cayce saw a congenital type of defect which might be described as a lack of a closure of certain parts of the nervous system in the coccygeal area, where he said the trouble with hydrocephalus arises. Then through these openings there are tendencies for the nerve impulse to seep in at the end of the spine. This then stimulates the incoordination in the lymphatic flow which brings about the excesses.

While this certainly is not entirely clear, this same picture is repeated in reading after reading and is perhaps best exemplified by the following extract:

Q-1. What caused her present condition originally?

A-1. Lack of closing of those ends when, in and through the period of gestation, that termed a tail drops off. . .the body. 3562-1

This reading was given for a five-year-old girl who, at the time of the reading, was able to talk and was intelligent but was unable to walk because of the size of her head.

Cayce does not mention anywhere obstruction as being an etiologic factor. He does mention in 3208-1 a karmic factor. This boy—17 years old—had cerebral palsy and hydrocephalus. Here it was implied that the illness would be more difficult to correct because of its karmic nature.

Assimilation of certain substances must be proper; and we would assume that the assimilation through the Peyer's patches principally has in some manner a relationship with the health and welfare of the lymphatic patches found in the nervous system itself. In the readings reviewed for this commentary, only one, 727-1, specified therapy which would be aimed specifically at the areas of assimilation.

There apparently is a relationship between the amount of lymphatic fluid produced through the incoordination described and the recommended use of atropine in the area near the coccyx, which Cayce described as often being "open" to the aberrant and trouble-making nerve impulses. There are apparently certain stages at which the atropine effect restores a balance in the production of lymph fluid.

Also interesting is the nature of change that comes about in this condition as therapy progresses. Apparently Cayce saw lack of actual nerve filaments in certain areas, which produce an inability for proper communication between the two major nervous systems already mentioned. As therapy progressed, then, he saw a gradual production of new nerve tissue where none existed before. If such a concept is tenable, then it is understandable why therapy designed to bring about the changes he suggests are needed must be continued over a long period of time. Nerve tissue does not grow rapidly. The following is a quotation which suggests just this particular concept.

While there is not outwardly a great deal of change, there is, in those centers indicated, the causing of better coordination between the sympathetic and cerebrospinal system and much better reaction. There are "feelers out" in the emunctory activity and the patches in the lymph activity, which causes and will produce the connections causing the action through the sensory system to be improved.   **3208-2**

II. Rationale of Therapy

In approaching therapy, we should remember that the body has a capability of *normal* function:

Thus, we would administer those activities which would bring a normal reaction through these portions, stimulating them to an activity from the body itself, rather than the body becoming dependent upon supplies that are robbing portions of the system to produce activity in other portions, or the system receiving elements or chemical reactions being supplied without arousing the activity of the system itself for a more normal condition.

1968-3

From the physiology already discussed, it becomes apparent that therapy should be aimed primarily at reestablishing a balance between the various emunctory patches in the spinal or autonomic areas which provide a relationship between the cerebrospinal and the autonomic nervous systems. When this coordination and the nerve tissue to carry proper impulses are reestablished, then the cerebrospinal fluid will be manufactured in the proper amounts and tissue will begin to establish a normal pattern.

It is questionable whether a head that has already enlarged will return to normal size, but this would probably be dependent upon the degree of calcification and the amount of enlargement that has already occurred.

One child, [3555], was given very little chance to continue his life in this experience, because of a karmic affliction, which would seemingly require very specific care that the parents perhaps were not mentally or emotionally adjusted to pursue and complete.

Thus the prognosis to be considered in any therapeutic program would depend upon many factors, even assuming that nerve tissue can and is being restored and rebuilt, and coordinations are brought back to normal.

In the younger individuals, manipulative therapy such as osteopathy and chiropractic was not advised in those cases reviewed. Osteopathy was suggested for a 17-year-old boy, [3208]. However, in the case of the five-year-old girl already mentioned, it was specifically suggested that osteopathy and chiropractic should not be used but that treatments should be neuropathic (apparently meaning a massage which is designed to affect the nerve endings of the cerebrospinal system and the autonomic—this through massage of those areas lying close to the spine and between the vertebral bodies where the connections would be made with the sympathetic ganglia). The massage thus should be concentrated in certain specific areas or "axes." This would mean probably the lumbo-sacral/coccygeal axis for the parasympathetic outflow; the seventh to ninth dorsal for the areas affecting the adrenals; and the first, second, and third cervicals which apparently have the greatest effect on the cranial parasympathetic outflow. Through the use of these massages or treatments, the nerves or the lymphatic patches are gradually restored so that coordination is improved between the areas which control the nerve relationships.

Atropine should probably be used in a hypodermic injection at the spine where L-5 joins the sacro-coccygeal segments. This should not be injected into the bone or into the spinal canal, but rather hypodermically. The rationale of this is rather difficult to postulate unless it is assumed that most of the activity of the drug occurred in this particular area where Cayce said it would cause a closing of those "ends" and a drying of the lymph which is being produced mainly from impulses in this area.

In summary, treatment should be directed at drying the lymph, bringing the cerebrospinal and autonomic nervous systems into better relationship, and bringing about a coordination of the various axes of the nervous system. Attention should also be given to proper assimilation.

III. Suggested Therapeutic Regimen

For the young hydrocephalic, who is still in the developmental stage, a small dose of atropine injected hypodermically at the junction of L-5 and S-1 should be the first therapy given. In a two-year-old boy who was karmically afflicted and probably did not survive for long, a large 1/60th grain dosage was given. However, in the five-year-old girl the dosage was 1/180th grain. She was larger but apparently the dose should be very small. For a young infant or one much smaller than a five-year-old, the dose should be significantly less than the 1/180th grain.

If the child is too young or restless to stand a long period of massage each day, massage should be centered on one axis one day, then another the next. Or else the entire massage three or four times a week might be a better procedure. The neuropathic adjustments or massages do not need to move the segments themselves, but there needs to be the coordinating of those patches of the emunctory flow between the lymphatic, or sympathetic-lymphatic and cerebrospinal system. The adjustments or massages in the last lumbar and in the coccyx segments should be also upon the brush end of the cerebrospinal nerves themselves. "To interpret this perfectly, x-ray the end of the spine—not the head, but where the source is—the last lumbar and the coccyx center." (3562-1)

In case [3208], osteopathic treatments were suggested as the only therapy. Also, diathermy to the lacteal duct area and the solar plexus area was suggested for an eight-year-old boy whose assimilation was improper; the diathermy was needed to break up the troubles in the Peyer's patches.

Thus it is seen that a course of therapy should be adopted which would fit the particular case and would center around an attempt to balance the incoordinations, close up the areas where abnormal impulses may arise, and bring about a regeneration of nerve tissue in the spinal cord or the sympathetic nerve system itself.

It must be reemphasized that patience, persistence, and consistency should be used when applying this therapy. Nerve tissue cannot regenerate quickly and a period of therapy aimed at perhaps two to three years should be anticipated when this is begun.

Do these, as we have indicated. . .Not as rote, but knowing that within self must be found that which may be awakened to the *building* of that necessary for the body, mentally and physically, and spiritually, to carry *its* part in this experience. For the application of any influence must have that which is of the divine awakening of the activative forces in every atom, every cell of a living body.   726-1

William A. McGarey, M.D.

Edgar Cayce readings referenced:
727-1
3208-1, 2
3555-1
3562-1

HYPERTENSION

I. Physiological Considerations

Hypertension is recognized as a common medical problem, the complications of which result in considerable morbidity and early mortality for many of the millions of persons affected in the United States. Apart from the occasional cases secondary to kidney disease, and the rare cases due to endocrine disturbances—such as hyperaldosteronism and pheochromocytoma—the cause of hypertension is not known. It is theorized that there is increased tonus or spasm at the arteriolar level of circulation. Excessive salt intake, nervous tension, and hereditary factors are felt to be involved in the pathogenesis of so-called "essential" hypertension.

II. Rationale of Therapy

In the Cayce readings, hypertension is ascribed in most cases to an "improper equilibrium of the circulation." In 3720-1, for example, a "strain" on the internal capillaries and emunctories (lymphatics?) was said to lead to a plethoric condition in the veins and arteries which, in turn, affects the "nerve forces" regulating the circulation. Excessive relaxation of nerve ganglia appears directly related to the increase in blood pressure. The end result is that the sympathetic and cerebrospinal nerve systems are unable to function in an integrated way to control the circulation. Incoordinations between the cerebrospinal and sensory systems result also; and symptoms are produced including languidness or weakness of the body and sensory disturbances.

A second area of etiology, related to the first, is anatomical lesions of the spinal cord or plexuses, sometimes traumatic in origin. For example, "increased pressure" in the area of the eighth and ninth dorsal vertebrae, a "strain" in the area of sixth and seventh dorsal, or "subluxations" of nerves were involved, leading to lesions of the nerve plexuses and ganglia controlling blood pressure. In one case, trauma to the coccyx area of the spine was said to have impaired the solar plexus, leading to a disturbance of the hepatic circulation, indigestion and derangement of the "blood supplying forces," resulting in hypertension. (5697-1)

In other cases, problems in the gastrointestinal tract were seen as the root causes of hypertension. Difficulties with elimination and "accumulations" in the colon were cited at times, leading to an "overquantity of blood." Malfunction of the Peyer's patches was said in several cases to lead to impairment of the hepatic circulation, with absorption of toxins into the system and adverse effects on the hypogastric and second cardiac plexuses. In several instances the impaired hepatic circulation was said to affect the kidneys, leading to overfullness of the capillary circulation.

In several cases the etiology of hypertension was found in the circulatory system itself, as in 3923-1, where there was an "overabundance of blood," but the system was "lacking those constituents needed to bring equilibrium." At other times an "overcharge of blood forces" or increase in blood supply or cells was claimed. In other cases hypertension existed because the blood was "slower in returning to the heart" than in going from the heart to the tissues (i.e., the venous part of the circulation was at fault).

Emotional factors were emphasized in 4255-1, where repression of anger and resentment were said to have affected the spleen, leading to hypertension.

III. Suggested Therapeutic Regimen

In general the therapies outlined for hypertension were intended "to produce perfect equilibrium" (3720-1) or to promote "equalization of the circulation" and "stability of the nerve forces" (3923-1). The readings emphasized the importance of patience, persistence, and faith in carrying out the treatments. In one case in which the mental attitude was said to have an important role in the condition, the patient was advised to "know first in what ye believe."

Diet was emphasized repeatedly; and patients were urged to avoid starch, sugar, spices, fats, pork, alcohol, caffein and carbonated drinks, and to increase their intake of bulbous vegetables, vegetable protein, and water. They were also advised never to eat when "wrought up or overtaken."

The wet cell battery appliance was recommended on several occasions, with the negative lead to the umbilicus and the positive to the ankle 30 minutes each evening for a total of 60 hours.

An interesting regimen was recommended to several patients. They were told to get out of bed as soon as awake; eat half of a lemon; take a long walk; eat the other half of a lemon with a pinch of salt; drink as much water as possible; then lie down until completely relaxed before breakfast. (4999-2)

Several types of tonic were recommended, including Calcidin (iodine-containing), and Kaldak (vitamin B-complex with iron). Also:

> Salt, three grains in 1 ounce water
> Peppermint, two drops
> Wintergreen, two drops

Take in the morning for three to five days. (4836-1)

To produce better eliminations through the kidneys, add to one gallon of water:

> Sarsaparilla root, 2 ounces
> Wild cherry bark, 2 ounces
> Burdock root, 2 ounces
> Mandrake root, 10 grains
> Beech leaves, 20 grains

Simmer till reduced to one quart, then add six ounces grain alcohol with two drams balsam of tolu. Take one teaspoon after each meal and at bedtime. (4288-1)

Another tonic was advised for one patient: Add simple syrup to the following to make 10 ounces:

> Tincture of valerian, 2 ounces
> Elixir of calisaya, 2 ounces
> Elixir of celerena, 2 ounces
> Potassium iodide, 3 grains
> Potassium bromide, 15 grains
> Elixir of capsici, 2 drops

The dose was one teaspoon once every three days. (5723-1)

Colonics were recommended several times, alternating with osteopathic adjustments. For those with spinal problems, osteopathic or chiropractic adjustments were advised, as well as vibrator massage (followed by peanut oil rub) or heat rays to the spine (in one case).

In cases involving the kidneys, a turpentine pack (10 drops to a pan of hot water) was to be applied to the kidney areas for 30-40 minutes, followed by Glyco-Thymoline packs to the same area. (5180-1)

An exercise was recommended to one patient, consisting of a circular motion of the upper half of the body with hands on hips. (3941-1)

Brian M. Boni, M.D.

Edgar Cayce readings referenced:

294-12	4345-1, 2	5180-1
3720-1	4836-1	5224-1
3923-1	4990-1	5697-1
3941-1	4999-2	5723-1
4255-1		
4288-1		

HYPOGLYCEMIA

I. *Physiological Considerations*

Hypoglycemia has been called the stepchild of modern medicine, for it is seldom indeed that a diagnosis of hypoglycemia is made or given any credence or importance by the modern physician. There are always exceptions, of course, and the doctors who do understand have continued to work toward acceptance of this condition as a significant illness in and of itself.

By use of a five-hour glucose tolerance test, which has been standardized for many years, a curve is developed on a graph. The curve indicates changes from the normal when hypoglycemia is present. This change concerns a lowering of the blood sugar level below the fasting state and may be demonstrated at any point after the 100 grams of glucose are taken by mouth. (Sample hypoglycemia curves are included in this commentary.)

Hypoglycemia merely means a lowering *(hypo)* of the sugar *(glyc*ose) in the bloodstream *(-emia)*. The opposite of this condition is *hyper*glycemia, more commonly known as diabetes mellitus. The two are closely related; it has been generally accepted among researchers in the realm of endocrinology that both the intestinal mucosa and the pancreas are related to at least the elevated blood sugar—and possibly the hypoglycemia as well. Many glucose tolerance curves show both conditions.

It is also well known that diabetes mellitus can have hypoglycemia as its precursor, thus giving more credence to the concept that the same portion of the body's functioning mechanisms may be involved in both conditions.

The adrenal glands seem to be abnormally functioning in many, if not most hypoglycemia conditions. The frequency is such that the Hypoglycemia Foundation several years ago prepared a booklet for physicians, entitled "Hypoadrenocorticism: An Endocrinologic Approach to the Etiology and Treatment of Functional Hypoglycemia." It is theorized that the adrenal cortex is substandard in its functioning and this lowers the blood sugar. It is well known, for instance, that in emergencies the adrenal cortex releases cortisone into the bloodstream, which in turn brings about a physiological rise in blood sugar to allow the body to meet the emergency by fighting or fleeing. Stresses which are not met in one of these two manners undoubtedly brings about disturbance to the entire body, including the adrenals, for the hormones are not used appropriately nor is the blood sugar. And, of course, stimulation of the nervous system and the alteration of the blood supply from the deep to the superficial circulation is only intended for the emergency, so failure to act creates internal discord.

Probably most of the hypoglycemia states are brought about through improper diet. These are called reactional or functional hypoglycemics. There are some individuals who have familial hypoglycemia, passed on as an hereditary tendency.

Much has been written in the popular literature and in medical journals over the years since hypoglycemia was identified as a syndrome and given its name in 1924 by Seale Harris, M.D., in the *Journal of the American Medical Association*. All factors involved in its etiology are certainly not yet known. This creates a difficulty, for most physicians feel uneasy when they cannot pin down the etiology in a disease process. Why hypoglycemia remains so unaccepted by the medical profession remains, however, a real mystery, for it is undisputed as far as the symptoms and the blood sugar findings are concerned. Also hypoglycemia is part of the picture of many other conditions of illness of the human body. So it behooves us to recognize what it is and what to do about it.

II. Edgar Cayce Readings on Hypoglycemia

Very little is given in the readings on what we call hypoglycemia. This may be simply because the condition was not readily recognized during the first half of this century, when the readings were given. Or perhaps those who had been diagnosed as having hypoglycemia did not seek out a reading. One 23-year-old man was having trouble calcifying the fracture site of a recent broken bone. (440-2) He was anemic and considerably underweight. There is not sufficient information to determine which of these conditions was basic and whether or not he actually had hypoglycemia. The second case indexed under hypoglycemia was for a 50-year-old woman who had been diagnosed at the Cleveland Clinic and was given a diet to follow. (3252-1) She was beset with fears and doubts, apparently, and was low on vitality; but it was simply suggested that she be given vitamin B_1 by mouth, follow the diet already prescribed, and to get lots of activity in the open air.

Throughout the Cayce material, however, there are suggestions for restoring the body back to a normal balance, as well as discussions relative to the manner in which the body becomes disturbed in its functioning.

From our experience working with these readings, it seems logical to conclude that hypoglycemia certainly has endocrine origins, and thus deeper causation in the attitudes and emotions of the individual affected. The adrenal, the thyroid, and certainly the pancreas and the small intestine—especially the duodenum—all are part of the picture.

The nerve supply to these organs comes from the spinal segments and the ganglia associated with those segments and from the celiac (solar) plexus which is closely related to the adrenal gland. In one reading, 3722-1, the 6th, 8th, 9th and 10th dorsal vertebrae were in need of specific manipulations or adjustments. This was for diabetes mellitus, not hypoglycemia, but the effect was to the pancreas and the duodenum and the spleen. These same organs are probably disturbed in hypoglycemia, also.

So lesions in the spine—osteopathic lesions—are probably a causative factor; the assimilation and elimination are problems; the attitudes need correction; and certainly the diet needs change to one that is constructive. And, of course, the glands need some kind of helpful attention. Rest is important; and the material suggests over and over again that patience, persistence, and consistency are ever part of the healing effort.

It is interesting to note that Cayce nearly always wove into the suggested physical applications a spiritual note—the Oneness of all things; the nature of the human being as body, mind and spirit; the importance of spending some time regularly in meditation; and the tremendous importance of the mind as the builder.

Thus it is mandatory, if we are going to be holistic in our approach, to look at this condition of hypoglycemia as an illness of all three aspects of our being and take steps to correct the condition at all three levels. Perhaps it would stimulate our enthusiasm if we looked at the healing of the body as an adventure in consciousness.

III. Suggested Therapeutic Regimen

In designing a therapy program for someone who has developed symptoms of hypoglycemia, a diagnosis must first be made, then the treatment should be individualized for that person. Modern-day medical techniques can be combined with the ideas of the medical heretics who understand that hypoglycemia exists and then the two of them can be merged with the concepts in the Cayce readings—in this way perhaps a more complete healing can take place.

The five-hour glucose tolerance test is a must in order to determine the degree and the nature of the hypoglycemia. It must be understood that any other co-existing condition of illness must also be under treatment of a constructive nature.

There are several steps in a therapy program that would probably be helpful for every person who has developed hypoglycemia:

1. A strict diet should be started. Basically, such a diet should include fish, fowl, and lamb for protein; lots of leafy green vegetables; plenty of fruit, fresh and cooked; salads; but no fried foods, no white flour or white sugar, no coffee or alcohol, no tranqulizers and no soft drinks containing caffeine. It is important to include both natural sugar (fruit) and protein as between-meal snacks.

Smoking is detrimental and should also be stopped, unless (as Cayce often remarked) the person is an addict. In that case, Cayce suggested five to six cigarettes a day. There are many aids today to help people stop the smoking habit, however.

2. As an aid to the diet, a soybean-protein-powder-blender mix made with either milk or fruit juice taken at night can often help the hypoglycemia patient sleep better and not have the nightmares that often accompany this condition.

3. Medication: B-complex vitamin once a day. At the A.R.E. Clinic, Inc., we use Adrex S.E.L. (an adrenal extract tablet) once a day, sometimes thyroid tablets, and sometimes Atomidine in a cyclic manner.

4. Osteopathic or chiropractic treatments once a week for a period of six to eight weeks with special attention given to the dorsal 6th, 8th, 9th, and 10th vertebrae. General treatments to the spine would, of course, be added to the specifics.

5. Regular and adequate rest is a must, as is exercise to keep the circulation and the nervous systems active. This is especially so for the sendentary person, who works much with the mind and not so much with the body.

6. Eliminations should be kept up normally with occasional

colonics, if they are available.

7. All of the above should be done with patience, persistence, and consistency. These qualities are spiritual in their activity and are often a requirement for healing to come about.

8. Meditation and regular study and interpretation of dreams are not mentioned in the medical schools, nor will one usually find these even in instructions of the medical heretic. However, the readings are adamant that these two disciplines are part of what every person must some day experience—so that his destiny may be realized.

There are other factors that may be added to a therapy program if it appears necessary. It must be realized that every condition of illness in the human body varies in its degree of severity. Thus the mild case of hypoglycemia will not need the attention and definitive care that the average case will. The severe problem demands even more extensive and painstaking therapeutic measures. Thus, the following treatments may be needed, if the conditions warrant:

1. Clary water was suggested in the Cayce material for diabetes mellitus. Since the two conditions are closely related, this formula may be helpful in hypoglycemia.

To relieve this condition, we would take that in the system that will give the balance of force to the body to create the assimilation and to give the excretory functionings of the emunctory forces their rejuvenating forces for the body, taking this in the system prepared in this manner:

To one gallon of rain water, add eight (8) ounces of clary flower (common garden sage). Reduce by simmering, not boiling, to one quart. Dissolve four (4) ounces of beet sugar in just sufficient hot water to dissolve it, then add, while warm, to other solution. Dissolve fifteen (15) grains of ambergris [currently banned by U.S. and Britain] in one (1) ounce of grain alcohol, add to solution, then add four (4) ounces of grain alcohol and fifty (50) drops or minims of oil of juniper, see, with three (3) drams of balsam of tolu cut with alcohol and added. The dose would be a dessertspoonful three times each day.   **953-1**

2. Extracts of the adrenal, pancreatic, and duodenal tissues are often helpful. (The adrenal has already been mentioned as Adrex S.E.L.)

3. The radio-active appliance described in the Cayce readings is suggested as an aid in helping the body to achieve a better balance. A simplified description of how it might work: When attached, the device picks up the electrical charges flowing through the body which

are in excess in one place and deposits them where they are deficient in another. On the basis of the concept that the human body is an electrical phenomenon, such a concept of action is not unreasonable.

4. As mentioned earlier, those conditions of the body which are not directly related to the hypoglycemia need attention and should be cared for.

We have placed information at the end of this commentary to make the description of the causation and the therapy of hypoglycemia a bit more understandable. It would be well to remember that true healing—as it has been described in the Cayce readings many times—is an event of the whole person and is an awakening of the forces within the body to their divine origin. So it is not something that may just come about for the person's convenience, but instead is a change, an elevation, an awakening of consciousness.

William A. McGarey, M.D.
Edna Germain, R.N., F.N.P.

Edgar Cayce readings referenced:
440-2
834-1
953-1
3252-1
3722-1

Hypoglycemia Diet

Upon arising . . . . . . Medium orange, half a grapefruit or 4 oz. fresh or unsweetened juice.

BREAKFAST . . . . Fruit or unsweetened juice. One egg with or without two slices of crisp bacon. One slice of whole wheat or rye bread or toast with butter. Beverage.

Mid-morning . . . . . Medium size fruit with a glass of milk.

LUNCH . . . . Moderate amount of meat, fish, cheese or fowl. Salad (large serving of leafy green vegetables and tomato) with mayonnaise or oil dressing. One slice of whole wheat or rye bread with butter. Dessert and beverage.

Early afternoon . . . Glass of milk (8 oz.). Cheese or nuts.

Late afternoon . . . . Fresh or unsweetened fruit juice (4 oz.).

DINNER . . . . Soup if desired. Liberal portion of lamb, fish or fowl. Vegetables. One slice of bread if desired. Dessert. Beverage.

2-3 hours after . . . . Glass of milk (8 oz.).

Every 2 hrs. until
  bedtime . . . . Small glass of milk (4 oz.) or handful of nuts or cheese.

ALLOWED:

Vegetables: Asparagus, avocado, beets, broccoli, brussels sprouts, cabbage, cauliflower, carrots, celery, corn, cucumber, eggplant, lima beans, onions, peas, radishes, sauerkraut, string beans, tomatoes, turnips.

Fruits: Apples, apricots, berries, grapefruit, melon, oranges, peaches, pears, pineapple, tangerines. These may be cooked or raw, with or without cream, but without sugar. Canned fruits should be packed in water. *Avoid* dried fruits such as dates, raisins, and apricots because of high sugar content. Large amounts of any fruit may contain too much sugar for you.

Beverages: Weak tea, decaffeinated coffee or substitutes. May be sweetened with saccharin or sucaryl. Juices: Any unsweetened fruit or vegetable juice, except grape or prune juice.

Desserts and miscellaneous: Fruit, unsweetened gelatin, junket (made from tablet, not mix), yogurt. Lettuce, mushrooms or nuts may be taken as freely as desired.

PROHIBITED:

All alcoholic and soft drinks, club soda, ginger ale, Pepsi, beer and wine. Alcoholic beverages usually have a high carbohydrate content. Sugar, candy and other sweets such as cakes, pie, pastries, pudding, ice cream and honey. Regular coffee, strong brewed tea or any other beverage containing caffeine.

TO BE AVOIDED:

Starchy foods—potatoes, rice, bananas, spaghetti, noodles, doughnuts, white bread, etc. Foods high in sugar—grapes, raisins, figs, dates, jams, jellies and plums. Pork—except crisp bacon. Large meals—frequent small meals of a high protein, low carbohydrate diet help maintain your blood sugar at a normal level which eliminates the unpleasant effects of hypoglycemia.

Five Case Histories of Hypoglycemia

Case 1

Lois, a 28-year-old woman with two small children, had been to a chiropractor who did a glucose tolerance test four years before she came to the A.R.E. Clinic. She had been told that she was hypoglycemic and had been given books to read. She decided that the chiropractor was a "health food nut" and abandoned any special diet. After three years of many symptoms—such as extreme fatigue, weakness of arms and legs, slurred speech, stumbling, numbness in arms and legs, slowed reactions (two car accidents during this time), severe anxiety attacks, incoordination, out-of-body experiences, confusion, lightheadedness, vertigo, arthralgia, muscle pain—she went to an internist physician. After many tests, at a tremendous cost, she was told that she was diabetic and to follow the Diabetic Association's diet—which made her feel worse. Disillusioned and confused, she came to the A.R.E. Clinic in October, 1981, after hearing about the Clinic at a Hypoglycemia Association of America meeting. After following the "hypoglycemia" diet planned to help her maintain an even blood sugar level, she felt "fantastic" in only eight days. She had no more nightmares and slept better.

Case 2

Julia, a 31-year-old woman, came to the Clinic two years ago. She had been previously treated elsewhere for depression and had had an acute reaction to some anti-depressant medication. After having a glucose tolerance test and starting on the hypoglycemia diet, she became capable of functioning in a normal fashion, caring for her children without need for tranquilizers.

Case 3

Jake, a seven-year-old boy, had had many nervous and overactive reactions from eating sweets. He had become inattentive at school, where he was becoming a discipline problem. He also experienced bladder control problems. After having a glucose tolerance test at the Clinic and following an individualized hypoglycemic diet, he began to do well in school and stopped having behavior problems. His mother spent a great deal of time explaining to his teacher and school nurse about the necessity of *no sweets* in his diet.

Case 4

Joan, a 40-year-old woman, found that candy, sweets, and especially wine upset her and caused headaches and extreme fatigue. She craved sweets. Her glucose tolerance test disclosed hypoglycemia with pre-diabetic tendencies. She felt much better after following the hypoglycemia diet.

Case 5

Mike, a 33-year-old man, had several symptoms—such as depression, fatigue, headaches and lack of concentration. He came to the Clinic after his wife had been diagnosed as hypoglycemic. After his glucose tolerance test and starting of the diet, he felt better and more energetic. He also lost weight that he needed to lose.

GLUCOSE TOLERANCE CURVE

NAME: _____

DATE: _____

300

275

250   SEVERE
             DIABETES

225

200

175

150

125   MILD
             DIABETES

100

75   NORMAL

50   ALL
            HYPOGLYCEMIC

25

FASTING ½ hr. 1 hr.   2 hrs.   3 hrs.   4 hrs.   5 hrs.   6 hrs.

INDIGESTION AND GASTRITIS

I. Physiological Considerations

Indigestion and gastritis are not entirely synonymous terms, but for practical reasons might be used together. The disturbance in the stomach and generally the upper portion of the intestinal tract falls short of that clinical condition known as peptic or duodenal ulcer but seems to be the precursor in many cases.

The physiological progression of events, as seen in the readings, seems to be fairly consistent. There is either an "acid" condition developed within the body as a result of infection of a chronic nature (which has its terminal effect on the liver, pancreas, and spleen) or an autonomic nervous system malfunction in the mid-dorsal region—from D4 to D9—which affects the functioning of the liver or directly upsets the normal activity in the stomach when digestion starts. Improper functioning of the liver, pancreas, and spleen in turn creates "used, refused energies" in the circulatory system; and these in turn suppress assimilation of necessary food substances in the lacteal duct area of the small intestine. This is the area of lymphatic tissue which is known as the Peyer's patch area.

With such accumulation of dross, so to speak, the disturbed impulses to the digestive area are magnified in their effect and gastritis and indigestion are a natural result. At this point the stomach refuses to digest food taken into it, there is further irritation of the walls of the stomach and the duodenum; and this by its local effect acts as a disturbance toward normal assimilation in the upper small intestine. Thus the effect is heightened and perpetuated.

Occasionally the condition described in the nervous system was that of a tautness, which would certainly imply a general nervousness of the body or what we know as stress or tension. Some of the complications, and certainly the cycle effect, continuing manifestation of indigestion, would not be present if the toxic and waste products were fully removed from the system. Thus the eliminations as a whole are involved in this lack of full function.

II. Rationale of Therapy

In approaching therapy, we should remember that the body has a capability of *normal* function:

Thus, we would administer those activities which would bring a normal reaction through these portions, stimulating them to an activity from the body itself, rather than the body becoming dependent upon supplies that are robbing portions of the system to produce activity in other portions or the system receiving elements or chemical reactions being supplied without arousing the activity of the system itself for a more normal condition.
1968-3

In view of the mechanisms involved in the production of gastritis or indigestion, it becomes apparent that the first aim in therapy is to neutralize and cleanse the stomach. This would effect a better possibility of adequate assimilation. Then the eliminations should be brought to a more adequate level so that overloading of the circulation could be relieved. It is important to keep the eliminations stimulated to some extent until balance is achieved.

The next aim is to balance the nervous systems, so that impulses which are being sent to the liver, the pancreas, the spleen, and the digestive organs themselves might be corrected and balanced. In this manner the inflammation present might be corrected more easily.

The final step is the restoration of normal assimilation and the rebuilding of those forces within the body which will act as a constructive influence in function.

It is important to be aware of the fact that this condition perpetuates itself through the influence exerted on the assimilation of the body. Thus we find the necessity of continuing therapy in cycles, to build up the entire body and break up the tendencies to continue the cycle of dis-ease.

III. Suggested Therapeutic Regimen

Cleansing of the stomach can be brought about by drinking quantities of pure water. However, Cayce suggested elm water to several people who had considerable irritation and suggested they drink only this as water intake. Elm water is prepared by taking a pinch of the powdered elm, putting it in a cup of water that has had an ice cube added. After allowing it to steep for three minutes, drink it cool. This apparently acts to combat the acidity present. Saffron tea—tea made with yellow or American saffron—was also suggested frequently, to "coat the whole of the stomach proper" just prior to the meal being taken. This should be used prior to each meal and can be made up by taking three teaspoons of saffron, adding it to 16 ounces of water and letting it steep for a half to three quarters of an hour. If an entire meal is made out of raw vegetables, no saffron need be taken beforehand.

A teaspoon of Milk of Magnesia is suggested after each meal. Alka-Seltzer should be used only after two or three doses of Castoria are taken. These measures would cleanse and quiet the condition of the stomach.

To stimulate the eliminations, colonics may be used in a planned series; Castoria or other mild cathartics; or in one case an oil colonic irrigation was suggested to soothe the tissues of the colon.

As the local conditions are being soothed, it becomes necessary to balance the nervous systems by the use of regular manipulations of an osteopathic nature, paying particular attention to the middle dorsal areas.

Assimilation is aided by changing the nature of the diet, tending more toward that of an alkaline-reacting nature. The diet suggested for [5545] is a good example. Beef juice may be taken. (See Appendix.)

Referred to as medicine, beef juice should be taken in most cases a tablespoon a day and it is to be sipped throughout the day.

Should we not attempt to awaken the inner forces to God's presence? "For, all healing comes from the one source. And whether there is the application of foods, exercise, medicine, or even the knife, it is to bring the consciousness of the forces within the body that aid in reproducing themselves—the awareness of creative or God forces." (2696-1)

William A. McGarey, M.D.

Edgar Cayce readings referenced:
18-1	1582-3	4841-2
1089-1	4332-1	5545-1, 2

Dietary Recommendations

Q-4. Should I continue taking Alcaroid? If so, when and how often?
A-4. So long as there's a tendency to belch or feel a fullness after the meal, take same. When this does not occur, leave off.   1710-2

Q-1. Should Alcaroid be continued?
A-1. If necessary. But if there are the applications made as suggested, these should take the place of much of that which has tended to cause the lack of proper assimilation.

If it is necessary, take the Alcaroid when there is feeling of indigestion or of too much greases in the digestive area. But adhere to the suggestions made as to the character of diet, and don't eat things you know you shouldn't eat and then expect to be relieved! 1710-7

We would begin taking internally the anti-acid digestant powder known as Alcaroid, at least two doses four hours apart; half a teaspoonful in two glasses of water at each dose.   558-4

Take an alkalizer, then; and here we will find that Alka-Seltzer will be very well. For the analgesic here will tend to ease the inclination for the spasmodic reaction in the stomach itself. One tablet; this not taken, though, until after at least two or three of the small doses of Castoria have been taken.   341-46

The water that is taken [by this individual in his condition]—most of same should carry those of elm and this should be prepared just before taking, but should *always* be cool, or cold.

Just before the *meals* are taken, [drinking] that of a *mild* tea of saffron should be able to coat the whole of the stomach proper. This will aid digestion. . .
Q-1. What quantity of elm and saffron should be used?
A-1. For each glass of water a pinch between the finger and thumb of the ground elm, stirred well, with a small lump of ice in same; prepared about two to three minutes before it is drunk. Of the saffron—this should be made as a tea, *steeped* as a tea—and *not* too strong. . .when this is taken, it should be preferably warm, and just before the meal, see? So that, that as first taken, in the system—or into the stomach—forms a coating over the whole of same. If these [drinks] are found to produce *distresses* at any time, *not* the *quality* of

the stuff but the *quantity* should be decreased; for these will be effective. . .in *changing* the conditions in the system. Charcoal tablets should be effective also, to reduce the amount of gas.   5545-1

Do give the body yellow saffron tea. This is the regular American saffron. Put a pinch between three fingers into a crock and pour a pint of boiling water over same. Let this steep as tea. Give the baby at least a teaspoonful of this two to three times each day. Make fresh every day.   2876-1

As for the properties to be taken, not a great deal of what would be called. . .medicinal properties; but have such as these:

To 3 drams of yellow saffron add about 16 ounces of water. Let this steep as tea for half to three-quarters of an hour; not boiling but just steeping, see? Use this as a drink three times each day. Take a *glassful* of it in the mornings before any meal is eaten, and before the evening meal (for we would have the raw vegetables in the middle of the day), and at night before retiring.   633-1

KIDNEY STONES

Kidney stones are termed *renal calculi* in medical language. When a stone passes down the ureter from the kidney to the bladder, the pain produced is perhaps the most severe of all pains man experiences in bodily illnesses.

When the stones remain in the pelvis of the kidney, however, there is often little or no pain. The problem facing the individual who has a kidney stone is either to leave it alone or to remove it by dissolution or surgery of one type or another.

In considering the cause and the treatment of these calculi found so frequently in the urinary tract, one should always look at the disease syndrome as a physiological process rather than as a static condition of a stone in place. For there are causative factors which gradually distort the physiology of the body in such a manner that over a long period of time a stone is formed, bit by bit—often without sign or symptom. When the condition is discovered, the aberrant functioning is finally recognized and must be either treated or left alone. There is always a choice.

Three stages of kidney stone pathology may be roughly defined: (1) tendencies toward calculi in the urinary tract—a condition wherein normal eliminations are breaking down (the trouble has its inception in the kidneys); (2) the acute or semi-acute stage, in which stones have formed and are in the process of passing or causing chronic trouble; and (3) the body has come to a relative balance and manages to maintain a homeostasis in spite of one or more stones in the kidney's pelvis. In this kind of a problem the stone may deteriorate at any point and cause acute pain and difficulty as it starts to pass down the ureter. On the other hand, some individuals live out their lives with a stone in place and may never be bothered by any discernible trouble.

The traditional course of events is to ease the pain, soothe the mucous membranes of the urinary tract, and either let the stone pass or remove it surgically. Sometimes, it is the better part of judgment to let it merely remain in the pelvis of the kidney if it is not causing a problem.

In the Cayce material, the viewpoint is taken that there is always a cause, and the correction of the condition involves restoration of a more normal physiology. Surgery is sometimes needed, but when undertaken inadvisedly can frequently cause more harm than benefit. The incoordinations, subluxations, destructive attitudes, and accumulations from inadequate eliminations must always be attended to and corrected if possible. And this job sometimes becomes more tedious than many sufferers are willing to undertake with enough persistence to be successful. However, this is the story that comes out of the Edgar Cayce readings given for those who were experiencing one degree or another of urinary calculus.

I. Physiological Considerations

The onset of symptoms from a kidney stone announces that a process has been going on for a long time during which sufficient precipitated or sedimented material has accumulated to form what we call a stone (although not the best name for it). The stone can be composed of a number of materials found in the body's bloodstream. However, the liquid excreted by the kidney as it performs its eliminatory function may be saturated to such a degree that portions are no longer in solution, and the crystallization process or sedimentary process begins. The length of time it takes to form a stone that would cause symptoms is really unknown; it probably differs with individuals and circumstances. But it most certainly takes weeks, months, or sometimes even years.

How does such a condition begin? Obviously, there are more substances to be eliminated by the kidney than is possible under existing conditions. Cayce describes the condition of the blood as having "refuse forces accumulated by the activity from the lack of distributing forces in the system." (843-7) Or said another way, "the toxic forces that are being carried in the system without proper eliminations through their proper channels" are among the causative factors. (1060-1)

But it is not simply the overflow of toxins in the bloodstream. From the standpoint of physiology as seen in the readings, circulation to the liver and kidney is impaired, thus causing a decrease and an incoordination in the eliminatory process. Because of the stresses on the kidneys themselves, accumulations begin. But this is still an intermediary step. The actual beginning of the problem is more basic.

In many of the readings, no specific reference was made to the causes of impaired elimination—although trouble in the alimentary process was always present. In other references, however, an injury to the spine, a fall, a blow—often forgotten—produced faulty neurological impulses to the liver and kidney (often also to the spleen, pancreas, and intestinal tract), which in turn brought on incoordination and disturbed functions. (141-1, 370-4, 1055-1) In one instance, lack of proper care of the kidneys and eliminations during pregnancy and following delivery brought on the stone six months later. Subluxations were causative in another instance.

In the physical readings, past lives are seldom mentioned, but in the life readings the Cayce source often stated that there are no accidents. So these so-called accidents to the spine might be viewed as karmic responses to past-life experiences and represent the other major etiological factor—destructive attitudes. In one instance, the kidney stone recurred. (843-7) Cayce suggested that the repeat performance came from mental attitudes of fears, oversensitivity, and anger, and from nonadherence to diets. The kidney, liver, gall bladder, pancreas, upper intestinal tract, and spleen are all under the influence of the adrenal glands (called in the endocrinology texts the "fight-flight glands"). These organs normally respond to any emotions or attitudes that activate the sympathetic nervous system through the adrenals or the hormones that arise in those glands.

We see, then, that the supersaturated conditions existing in the kidney excretions, the incoordinations between the liver and the kidneys, the toxins accumulated in the bloodstream, and even the injuries which might bring about some of the problems may all have as an underlying essence, as a primary cause, the attitudes and emotions that cause destruction in the body.

Remember that the attitude of the body—towards circumstances, towards individuals, towards conditions—ever has much to do with creating an environment for disturbing or for helpful things as related to the bodily functions. . .

Know that there are ever those experiences to be met in the experience of each soul, that must be met. Meet these, not in anger, not in wrath but in

gentleness and the fruits of the spirit; not in swearing vengeance or any of those attitudes.   **370-5**

II. Rationale of Therapy

Throughout the Cayce readings, repeated references are made to the importance of persistent follow-through in therapeutic measures. In this particular problem, the theme is the same. For a 53-year-old man, [370], with passage of a stone and a deteriorating physical condition, Cayce saw the possibility of building the body back to normal, "if there is the persistence and consistence in the activities, the application and the attitudes of the body towards a *constructive* influence throughout its bodily functioning itself, as well as its applications to those things that may make for helpful influences." (370-4)

In cases in which the problem is quite complicated physiologically or the physical condition can easily turn into a critical situation, then *all* of Cayce's suggestions must be followed—these were the instructions. To [1054], a 37-year-old woman who had a calculus, it was pointed out that the problem could be eliminated; but, he warned her, unless they are "done *consistently* and *persistently,* for a sufficient period to insure that the causes in the first, and the effects that have already been produced, have been rejuvenated and resuscitated for their normal activity, then don't begin them!" (1054-1) And another, a 53-year-old man, [1060], was told he would run into extreme measures of therapy [surgery?] "unless all are done. . ." But, he added, if those suggestions would be done cooperatively and in a way that would aid the body to produce helpful influences, "resuscitating forces, revivifying energies, may be brought about in the body." (1060-1)

In applying these suggestions to individuals today, it must be kept in mind that every person is different. No two readings contain exactly the same directions. Thus with mild, severe or asymptomatic renal calculi, a given course of therapy—including consideration of attitudinal changes—must be followed with patience and persistence. It is always a process of aiding the body in altering its functioning physiology in such a manner that balance is maintained and constructive influences are always kept. And it is well to remember that healing the body physical without giving it hope in the spiritual is to save a body for destruction in materiality.

Therapies for Renal Calculus

In the readings studied, including all those currently indexed under kidney stones, the following suggestions were identified as being helpful:

1. *Turpentine stupes:* These were prepared in different strengths. For [843], ½ pint of spirits of turpentine was added to one to one-and-a-half quarts of hot water. Heavy flannel, five to six thicknesses, was dipped in the solution and applied over the bladder and pubic area, "so that there may be the relaxation of the urethra and the penetrating forces of the turpentine to alleviate." (843-4) Cayce gave some interesting information to this man: ". . .we find that the application of the turpentine stupes over the area as indicated would offer a means for causing a disintegrating of the stone sufficient for its passage without operative forces; because of the very nature of the penetrating influences of the turp." (843-5)

For a 35-year-old woman, [540], a milder solution was suggested: two ounces of turpentine to a quart of water. The pack was to be placed over the kidney area, and a massage done afterward to the abdomen with a mixture of equal parts of mutton tallow, spirits of turpentine, and spirits of camphor.

And in reading 1472-16, an even more dilute solution of spirits of turpentine was suggested—one teaspoonful to a gallon of water, heated to 90 degrees. The flannel cloth dipped in this solution was to be applied for an hour across the kidney area twice a week, followed immediately by massage with a solution of peanut oil (one ounce), olive oil (one ounce), and melted lanolin (one-half teaspoon).

2. *Osteopathic manipulations* were suggested frequently. Most often those areas of the spine below the shoulder blades and down into the lumbar and coccygeal vertebrae were designated as needing most attention, but the upper dorsal and the cervical were frequently mentioned. Treatments were to be given sensitively, deeply for some and very gently for others, depending on their need and, of course, their physical condition.

3. *Massage* has already been mentioned. Various combinations of oils have been suggested. In 843-6, for instance, Cayce suggested a combination made up of equal parts of olive oil, tincture of myrrh and compound tincture of benzoin, this to be massaged across the lower back from the kidney area to the sacrum. Instructions were to heat the olive oil, then add the other two constituents. The massage was to

prevent "the body from tiring so" and to relax the patient. Another common massage formula is equal parts of mutton tallow, spirits of turpentine, spirits of camphor and compound tincture of benzoin.

4. *Diet* is a factor in all instances. Only foods that are easily assimilated should be eaten. If foods are taken at all, cooked vegetables and cooked fruits could be eaten when the problem is acute. As a general maintenance diet one should eat one meal consisting of only fresh raw vegetables or fruit, a simple breakfast (avoid combining citrus and cereal at the same meal), and a dinner of principally vegetables. Baked potato peel is very good; pears or grapes are perhaps the best fruit. When able, such patients may eat fish, fowl or lamb as protein. It must be kept in mind that the diet should always be such as not to add more to the body than the body can tolerate and use adequately. This means no alcohol, pastries, or desserts; avoid sugars and to a great extent starches. Cayce reminded one person that chewing food well would activate the salivary glands to supply the "lactics—or the alkalines—as they enter the system." (1060-2)

5. *Mullein stupes and mullein tea* were both recommended, but infrequently.

6. *Watermelon seed tea* (made like any herb tea) has been found in the readings to be beneficial in all kidney conditions, so it is not surprising to find it mentioned where stones have been formed. It was not a frequently recommended suggestion, however.

7. *Colonics and enemas* are suggested, for both these procedures increase the elimination of toxins from the bloodstream, giving relief to the kidneys in their attempts to return to normal conditions.

8. *The wet cell battery,* radio-active appliance, and diathermy were all suggested to at least one of these individuals for whom readings were given, but it cannot be determined for certain that they were specifically for relief of the kidney condition. In one instance, reference was made to "vibrations" which would help to disintegrate the stone, and we might assume that that *was* meant to refer to the wet cell battery.

9. *A prescription of oils* to be taken orally was suggested for a man with nephritis and a kidney stone. To stimulate the dissolving of the "sediments" and to bring about better eliminations through the liver and kidneys, the following (in reading 149-1) was suggested to be taken in a capsule once daily, along with osteopathic treatments:

      Eucalyptol, 1 minim
      Rectified oil of turpentine, ½ minim
      Oil of juniper, 1 minim

    10. *A pack of baking soda,* saturated in hot water and applied over the bladder area, was suggested in one case (149-1) to ease stresses in the bladder and urethra.

    11. *Castor oil packs* were recommended to aid elimination of toxic forces that had gradually built up destructive influences in the body. Laxatives for [1060] at that time were not good; rather he needed something that would not only aid eliminations but also build up vitality and resistance within the body. It was suggested that the packs be used for three-and-a-half to four hours, changed every 20 to 30 minutes, using two to three to four thicknesses of heavy flannel. They were to be applied as hot as could be endured and gentle osteopathic manipulations were to be done during the period when the packs were being used. Two days later, another reading was taken on the man, who had by then greatly improved (he had gall bladder gravel as well as kidney stones). Cayce's psychic report was that the sedimentary conditions in the gall bladder and the hardening in the kidneys "have in a manner been dissolved by the use of the oil packs and the manipulations that have aided same to be *expelled* from the body itself." The one session with the packs was all that was needed. After that, colonics and enemas provided cleansing for the intestinal tract.

    12. For a teen-ager (427-2) who was diagnosed as having stones, or "sediments" in the kidneys as Cayce called it, a prescription was given to be taken "every second day" in the morning before breakfast:

      Phosphate of soda, ½ teaspoon
      Syrup of sarsaparilla, 2 minims
      Oil of juniper, 1 minim

And, every fifth day, one minim of sweet spirits of nitre was to be added to the mixture.

    13. *Attitudes* were always directed toward constructive thinking and helpfulness. Anxieties were to be replaced by faith in the knowledge that help is available. The 14th chapter of St. John was recommended at least once in these particular readings, to be read every night before retiring.

    14. For a man of 34 years who was experiencing an acute attack of kidney stones, Cayce suggested (in reading 5580-1) osteopathy and the following herbal remedy: To one gallon of rain water, add

> Sarsaparilla root, 4 ounces
> Wild cherry bark, 2 ounces
> Yellow dock root, 2 ounces
> Calisaya bark, 2 ounces
> Black root, 2 ounces
> Mandrake root, 30 grains
> Buchu leaves, 10 grains

Reduce by simmering to one quart. Strain while warm. Add three drams of balsam of tolu cut in four ounces of grain alcohol. Give two teaspoonfuls four times daily.

15. *Finally, surgery* was occasionally prescribed. For a 56-year-old woman with a large stone, Cayce saw "accumulations in the kidney itself from conditions where incoordination between the circulations of liver and kidneys has caused sediments to form, irritations that, as to size and condition, will require operative measures. . .We would operate." (3623-1)

III. Suggested Therapeutic Regimen

For prevention of stones, the Cayce readings suggest that one should always look first to one's attitudes and emotions. Make corrections there, if needed. Then adopt a good basic diet which avoids fried foods, red meats (for the most part), white flour and white sugar products, and certain combinations of foods (such as cereals and citrus at the same meal). There are many publications on the market now dealing with Cayce's suggestions about diet, and these should be consulted. Lots of green vegetables and fruits are good, with fish, fowl and lamb supplying the protein.

Exercise regularly. Osteopathic or chiropractic treatments at intervals, even when one feels normal, are good procedures to follow. Full-body massages are good alternatives to the manipulations, especially if the latter are not available.

For the acute case of kidney stones, it is vitally important that relaxation be induced, so that the stone can pass without surgical interference. Here, the turpentine stupes can be used as well as the castor oil packs. Both of these tend to help break up the stone, and so are helpful. Osteopathic manipulations are very important in these instances; they aid in the relaxation of the tissues and help in the coordination of the liver and kidneys. Colonics or enemas are also helpful. The eucalyptol prescription in step 9 above might be helpful and, of course, it is very important that the patient help all he can by allowing his body to relax. (While biofeedback had not even been thought of when Cayce gave his readings, it is one way of training people to relax portions of their bodies.)

Attitudes should be of the nature of believing that the condition can be overcome. But it should be remembered that acute renal calculus is a very severe condition, and the aid of a narcotic to relax the ureter and the possibility of surgery as a final necessity should not be ruled out.

For the chronic case of renal calculi, all of those measures suggested for prevention should be utilized, keeping the body in a constructive phase and letting dissolution of the stone come about gradually—if it does come about at all. If the stone is large, such as a "staghorn" calculus, pieces may break off as dissolution occurs; these could cause acute problems as they try to pass down the ureter. Turpentine stupes may be used over a long period of time—and other measures that have been suggested in this commentary—but it must always be recognized that each person must make choices for himself. A large stone residing in the pelvis of the kidney is not an easy thing to correct. In many instances because of the psychological makeup of the individual, it may not be easily possible for the condition to be corrected. On the other hand, if the Cayce readings are to be taken at face value, it is *always* possible to clear up any condition. Choice is necessary as well as prayer, then definitive action to arrive at the method and the correction.

But no matter what the problem one faces regarding kidney stones—their formulation or their presence—the instruction that Cayce gave to a 53-year-old man suffering from a kidney stone should be kept in mind:

And let thy prayer oft be, in thy deeper meditation:
Father, God, Thou art life! Thou art hope! Thou art justice! Thou art mercy! In these may I, Thy servant, claim Thy care, Thy love; that my body may be cleansed as my mind may be cleansed, that I may be before Thee holy and acceptable unto Thee to do service to my fellow man in Thy name; and that the glory of Thy love as manifested in the Christ, my Savior, our Savior, may be manifested more and more in the earth. . .

And be consistent as to the applications of those suggestions and those activities that may bring about this; for every force and every power in the earth is of Him. Will you use it in His service or in defying Him in thy vainglory?   **370-5**

William A. McGarey, M.D.

Edgar Cayce readings referenced:

64-1	1103-4	4612-1
141-1	1152-7	4892-1
149-1	1333-1	4989-1
370-4, 5	1472-1, 16	5137-1
416-17	1547-1	5267-1
427-2	1588-1, 2	5404-1
540-9	1745-5, 6, 7	5420-1
601-25	1811-1	5495-1
843-4 through 8	1839-1	5499-1
1051-1	2392-1	5580-1
1054-1, 2	3442-1	
1055-1	3623-1	
1060-1, 2	4281-1, 11	

LEUKEMIA

The purpose of the research which formed the basis for this report was to study all known cases of leukemia in the Edgar Cayce readings in order to summarize the program of treatment suggested as well as to set forth any etiological factors mentioned. These data can then be used as the basis for further research in the form of controlled experiments by qualified physicians to determine the worth of the suggestions. The summary of treatment is not to be taken as an endorsement by the writer. The validity of the data must be decided by careful subsequent research. The etiological mechanisms described are meant to be considered as theories to be proved and not facts already established.

In the indexing of the Edgar Cayce readings, 23 readings given for 11 people have been classified as leukemia. However, after careful study of the material with subsequent follow-up research, only seven cases (16 readings) show a reasonable certainty of having been leukemia by confirmation with certified photostats of death certificates or hospital record summaries or in the file correspondence with doctors or patients. The following discussion is based on these seven cases:

[13]: Acute monocytic leukemia (death certificate), two readings.

[534]: "Leukemia" (newspaper report), one reading.

[1174]: Lymphatic leukemia, aplastic stage (hospital record summary), one reading.

[2456]: Acute lymphatic leukemia (doctor's letter), six readings.

[2488]: Acute lymphatic leukemia (hospital record summary), two readings.

[3000]: Leukemia (patient's letter with history and doctor's diagnosis), two readings.

[3616]: Lymphatic leukemia (patient's letter with doctor's diagnosis), two readings.

In passing it might be noted that four of the cases studied (seven readings) were designated as Hodgkin's disease rather than leukemia:

[177]: (Death certificate), two readings.

[2621]: (Death certificate showing results of post-mortem), three readings.

[3007]: (Doctor's letter), one reading.

[5360]: (Patient's letter giving doctor's diagnosis), one reading.

Case [2621] presented etiological mechanisms and treatment similar to many of the leukemia cases (see below).

Etiology of leukemia in human beings, based on present evidence, appears to involve viruses, environmental factors, cell mutations produced by irradiation, chemical agents, genetic influences, and abnormalities of host resistance. None of these factors has been conclusively shown to be causative, thus the real cause of leukemia remains shrouded in mystery.

I. Physiological Considerations

The readings approach the cause of leukemia in a manner that implies more than it says. Life as we know it is a manifestation of spirit insistent on its being active in a manner determined by the nature of the mind and physical structure of the cells themselves— meaning that life is already present and active. Implied, then, is that the disturbances which arise are disturbances of the ways in which this life force is manifesting in single structures and in systems throughout the body. Thus, the readings' approach to etiology of diseases is a physiological one but it assumes initially that the inner forces within the body are spirit in action.

Thus some of the comments in these readings on leukemia seem to imply that deficiencies of certain elements assimilating into the body are basic causative factors. In other places attitudes of the mind are said to be essential in directing either the recovery in a complete manner or as being causative of the loss of life. In case [2456], for instance, the individual is told, ". . .for, without the desire for the recovery for a purposefulness, little may be fully accomplished." The mind then helps, as Cayce sees it, in directing the final outcome of a given case, as it directs even the function of an individual cell.

Not a large enough number of cases were available to be able to discern any outstandingly significant pattern in the types of treatments recommended. In the seven cases some type of liver was suggested in four (2456, 2488, 3000, 3616); UV light with a green glass in three (2456, 2488, 3000); infrared light in two (1174, 3616); beef juice in three (534, 3000, 3616); orange juice in three (2456, 2488, 3616); and Atomidine in three (534, 2456, 3616). All that can be concluded is that these are the types of treatment most frequently suggested in the small number of cases present in the readings.

The cause of leukemia was not given in a detailed way, but some general suggestions were advanced. A disturbance in body catabolism was noted in [3000] and loss of the energies of anabolism (assimilative forces). "Infection" through the spleen was linked with an excess of destructive forces in the lymph in case [2456]. The nature of this "infection" was not spelled out—whether bacteriological, viral, or some other type of destructive force. Infection as a medical term would imply some type of disease process able to be transmitted from one individual to another, but the readings did not elaborate. It is a medical fact that the red cell count decreases and the white blood cell count mounts in leukemia. In the readings, this destructive process chiefly of red blood cells was linked to an overactivity and "infection" of the spleen. This "infection" could mean mainly an overabundance of white blood cells, although in [1174] a "strep in the blood supply" was mentioned.

The whole process of the disease was said to be caused by a glandular disturbance from unbalanced chemical reactions in the body (2456, cf. 2621—Hodgkin's). This could point toward a biochemical cause of the disease. The reading specifically mentions iodine deficiency. This could be the rationale for advising iodine trichloride (Atomidine) as a gland stimulant. In 1174-1 the thyroid gland was mentioned in particular. A lack of proper activity of the structural portions of the body (3000-3) could refer to the red blood cell-producing capacity of the marrow, especially the ribs (which are mentioned specifically). These portions of the body could in turn be affected by the glands. Mention was also made of the activity having become static in the cerebrospinal system centers which control the marrow production from the ribs (2456-2). Apparently an attempt was made in the treatment to stimulate these centers through ultraviolet and infrared light as well as manual massage.

The order of cause and effect was indicated most clearly in [2456], in which a lack of iodine in the system was said to cause an imbalance in the glandular forces which in turn caused an "infection" (or over-abundance of white blood cells) in the spleen. This "infection" in turn caused a disruption of the anabolic-catabolic balance of the body and what the readings described as a "dryness or hardness" of the lymph along the ribs and spine. Disturbance of the anabolic-catabolic balance then presumably was what affected the marrow and the control of the production of red blood cells via the cerebrospinal centers. The liver was supposed to provide factors which aided the manufacture of red blood cells. The mechanism of these cause-and-effect relations was not described.

It is interesting to note that in one of the four cases of Hodgkin's disease in the readings ([2621], which was called Hodgkin's in the reading itself and confirmed by autopsy) the etiology and treatment is very similar to that discussed above—e.g., etiology: biochemical imbalance; treatment; ultraviolet light with green glass, Atomidine, liver, beef juice. Reading 1779-5 (monocytic anemia with white blood cells mounting toward leukemia), which was rejected from the above analysis because of insufficient supporting evidence for a definite diagnosis of leukemia, emphasized the spleen and suggested Atomidine as part of the treatment. These similarities hint at the possibility that perhaps there are some similar underlying biochemical mechanisms having to do with the endocrine glands and the spleen in various diseases of the blood.

II. Rationale of Therapy

Throughout the cases included here is developed the concept that the cells of the body, even the red blood cells, are brought into structure or are built through several influences. These influences are those of assimilation, those derived from glandular tissue throughout the body, and probably those taken in through the lungs as what he called once "ozone and carbon forces." The assimilative faculty is primarily those patches of lymphatic tissue which are known as Peyer's patches and associative structure and function. In other words, the lymphocytes formed in the patches, as they absorb factors from digested food, take as part of their various structure globulins (and other as yet unknown factors) as substances to rebuild the body—as "structural activity." These materials are acted upon by hormones released by glandular tissue, which have been in turn activated by vitamin substances. These two forces combine with the energies that I would assume were those from the lung, to bring about rebuilding of cells throughout the body.

Iodine is one of the basic substances which the readings saw as essential to the body and its function. Thus in [2208] we see the "lack of the cells becoming activated upon by the iodine—that is a part of the structural activity through the system." And in [3003] this particular leukemia arose "from the lack of proper activity of the structural portions of the body, especially through ribs and the spleen and pancreas to react with the digestive activities of the body."

Again in line with the view of the body as the sum total of physiological processes either coordinated or uncoordinated, the readings saw excessively high white count as an attempt on the part of that portion of the body—the white blood cell forces—to meet the needs in rebuilding the structure as rapidly as it was being destroyed. Obviously, without the necessary element no adequate solution can be arrived at no matter how many cells are thrown into the bloodstream in such an effort.

Such an etiology is just a hypothesis, and adequate explanation of a comprehensive nature in one place in the readings is lacking. However, bringing these various bits of information together helps us understand in what manner and for what purposes therapy was directed.

III. Therapeutic Regimen (New Area for Research)

On the basis of the hypothesis just suggested, a method of treatment which was proposed in reading 2208-1 becomes of interest. One cc of tincture of iodine mixed with some blood taken from the patient and this added to the next transfusion would bring about a cure, if it were to be repeated in the proper sequence. Animal experimentation is suggested in order to establish proper dosages and proper balance for therapy, but the reading indicates that these methods would be effective in treating any individual case of such nature (myelogenous leukemia). If such a therapy were to be developed "it will be found that there will be the ability to reduce the percentages of such cases more than 50%."

With the validity of the readings already established in so many different directions, this last statement is quite exciting and should stimulate interest in testing such a therapy.

A. Electromagnetic Vibrations

    1. Ultraviolet light. UV light (mercury quartz) was to be

used 40 inches from the body with a green-stained glass plate (at least 10 x 12 inches) suspended between the source of UV light and the body (2456, 2488, 3000, cf. 2621—Hodgkin's). The treatments were to be administered over the dorsal aspect of the body for not more than a total of five minutes and not more than one to one-and-a-half minutes in any one spot with special emphasis to the spleen and rib area. This treatment was to be given one to two times per day.

2. Infrared light. In [2456] it was indicated to apply this for 35 to 40 minutes every other day to the cerebrospinal area as a stimulation for the deep therapy produced to the structural portions (bones) along the rib area. Also in 3616-2 infrared was recommended for the back and the area over or opposite the spleen.

B. Physiotherapy

1. The body was to be massaged with a mixture of grain alcohol and peanut oil along the spine, especially D5, D6, D7 after the ultraviolet treatment. (2456, cf. 2621-1—Hodgkin's)

2. Osteopathic manipulations were to be given to coordinate D9, the brachial plexus, and the upper cervicals with the sacral and lumbar areas. (2488-1)

3. The wet cell appliance was recommended in the manner that the radio-active appliance was ordinarily used. (See 3000-3.)

C. Drugs

1. Iodine trichloride (Brand name: Atomidine): The dose was to be started with one to two drops in half a glass of water and then increased stepwise until 5 to 15 drops were being given. The drug was then stopped for 5 to 10 days when the process was to be repeated. (534, 2456, 3616, cf. 2621—Hodgkin's)

2. Ventriculin (the intrinsic factor made from animal gastric mucosa and ordinarily used in the treatment of pernicious anemia): No specific dose was mentioned; therefore, the usual adult dose was assumed. (534)

3. Atropine in a dose of 1/80 grain was to be given 3 to 10 minutes before any transfusions. (534)

D. Transfusions (534, 1174, 2456)

E. Additions to the Diet

1. Beef juice was to be prepared as follows: Cut a pound of

lean round beef into small cubes. Put the cubes (only the lean, remove all fat) in a covered fruit jar. Put jar inside a pan of water (water coming to about half the depth of the jar). A cloth may be put in the bottom, around the outside of jar, to insure not breaking or cracking the jar. Boil until chunks of beef are thoroughly done. Strain. Keep juice in a cool place. The quantity recommended was two to four teaspoons per day to be taken one teaspoon at a time and sipped slowly so that each sip of the juice could be mixed thoroughly with the juices of the mouth before swallowing.

2. Liver was to be prepared in many different ways but as a general rule as rare as possible. Also it was supposed to be better to take it by mouth rather than by injections (although liver extract was advised in [2488], cf. 2621—Hodgkin's).

a. Broiled rare. (3616)

b. Ground and steamed in Patapar paper. (2456-4)

c. Liver pudding (2456-1, 3000-3, cf. 2621-1—Hodgkin's). To be prepared as follows:

One-half pound ground calf's liver

One-half cup blood (which you can get butcher to save from grinding the liver)

Butter a pan six inches square and two inches deep. Season the liver with salt to taste and a piece of butter the size of a walnut. Melt and mix with the liver, then pour blood over the liver. Run in hot oven about 10 minutes.

d. Cf. 2621-1—Hodgkin's, where liver juice was recommended: To be prepared in the same way as beef juice, but using calf's liver and to be taken in as large quantities as the body could tolerate.

3. Orange juice. (2456, 2488, 3616; cf. 177—Hodgkin's) The juice was to be squeezed and drunk fresh from tree-ripened Florida oranges—all a person could drink in a day (at least 6 to 10 glasses).

IV. Summary

1. The small number of cases (seven) does not constitute an adequate sample upon which to base definite conclusions about the worth of the various treatments suggested or the validity of the etiological mechanisms described or implied. In the cases studied

there was poor follow-up in regard to what extent the recommended treatment was actually followed. Also many of these cases were terminal when the readings were obtained.

2. Although the number of cases is too small to show a statistically significant pattern of treatment which may be taken as normative or average for the readings, hints may be suggested for future medical, scientific, and clinical research which may yield more definite results in regard to etiology and treatment. One of the most interesting ideas is that a basic lack of iodine interferes with the proper functioning of the endocrine glands and, therefore, affects the biochemistry of the body to cause the disturbance of the spleen and bone marrow which in turn affect the numbers of both red blood and white blood cells. This suggests a basic biochemical cause of the disease. Controlled clinical experiments could be conducted to test the value of a treatment regimen consisting of combinations of the most frequently suggested types of treatment in the leukemia readings: ultraviolet light with green glass, infrared light, Atomidine for gland stimulation, and additions to the diet (i.e., liver, beef juice, and orange juice).

3. All of the readings dealing with diseases of the blood, such as the various anemias and Hodgkin's disease, should also be studied in detail to provide a basis for comparison with the treatments recommended and the etiologies suggested for leukemia.

Understanding of any disease process is certainly a multifaceted problem, but the more light shed on any problem, the better one is directed toward the answer. The ideas from the readings, the suggestions for further research, these remind us that the body really is made up of atoms which are units of force and that we are in reality a structured representation of forces in action. True healing might then be an activity quite foreign to our present concept.

For all healing comes from the one source. And whether there is the application of foods, exercise, medicine, or even the knife, it is to bring the consciousness of the forces within the body that aid in reproducing themselves—the awareness of creative or God forces.   2696-1

Walter N. Pahnke, M.D.

Edgar Cayce readings referenced:
71-3
1270-1
2208-1
2456-1 through 6
3000-3
3616-1, 2

LEUKOPENIA—LEUKOCYTOSIS

Much is known about the white cells of the bloodstream, their function in the defense of the body, and their origin in the lymphoid tissue of the body and bone marrow. The reader is invited to review the anatomy and physiology of white blood cells. Not so commonly known is that the lymphocytes carry beta- and gamma-globulin within the structure of their cells and release it in various places within the body. The fate of these same lymphocytes, however, is and has been a puzzle for many years. Sanders and associates in 1940 estimated that the entire population of lymphocytes in the circulation of the cat is replaced five times daily. The destiny of the lymphocyte in the human being and the numbers apparently destroyed each day have not been accurately estimated. This information, however, is interesting in relationship to the material which follows.

This commentary is based on a random selection of readings in which a decrease (leukopenia) or an increase (leukocytosis) in the number of white cells is, in a sense, concomitant with other disease processes. Thus the concepts will remain rather limited and not a true picture of what the readings as a whole would present. Changes in the circulating blood are found in nearly all physical conditions and Cayce commented upon this often.

We are always faced in these readings with the concept that cells and organs and tissues, systems of the body, all have consciousness. Apparently this consciousness is an awareness of conditions that exist within the rest of the body. Typical of the activities seen as existing within the body—very much like conditions as might be seen in a city or a state or a nation—are those found in 5575-1 where leukocytosis accompanied disturbances in the functioning organs of the body. In this case the excess numbers of white cells have "been created to meet the needs of the conditions." The needs apparently were recognized and what we usually call trouble—leukocytosis—is represented here as an attempt to correct the imbalance of the body. Later in the same reading a fullness was described as having been "created in the circulatory system, attempting to meet the needs of the condition." It would appear that the lymphatic tissue in all portions of the body and the bone marrow centers of white blood cell production act as units with some sort of central awareness and control.

The function of the lymphocytes (5697-1) might be more obvious when they are deficient, "for they are called on often to rebuild, especially in the cell force having to do with the action of the nerve centers." This is pointed up a bit differently elsewhere (4790-1) in there being "not sufficient then of those elements in the system to give the needed white blood or the leukocyte forces to meet the needs in coagulation in the system."

Other references in the readings indicate that the Peyer's patches are a principal supplier of lymphocytes to the small patch-like areas of lymphatic tissue within the autonomic ganglia where connection and coordination is maintained between the autonomic nervous system and the cerebrospinal nervous system—the unconscious and the conscious minds. These Peyer's patches are also centers of assimilation of various substances including vitamins. These are taken then through the bloodstream to the glands and used as energies in the process of coagulation. Coagulation is the rebuilding of cells throughout the body.

It is interesting that in case [4182], Cayce indicates that there are disturbances in the Peyer's patch area with a deficiency occurring in the white blood cells, apparently the lymphocytes. Coagulation, however, takes place in the system with exertion. This would indicate that activity of the muscles and the bone centers of cell reproduction would bring about an activity within the system which is normally supplied by the lymphocytes. In this individual, asthenia was the diagnosis and an easily fatigued condition came about from either physical or high mental exertion. This was from weakness within those cellular forces associated with the lymphatic rather than bone marrow centers. Here in [4182] the Peyer's patches were overactive and produced too much lactic fluid but not the white cells associated with it. This produced an alkaline condition within the body. In [3279], on the other hand, a case of tuberculosis, there was also a leukopenia but not the associated overactivity of the Peyer's patches. Thus here an acidity developed within the system.

It appears that the Peyer's patches are a focal point of control and influence within the defense forces of the body. A third condition is found in [5580], diagnosed as renal calculus, with associated high white count. The primary pathology here was a toxic condition throughout the Peyer's patches—described as a lack of coordination in the Peyer's patches, creating all manners of troubles. Accumulation of toxic products through the whole system gradually created a toxicity in the ascending colon and the hypogastric nerve plexus. This finally affected the kidneys and bladder and gradually produced the condition. These comments given many years ago are interesting in view of most recent findings concerning the functioning of Peyer's patches. (See Circulating File.)

A tentative generalization might be made here regarding deviations from the normal white count. A decrease in the lymphocytes particularly or in the total white count might well indicate a lack of assimilation in its proper activity to produce those substances necessary for cellular rebuilding and maintenance of balance within all the cells in the body. An increase in white blood cell count or leukocytosis, on the other hand, could indicate a building up of toxins with a reaction from the cells which would rebuild and keep things normal as they attempt to meet the increased liability incurred to all of the cells through the accumulation of toxins, waste, used and refused energies in the body.

The actual production of leukocytosis can be traced much like the events that lead up to a conflict between countries. In case [18] the primary incoordination which came about between the eliminating and assimilating systems created an accumulation of drosses in the system and toxic forces, plus a disturbance in the circulation of the liver. This disturbed hepatic circulation and inadequate liver function in turn brought about an impoverishment of the blood supply and more drosses added to the circulation. In the lower hepatic circulation, the kidneys attempt to function where there should be more activity of the liver. This in turn causes indigestion and a strain and stress in the area of digestion and assimilation with reflexes to the nerve centers, controlling these which then became overtaxed in their functioning. These in turn produced low pulsations of nerve energy and thus came a call to the bloodstream to meet the needs. A strange story perhaps, but one that demonstrates the interrelations of dynamic functions and physiologic activities.

Therapy for leukopenia or leukocytosis should be aimed at the particular condition which is dominant. There are several interesting suggestions in therapy to be found in this file however. (See 3883-1, 4182-1 and 4790-1.)

William A. McGarey, M.D.

Edgar Cayce readings referenced:
18-2
1516-1
3279-1
3883-1
4182-1
4282-1
4790-1
5487-1
5575-1
5580-1
5697-1

MENOPAUSE

I. Physiological Considerations

It is well known and understood that some women pass through the "change of life" without serious symptoms or difficulties, while others have a long, drawn-out menopause that becomes a major health problem and requires medical attention—often, however, with little response.

During menopause, the woman moves from the child-bearing age to a balance of the body wherein much less estrogen is available to the body cells, resulting in the inability to become pregnant. The symptoms of menopause begin sometime during the latter years of the third decade, but more commonly around the age of 40 to 45. Again, it is uncommon for menopause to continue beyond age 50, but some women experience symptoms well into the late years of their 50s and occasionally into their 60s.

Surgical menopause comes about when a woman's ovaries and uterus are removed. This may occur at any age and is much more sudden and frequently more disastrous in its effect.

Symptoms can be multitudinous and, therefore, lead some observers to credit the problems to a psychosomatic origin, so that the woman is referred to a psychologist or psychiatrist. However, physicians who clearly observe the nature of the body—its unity, its coordination or lack of it, and the manner in which function in the body comes about through the nervous system, the glandular influences, and the activities of the body's life-support systems— understand that most symptoms have their bases in the physical body and its workings.

Symptoms observed most frequently are hot flashes, insomnia, fatigue, headaches, constipation, general aches and pains, tensions, nervousness, visual changes, tachycardia, discomfort in the heart area, indigestion, and a variety of mental/emotional disturbances ranging from mild to very severe. The Cayce readings regularly refer to the nature of the human being as body, mind, and spirit; so it is not strange that they lead us to understand some of the disturbances in these relationships.

The readings suggested to [1100] that the distresses she was experiencing had to do with the organs of the pelvis and with those of the eliminating system. (1100-28) And in nearly every instance in those readings studied, there was an incoordination between the autonomic and cerebrospinal nervous systems. The organs of the pelvis, of course, produce estrogens, so the glandular imbalance is disturbed.

Hypochondria was a problem in reading 2054-1, but this was not an unrelated condition. Instead, it was—at least in this instance—due to circumstances within the body while under the influence of the menopausal changes. These brought about an "indeterminate reaction of impulse between the two systems. . ." (autonomic and cerebrospinal), causing a glandular incoordination and "at times the losing of self almost to the incoordination between the reflexes from the sympathetic system, and the coordinant reaction through the cerebrospinal system." Thus, in this instance, hypochondria resulted, so that the body reacted "not always to the suggestion but always to the suggestion there *is* a reaction." (2054-1)

The Cayce source also saw some of the difficulties as arising from a disturbance through the upper hepatic circulation that needed to be normalized.

With the variety of problems that accompany a "change of life," so to speak, it needs to be understood that mental/emotional/spiritual attitudes and influences lay the groundwork for changes that accompany the decrease in estrogen level—often the only chemical change that can be demonstrated. Thus, every woman can have a different kind of menopausal experience, depending upon what she had done with her life experiences, her stresses, her heredity, her diet, her beliefs, and the manner in which she faces life and her purpose for being here.

The readings had this to say about the glands and their activity: ". . .the glandular forces make for disturbing activities at times, but keeping the mental and physical balance as has been outlined, with the adjustments, the activities in the physical and mental fields, the glands respond.

"For the glands are that through which the relationships are kept established as it were between the spiritual body and the mental body." (1158-13)

Is it any wonder, then, that there are differences between the manner in which women go through the change? All symptoms have an origin, and most of the underlying difficulties can be dealt with constructively. This is the message of the Cayce readings.

II. Rationale of Therapy

In understanding therapy for menopausal symptoms and in obtaining the best responses, one needs to pay attention to the ongoing process in the physical body and also to recognize that every woman probably has a set of physiological imbalances completely different from the next.

The process in the menopausal woman is an adjustment to the gradual (or sudden) decrease of female hormones circulating in the system. This adjustment can occur in an individual whose body is already disturbed by a variety of imbalances or it may come about in a completely normal person. The reaction in these two instances is always markedly different. This may explain why some women experience little disturbance during the "change of life" while others undergo all sorts of problems.

In the readings given for different women, the suggestions for re-establishing a balance in the body were grouped into six different categories—the specifics always dependent upon the needs of the individual for whom assistance was offered.

1. *General Care of the Body*

Adequate rest, a diet that is balanced yet corrective in its nature when needed, and exercise. These three therapies were always suggested when there seemed to be a deficiency or a need.

One woman was instructed to spend six to eight weeks relaxing and resting in the sand and sunshine in Clearwater or Clearwater Beach, Florida, for a couple of hours each morning and each afternoon, when the ultraviolet rays from the sun are not too strong. (2966-2) This, combined with her massages and shortwave therapy, was intended to relieve the headaches, the hot and cold flashes, the irregularity of the heart, and the feelings that portions of the body were going to sleep too easily. Another woman was told that she needed to keep more balanced, more rested, and not to bring about an "overactivity or overstimulation of the vital forces of the body, *especially* as related to the activities of reproduction." (1158-17) So rest is often highly important.

A diet oriented toward alkaline-reacting foods was most frequently recommended for menopause. No fats, no fried foods, rarely beef— this was the injunction given to a 38-year-old woman who had undergone a complete hysterectomy. (3386-1)

A special diet was recommended for a woman whose digestive system was giving her problems of gas and regurgitation. Her reading (1713-21) suggested a cleansing regimen: oranges only or oranges and lemons for five days, as many as desired; or apples (Delicious) for three days; or grapes for four days. Any of these would be helpful for cleansing the system from impurities and thus prevent inclinations for gas formations, etc. After the cleansing diet, then half a teacup of olive oil was suggested to be taken. **A note of caution:** If one has gall bladder problems, this amount of olive oil may cause a surgical emergency, forcing stones down into the bile or common duct. Lesser amounts of oil are recommended in most of the instances wherein this kind of cleansing is given.

Exercise—plenty of it—was a frequent recommendation. It is understood from the general tone of the readings that regular exercise, preferably walking, was a basic undergirding of a therapy program leading to health and balance.

Specifics aside, it can be seen that a woman going through the difficulties of menopause would best care generally for her body with rest, a good diet, and exercise.

2. *Working with the Structural Portions of the Body*

Grouped under this heading are osteopathic treatments, chiropractic adjustments, massages, electric vibrator treatments, and hot packs on the back. All of these are in a very real sense related, since they relax or adjust or move the muscles or vertebrae of the spine and bring about a more balanced function of the portions of the body which these areas (in relation to the spinal cord and its functions) actually supply. Primarily in the instance of the menopausal woman, the ovaries, the uterus, and the thyroid are the most important structures involved in this kind of therapy. However, the circulatory system, the nervous system, the assimilation and elimination, and the entire glandular system are affected and may become more normalized through such assistance.

The following extract tells the story of what goes on with manipulation, massage, etc., and the importance of these therapies:

Q-2. Should other glands be stimulated which have not been?
A-2. As just indicated, these should be stimulated, but from the centers from which the *impulse* for their activity emanates!
Let's describe this for a second, that the entity or body here may understand, as well as the one making the stimulation:
Along the cerebrospinal system we find segments. These are cushioned. Not that the segment itself is awry, but through each segment there arises an impulse or a nerve connection between it and the sympathetic system—or the nerves running parallel with same. Through the sympathetic system (as it is called, or those centers not encased in cerebrospinal system) are the connections with the cerebrospinal system.
Then, in each center—that is, of the segment where these connect—there are tiny bursa[e], or a plasm of nerve reaction. This becomes congested, or slow in its activity to each portion of the system. For, each organ, each gland of the system, receives impulses through this manner for its activity.
Hence we find there are reactions to every portion of the system by suggestion, mentally, and by the environment and surroundings.
Also we find that a reaction may be stimulated *internally* to the organs of the body, by injection of properties or foods, or by activities of same.
We also find the reflex from these internally to the brain centers.
Then, the *science* of osteopathy is not merely the punching in a certain segment or the cracking of the bones, but it is the keeping of a *balance*—by the touch—between the sympathetic and the cerebrospinal system! *That* is real osteopathy!
With the adjustments made in this way and manner, we will find not only helpful influences but healing and an aid to any condition that may exist in the body—unless there is a broken bone or the like!   1158-24

3. *Influencing the Electrical Systems of the Body*

Treatments to the body's structural portions certainly have an influence on the neurological system and thus on this portion of the body's electrical system. In the readings, however, a flow of energy was described that moves through the body in the form of a figure eight. It crosses at the umbilicus and forms the basis for another kind of therapy—the radio-active appliance, whose manufacture and use are described in the readings. It should be noted here that this device theoretically functions by taking electrical charges too numerous in one area of the body and moving them to other areas which are deficient. One individual, [1457], was to use this appliance with one attachment on the 12th dorsal area and the other on the pubic center (directly over the pubis). In this instance, the appliance would be used daily for a month, or through the menstrual period, left off for a few days, and then perhaps repeated.

In case [3386], the violet ray was recommended for use alongside the spine just before retiring, apparently to bring a degree of relief to bodily tensions and to balance the neurological system more adequately.

The violet ray was also recommended for [4280]. She had severe difficulties in her menopause, which affected her pineal gland and caused periods of near mental blackout. She was given the formula for a bitter syrup to take internally. For the hot and cold flashes, cold feet, and general irritation, an Epsom salts hot sitz bath was to be taken, followed by a thorough rubdown, and then the violet ray treatment, both along the cerebrospinal system. And she was told to walk or ride in the open air, to keep pleasant company, and "*be* pleasant to others.*"

4. *Local Therapy*

It is always helpful to treat the body locally where the problem lies. The helpfulness may have to do with the consciousness, as stated in the readings, that lies within each cell, each atom of the body. Perhaps these cells need comfort, need to know that they are being cared for and recognized because they have problems. For whatever reason, local therapy always helps. In menopause, the sitz baths just mentioned can be of aid in increasing the circulation to that area of the body.

Between—not during—menstrual periods, douches with Atomidine were often suggested for pelvis problems. A 41-year-old woman was given directions to take such douches, apparently to aid in alleviating the problems of the beginning changes in the system— the readings' description of early menopause. (1713-21) First she was told to take Atomidine douches, a teaspoonful to a quart and a half of water. Later on, in another reading—at this point menopause was really upon her—she was instructed to take also Glyco-Thymoline douches, a tablespoon and a half to a quart of water.

One woman was told to use the violet ray with a vaginal applicator. (528-28) Massage to the lower back and osteopathic treatments in that area can also be classified as local therapy, although they bring about a different kind of response.

5. *Medication*

Of all the medications used for menopause, oral and intramuscular injections of hormones probably rate as number one. The readings recommended them frequently. Atomidine, taken orally, was nearly standard therapy, for it is intended to normalize the function of the glandular structures in the body. Calcios—a calcium product—was often added to the regimen. During those years when the readings were given, Tonicine was suggested as a hormone additive to be taken orally; it contained extracts from the ovary and the thyroid. Other medications were seldom suggested.

6. *Constructive Use of the Mind*

The mind needs to be kept in a constructive phase. The reality of the human being as a body, mind, and spirit is constantly reaffirmed in these readings. To one woman Cayce had this to say:

Do these; keeping the body mentally constructive. That is, as the very nature of the mental influences of the body would be as constructive forces, know that their application does not consist of formulas or ritual but just being kind, gentle, patient, even with those that apparently would torment thee. This is *magnifying* those influences that keep a body mentally, physically, spiritually balanced. For the mind is the builder. Hence it is both material and spiritual.

If spiritual constructiveness is used, then, that builded into the experience must be of those very constructive natures.   1457-1

To another, he said, "Sing a lot." (3386-1) To still another, ". . .be pleasant to others!" (4290-9) In 1540-3, Cayce pointed out that "As to the constructive forces—know that the *spiritual* is the source of health, of light, of understanding; and necessarily the source of *all* happiness."

III. *Suggested Therapeutic Regimen*

Lacking the psychic ability to look into the body and ascertain what incoordinations exist, where the body is malfunctioning, what attitudes are not constructive, and how severe the menopause really is, one must rely on a general approach toward correcting the menopausal syndrome.

Always a direction should be taken toward balance: balance in the nerve supply, in the circulation, in the hormonal system, in the structural setup of the body, and between assimilation and elimination. And much attention should be paid to the attitudes, emotions, and beliefs of the individual.

So what would be a general therapy program for such a person? Perhaps the following would be helpful, no matter how mild or severe the conditions may be:

1. A basic alkaline-reacting diet, eliminating fried foods, fats, white flour and white sugar, pork, with only occasional beef. Protein as in fish, fowl, or lamb. Lots of salads, fruit, cooked vegetables;

2. Adequate eliminations;

3. Adequate rest;

4. Osteopathic manipulations. Massages and use of violet ray if these are not available;

5. Atomidine, taken orally in cycles;

6. Alternate Atomidine and Glyco-Thymoline douches—one of each every week for the space of several months, avoiding the douches when periods come. One teaspoonful of Glyco-Thymoline to a quart of water;

7. "...keep the mental attitudes towards all helpful influences..." (1100-28) Use the mind constructively, meditate regularly, seek to apply the fruits of the spirit in one's life day by day.

In all likelihood, the individuals with menopause for whom Cayce gave readings were not exactly in the same condition as anyone else you might meet. However, there are enough similarities in the symptoms experienced that a regimen such as that shown above might be utilized, and other treatments Cayce suggested (as listed earlier in this discussion) might then be added if applicable.

Menopause is a changing of the life situation, and it can be met with equanimity if the body is balanced in its function. Life's daily experience can be encountered with a smile and a song, but the body must be attended to and the attitudes must be looked at and corrected.

William A. McGarey, M.D.

Edgar Cayce readings referenced:	1713-21, 22	3272-1
538-28	2054-1	3386-1, 2
1100-28	2463-1	4105-1
1158-13, 16, 17, 18, 20, 23, 24, 31	2581-1	4280-9
1457-1	2966-2	5089-1
1540-2 through 5	2988-5	

MENTAL ILLNESS

Presented to the Second Annual Symposium of the Medical Research Division of the Edgar Cayce Foundation in Phoenix, Arizona, January 13, 1969.

Introduction

It is a pleasure for me to have this opportunity to share with you some of the ideas expressed in the Edgar Cayce readings on mental illness.

My paper is in no sense final, but is rather a report of research in progress with some indications of the trends we have found thus far. It is based on a study of 365 cases directly related to the subject, and numerous other cases to which I was led for supplementary information.

As a psychologist, it was rather disconcerting to note that Edgar Cayce did not recommend the services of a psychologist or psychiatrist in a single case.

In one case (1428-1, M.30) Edgar Cayce was asked, "Should the advice of any of the previous physicians be followed?" He replied, "As we find, rather these suggestions that have been made here. . ."

Another question was "Would he be benefited by weekly visits to Dr. Stewart of the Meadowbrook Hospital?" Cayce answered, "As we find, if these are applied in the manner indicated, it will be better than hospitalization, better than weekly visits. . ." Dr. Stewart was a psychiatrist.

It was interesting to note also that Cayce saw a person as a whole, with mind, body and spirit as a single unit, all so closely tied that it was not possible for one aspect to be diseased, either physically or mentally, without the whole person suffering the consequences. Hence, I have entitled my paper, "A Holistic Theory of Mental

Illness." This point of view is expressed in the following statement from one of the readings:

For, the body-physical becomes that which it assimilates from material nature. The body-mental becomes that which it assimilates from both the physical-mental and the spiritual-mental. The soul is *all* of that the entity is, has been, or may be.   2475-1

In one case (5210-1, F.22) the patient asked, "Am I slightly mentally ill?" Edgar Cayce's answer was, "No, save as to who would be the judge. Every individual is slightly mentally ill to someone else."

With this general perspective in mind, let us now turn to his diagnoses.

Diagnoses

The symptoms of the patients I will describe were the typical symptoms of the psychoses: disorganization of thought, disorientation in time and space, withdrawal and autistic behavior, depersonalization, extremes of mood, hallucinations, delusions, etc. Most of the cases were diagnosed, in the language of the day, as dementia praecox or insanity. Using a more current system of classification they would be labeled schizophrenic, manic-depressive, or paranoid.

Most of these patients were brought to the attention of Mr. Cayce as a last resort. They were grossly disturbed, and some had been in institutions for many years.

In diagnosing a condition, Mr. Cayce seemed to be able to tune in to the autonomic and central nervous systems of the person. He believed that each cell in the body had an awareness of its own, and that the totality of this awareness constituted *mind,* with which he was in communication.

It was apparent at times that he had a form of visual perception which extended over the miles. Not only did he perceive the conditions of internal organs but also external environmental features.

In one case (5167-1, M.30) in which there were lesions in the brain caused by accidents, Cayce remarked, "My! What a mess!" In another case (2248-1, F.24), he said, "Yes, the big house is here, too!"; and in another, (5228-1, M.31), "That's where the railroad crosses." With this description of the physical, mental, and spiritual health of his patients.

In order to share with you as broad a perspective as possible in a short period of time, I thought that instead of discussing a few cases in detail, it might be more productive to survey the highlights of many cases and then summarize at the end.

I have abstracted 32 diagnoses which are representative and contain examples of different aspects of Edgar Cayce's view of mental illness. They will orient you to his point of view.

1. Prenatal condition which affected glands—especially pineal and pituitary. Improper coordination between autonomic and cerebrospinal systems. (4853-1, F. Adult)

2. Growth which causes pressure on pineal gland, thus affecting several organs. (4849-1, F. Adult)

3. ". . .the seat of the trouble [is] where the entrance of the sympathetic with cerebrospinal and pineal nerves enter the brain. . ." Brain impressions do not coordinate with sympathetic impressions from the sensory system. (4800-1)

4. Lacerations to womb; also adhesions which affect the nerve system and bring on hallucinations. (4624-1, F. 45)

5. Blood deficient in its rebuilding force, thus hallucinations. (4519-1, M. Adult)

6. Overtaxing caused incoordination of the sympathetic and cerebrospinal systems. Engorgement in the 1st and 2nd cervical areas of the spine and at pineal gland. (4432-1, M. Adult)

7. Birth injury to lumbar and sacral regions of spine—breech birth. "In later years. . .an accident to the end of the spine (four years ago [on the] sixteenth of September. . .)" which damaged coccyx. (4342-1, F. Adult)

8. Incoordination in the glands of reproduction because of the fall she had at six years of age which injured the spinal center and produced reflexes in the pineal gland. (4433-1, F. Adult)

9. Poisons have entered the system from infected tonsils. (4290-1, F. 58) (Cayce said of this patient's nerve system: "This we find, as would be slangily said, 'all shot,' see?")

10. Injury to spine to coccyx area which destroyed the connections between systems. (Patient's problem began right after an accident on bicycle 10 years before.) (3223-1, M. 31)

11. "The conditions here, as we find, have been so aggravated by animosities, and by hates, that we have a deterioration in the nerve force along the spinal system; so that this is dementia—and now possession, such that this may appear near to hopeless in this

experience." (Edgar Cayce suggests that emotional stress may destroy nerve tissue, and also that the patient will have another incarnation in which to improve the situation.) (3315-1, F.40)

12. "Extreme nervous tension that overtaxed the system as received through the sensory forces, until the cells broke here at the 1st cervical." (4097-1, M. Adult)

13. Illness of mind, not so much of body. He cannot respond to kindness because of experiences. Study and strain. (Patient age 22, completed one year of college.) (5405-1, M. 22)

14. Pressures left in the coccyx, lumbar, and dorsal areas after infection in the genitive system. Not true dementia, but incoordination. "Also those surroundings, the environs, those activities have brought about much of that which is a relative condition." (1428-1, M. 30)

15. "These are the result of chemical and glandular reactions in the body; producing a deteriorating reaction in nerve impulses." (2614-1, F. 37)

16. Accident impinged the centers about the 3rd lumbar. This affected the kidneys and caused uremic poisoning. (4186-1, M. Adult)

17. "An injury to the coccyx from a fall when only about three and a half to four years old." This caused glandular dysfunction. (Patient was age 18 at time of reading.) (2721-1, F. 19)

18. Disconnection or disassociation of sympathetic and cerebrospinal systems which caused lesions in the brain. Those on whom he is dependent must bear the burden. There is no hope. (Patient was a 20-year-old male.) (4991-1)

19. Coordination has been severed. There is no hope. (586-1, F. Adult)

20. Overtaxation of the system, physically and mentally, caused eruptions in blood cells. Pressures are "*functional,* rather than organic in their nature." (2359-1, M. Adult)

21. A lesion in the lacteal duct and that as coordinating with the organs of the pelvis. "The reaction to the pineal becomes so severe as to short-circuit the nerve impulse; carrying or producing a fluttering, or an engorgement in static waves to the base of the brain." (2465-1, F. 28)

22. Pressures on spine from childbirth of her first child.

23. "The body-mind lost control of itself through overtaxing of the body-mind, combined with a type of fever that was part of the experience when the body so taxed itself; reducing the body forces to

such an extent that in many centers along the spinal column there came to be less and less ability for the centers to coordinate between sympathetic and cerebrospinal nervous systems." (2865-1, F. 31, M.D.)

24. Causes both psychological and pathological. "Psychologically, these have to do with the karma of this body, and those responsible for the physical body." (3075-1, M. 24)

25. Patient at age 13 joined the Missionary Baptist Church. "When he was baptized he was stricken with a headache which lasted for years." A physician said that the headaches were caused by masturbation. Edgar Cayce said that a lesion in the brain centers caused a loss of control. "The voluntary and involuntary reaction or impulse, as carried in the white and gray matter of the nervous systems tends in certain centers to run together and become confusing to the body." (3158-1, M. 37)

26. "It is purely a physical condition, from a pressure existent in the coccyx end of the spine, affecting directly the organs of the pelvis." (3415-1, F. 22)

27. Injury to coccyx area and pressure on the brush end of the cerebrospinal system affects glandular forces. Glands of assimilation not functioning well. This causes undue development of breasts and other areas. (3609-1, F. 35)

28. Cellular waste materials not being carried out of the brain.

29. ". . .adhesions in the pelvic organs, as directly connected or associated with the lyden (Leydig) and the pineal glands." (4002-1, F. 28)

30. "With the mental exhaustion of body, through taxation physically and mentally, there came that almost complete disassociation between sympathetic and cerebrospinal nervous systems. . ." (5467-1, M. 45)

31. Hereditary tendencies to physical defects in the cerebrospinal nerve system, so incoordination of systems. (Parents were first cousins.) (5690-1, M. 27)

32. "There has already been departure of the soul. . .no physical help. . .may be administered. . ." (5344-1, F. 35)

To summarize the diagnostic material, the following points seem pertinent:

1. Cayce spoke of mental illness as basically a physical problem once it is manifested. It could be caused by injury, glandular

dysfunction, or emotional stress; but the result was incoordination or a lack of balance in the system.

The most frequently mentioned incoordinaiton was between the autonomic and central nervous systems. (Cayce used the term sympathetic for autonomic.) This was physical, or perhaps chemical, in nature and occurred most often along the spinal cord in those centers where the two systems join. The readings are not specific about the details, but they imply a separation or dysfunction of the synaptic connections.

Cayce mentioned spinal injuries as the cause in many cases. In several instances, these injuries were confirmed by letters from the patient or a relative. But he also stated very clearly that emotional stress could produce the same effect. "This produces, through these pressures, those spasmodic conditions to the reaction between the sympathetic and the cerebrospinal system—which has been termed a *mental* disorder. The reaction is not mental, but a physical—that acts to, or on, the mental—so that the reflexes that come through the sympathetic system are those that prevent a normal impulse from their reaction, causing that pressure, that condition. . ." (2200-1)

In another reading he was even more specific: "And thus the nerve forces for the body, this body as any body, any individual, who makes destructive thought in the body, condemning self for this or that, will bring, unless there are proper reactions, dissociation or lack of coordination between [the] sympathetic and cerebrospinal system, and it may develop any condition which may be purely physical by deterioration of mental processes and their effect upon organs of the body." (5380-1, M. 54)

One could not wish for a clearer statement of the basic premise of psychosomatic medicine, and it was spoken long before the recent rapid growth of this discipline.

In a few cases, Cayce was asked about the cause of hallucinations. He described synaptic dysfunctions which resulted in the reception of messages by the central nervous system which were not sent by the sensory system. "We have just described how that the supersensitiveness of the nerve forces opens the body to such influences; or the body becomes what might be termed a human radio, but in giving expression to what is heard may often deflect what is actually said, felt or thought. For, thoughts are things! and they have their effect upon individuals, especially those that become supersensitive to outside influences! These are just as physical as sticking a pin in the hand!" (386-2)

When we discuss, in a moment, the treatment programs Cayce prescribed, we will see even more clearly what he meant by incoordination between the autonomic and central nervous systems.

2. Another frequently mentioned condition was glandular dysfunctions. These were caused by prenatal developmental problems, infections, injuries, incoordination in the autonomic nervous system, etc. The pineal gland, in particular, was mentioned numerous times.

Cayce implied that this gland included both autonomic and central nervous system pathways and served a coordinating function.

3. Functional disorders, such as emotional stress, nervous tension, or "overtaxing" were suggested as common causes of mental illness, but they were manifested in a physical disorder.

Mental illness then, according to Edgar Cayce, is caused by either physical, mental, or spiritual imbalance. But regardless of the precipitating factor, all aspects are affected adversely. The person is a complete unit which can only function as a whole.

Let us look now at his treatment program.

Treatment

In order to provide a broad perspective, I have, as above, abstracted several examples of treatment procedures. Each was specifically formulated for the particular case. But before I present these examples, I want to mention that Cayce suggested, in the majority of cases, that the patients use either a wet cell appliance or a radio-active appliance as a part of therapy. (These were instruments which he described in several readings.) It is sufficient for our purposes here to point out that these appliances provided a low-voltage electrotherapy. In the wet cell appliance the current passed through a solution which was usually chloride of gold. Specific areas on the body were designated for the attachments.

Now, a few examples of prescribed treatments:

1. Wet cell appliance carrying vibratorially the chloride of gold solution. (Formula was given and attachments described.) Appliance to be used three times per week for 30 minutes.

Massage with equal combination of witch hazel and peanut oil. (Specific areas of massage were indicated.) (1513-1, M. 47)

2. Wet cell appliance with chloride of gold and also radio-active

appliance. Massage whole body and suggest "quiet," "peace," etc., when the patient is almost asleep. Follow a body-building diet. Almonds, in small quantities, are good for the body. (271-1, M. 34)

3. Correct adhesions as related to the organs of the pelvis by an osteopathic gynecologist or the condition may cause deterioration of nerve plasm. (3475-1, F. 22)

4. Wet cell appliance with nickel plate, massage with olive oil and tincture of myrrh. One drop of Atomidine two days per week to purify and cleanse the glandular system. (5014-1, M. 11)

5. Take the patient to a place near sun, sand and sea, with pine woods, and wear as few clothes as possible. (386-1, F.20)

During massage the following suggestion was to be repeated to the patient. I want to share this statement because it explains, in part, the function of the appliance.

Now there is being created in the impulses from the ganglia in the system the normal reaction to the sensory and sympathetic systems of the body. And this is being normally *acted upon by the vibrations, and the reactions will be a perfectly normal balancing in the mental, physical and spiritual being of the body. . .*

. . .It is glands' reaction, and we are changing these through the vibrations that have been set up; as indicated in nerve impulses from the ganglia along the cerebrospinal system to functioning of organs throughout the body.

386-3

6. There is complete disassociation of sympathetic and cerebrospinal systems. This has caused lesions in the brain and there is little hope. (Cayce advised those on whom the patient was dependent to bear the burden.) (4991-1, M. 20)

7. Castor oil packs over the liver and umbilicus plexus. This will relax the system. Deep massage in sacral and lower lumbar areas. Take Codiron tablets daily until several hundred have been taken. Radio-active appliance each day for 30 minutes. Use period of appliance for meditation. Read John 14, 15, 16, 17. (A follow-up letter said that Codiron tablets had been taken off the market. Edgar Cayce suggested White's Codliver Oil Tablets.) (1614-1, F. 38)

8. Osteopathic adjustments were prescribed regularly. A typical case was that of a female patient, 27 years old, who had suffered an injury to the area of the 4th lumbar which caused pressure on the pineal gland. This was Cayce's diagnosis. The patient was in St.

Elizabeth's Hospital in Washington, D.C. Cayce prescribed osteopathic adjustments to relieve pressure in the lumbar area of the spine.

Numerous cases were similar to this one. Some received results they
considered "miraculous." Many others never tried the treatment.

9. Animated ash internally. Also ultraviolet ray and massage.

10. "Or the gold may be taken internally in very minute doses, for
the stimulation of those gland secretions that make for creative
energies and forces through the activity of all the glands in the
body..." (915-2, M. 62)

11. Other treatments prescribed were:

   a. Extract of the passion flower to quiet the body
   b. Surgery
   c. Colonics to aid eliminations
   d. Kindness
   e. Injection of liver abstract
   f. Submerge in hot water 15-20 minutes, then massage
   g. Mayblossom bitters
   h. Turpentine packs over kidneys and pubic area to drain
bladder
   i. Concentrated beef juice
   j. Jerusalem artichoke—to provide insulin
   k. Glyco-Thymoline
   l. Milk and grape diet for three days
   m. Colors purple and lavender about the body; also provide
music on strings or organ.

I have not exhausted the examples of the various treatments
suggested by Edgar Cayce, but I have mentioned enough of the most
common ones to give you some orientation to his method. Now let me
summarize and comment briefly on the section on treatment.

First of all, let me point out that although there were frequently
many common elements in the treatment programs, they were very
specific for that individual. The *exact* location of the castor oil pack
was described. The *precise* amount of medicine was prescribed. These
varied from patient to patient.

Cayce emphasized the importance of carrying out his instructions
to the letter. In subsequent readings on a patient he would frequently
reprimand those in charge for not following instructions precisely. He
knew when they had not, and those who responded acknowledged
that he was right.

Cayce also suggested particular doctors to his patients. Some of these doctors had never heard of Edgar Cayce, and he, in his waking state, had never heard of them.

You will remember that Cayce came to believe that all of us live many lives. He was convinced by the data from his own readings. In a few cases in which he suggested that the suffering of the person was karmic—that is, related to other lives and for the benefit of the person—he seemed to reluctant to prescribe a cure. (3700-1, M. 28) He also said that we must pay the price necessary for our soul development.

Let me summarize the specific treatments Cayce recommended:

1. The wet cell appliance. This was suggested in almost all cases of mental illness.

2. Osteopathic adjustments to the spine. This was very frequently recommended.

3. The radio-active appliance. This was recommended primarily for patients who were agitated or aggressively acting out.

4. Massage. Both deep massage and gentle massage with specific areas designated and the appropriate oils prescribed. Usually these were olive oil, peanut oil, and lanolin.

5. Cayce strongly emphasized that those who treated the patient must be sympathetic. He said, ". . .the greatest thought that comes to the mind of man [is] 'somebody cares.' " (3365-1, F. 17)

6. Then finally, he recommended numerous specific medicines to suit the particular needs of each individual patient.

The most important treatment seemed to be the wet cell appliance, so let me comment briefly on its theory.

This appliance provides low-voltage electrotherapy. The current passes through a wire immersed in a solution of chloride of gold. On rare occasions, the readings suggested chloride of silver or some other solution. Typically, the patient was told to use the appliance for 30 minutes, three times per week.

Since most all cases included a condition of incoordination between the central and autonomic nervous systems, the appliance was recommended to deal with this problem primarily. Edgar Cayce explained its purpose in the following paragraph from the reading of a 30-year-old woman:

As we may see in a functioning physical organism, electricity in its incipiency or lowest form is the nearest vibration in a physical sense to Life itself; for it is the nucleus about each atom of active force or principle set by

the atomic activity of blood pulsation itself, that begins from the very union of the plasm that creates life itself in a physical organism. **3950-1**

In another reading he said that the appliance was the instrument "that would build, as it were, nerve ends so as to form, in those areas as indicated, connections in nerve plasm." (5088-1, F. 67)

The effect is to create better connections at the synaptic centers, especially where the central nervous system and the autonomic system join. The electricity apparently creates nerve plasm or tissue which enlarges the synaptic knobs and thus improves the connection.

Perhaps this is what happens on a more temporary basis in electro-shock therapy.

This theory makes perfect sense and does not contradict current thinking relative to neural and synaptic transmission.

It is particularly interesting in light of Cayce's explanation of hallucinations which I mentioned above. You remember that he suggested that a misfiring, or spontaneous firing, of a nerve impulse delivered a message to the central nervous system which was not sent by the sensory system.

Most doctors are familiar with the phantom limb phenomenon in which a person "feels" pain in a foot that has been amputated. Apparently this is also a case of a spontaneous firing of a nerve impulse or a bad connection somewhere higher in the system.

Space does not permit us to look more closely at some of the other aspects of the treatment program, each of which must be thoroughly researched. I believe, however, that the wet cell appliance is the most important.

Please note once again that Cayce's treatments involved the whole person. He provided for the building of nerve tissue, the cleansing of the system, the stimulation of glands and blood circulation, proper diet, sympathetic attendants, and also a time for meditation and prayer.

Prognoses

What about the outcome of these cases? Was treatment successful?

Edgar Cayce, after 33 years of readings, said the following in a letter to one of his patients: "Wherever there has been the whole-hearted cooperation of everyone concerned, we have not found a single instance where a definite change for the better hasn't been wrought as promised."

This is a remarkable statement, but it appears to be true. The first part of the sentence, however, is very important. "Wherever there has been the wholehearted cooperation of everyone concerned. . ." This was the problem.

Those who precisely followed Cayce's instructions got immediate results. Some of these patients and their doctors wrote and used the term "miracle" to describe the patient's progress or cure. Other patients who followed the instructions half way got half-way results. Many patients, or their relatives, for a variety of reasons, did not even attempt to follow Cayce's suggestions. Some were unable, some had no faith in his prescriptions, and many were advised not to by skeptical physicians with whom they consulted.

Over the years, when the Association has tried to follow up with letters and questionnaires, the response has been very poor. In most of the cases, we do not know whether or not the reading was followed, or whether or not the desired results were obtained. This is most unfortunate, because many of the patients for whom the readings were given have died or are getting old. The number grows smaller each year.

Despite this lack of "wholehearted cooperation," enough patients did report their experiences to enable us to make some tentative judgment relative to the success of the treatments. Cayce's statement holds up very well. Where there was cooperation, "changes for the better were wrought as promised."

Conclusions

If Edgar Cayce had been right about nothing, we could dismiss him easily; but the more his readings are researched and tried in the clinic, the more impressive this data becomes. There is a lifetime of exciting inquiry for all of us if we will but accept the challenge of the tremendously productive life of this man.

He said, "To be sure, these interpretations would not be accepted by some as an explanation. And yet there will come those days when many will understand and interpret properly." (3075-1, M. 24)

Mental illness is our number one health problem. It may well be that Edgar Cayce has provided us with the basic information which is essential to the understanding that we need and do not have.

In any event, he was a man who set an example worthy of being followed, for he was dedicated to relieving the suffering of his brothers. He said, "Communicate then, in prayer, in meditation, in thoughtfulness—not as to how ye may be this or that but as to how ye may do this or that for thy Maker, for thy fellow man." (3691-1)

Cayce also said, "So does it behoove every soul to so live and so act, in its contacts with its fellow man in its business and commercial life, that it will not be afraid to stand on the corner and watch self pass by—in relationship to its activities with its fellow man." (531-1)

These quotes sum up Edgar Cayce's formula for good mental health. He puts it into a single sentence with which I will close. "Keep the eye single to a service for *spiritual* understanding, and a mental aberration. . .may not touch thee!" (1442-1, M. 14)

James C. Windsor, Ph.D.

Bibliography

1. Brozier, Mary A.B., *The Central Nervous System and Behavior,* Madison Printing Company, 1959.

2. Cayce, Edgar, *Readings,* A.R.E. Library, Virginia Beach, Va., 1945, 1971.

3. Deutsch and Deutsch, *Physiological Psychology,* The Dorsey Press, Homewood, Ill., 1966.

4. Gantt, W.A., *Physiological Bases of Psychiatry,* Charles C. Thomas Press, Springfield, Ill., 1958.

5. Greenfield, N.S. and Lewis, W.C., *Psychoanalysis and Current Biological Thought,* University of Wisconsin Press, 1965.

6. Harlow and Woolsey (eds.), *Biological and Biochemical Bases of Behavior,* University of Wisconsin Press, 1958.

7. Hebb, Donald Olding, *The Organization of Behavior,* Wiley-Interscience, New York, 1949.

8. Hebb, Donald Olding, *A Textbook of Psychology* (2nd ed.), W.B. Saunders Company, Philadelphia, 1966.

9. London, P. and Rosenhan, D., *Foundations of Abnormal Psychology,* Holt, Rinehart and Winston, Inc., New York, 1968.

10. McGarey, W.A., M.D., "Edgar Cayce and the Palma Christi," *The A.R.E. Journal,* Vol. II, No. 2, April, 1967.

11. Morgan, Clifford, *Physiological Psychology* (3rd ed.), McGraw-Hill, New York, 1965.

12. Pauling, Linus, "Orthomolecular Psychiatry," *Science,* American Association for the Advancement of Science, Washington, D.C., 19 April, 1968, Vol. 160, No. 3825.

13. Rinkel, Max (ed.), *Chemical Concepts of Psychosis,* McDowell/Obolensky, New York, 1958.

14. Roessler, Robert, and Greenfield, Norman (eds.), *Physiological Correlates of Psychological Disorder,* University of Wisconsin Press, Madison, 1962.

15. Sheer, Daniel E. (ed.), *Electrical Stimulation of the Brain,* University of Texas Press, Austin, 1961.

16. Stearn, Jess, *Edgar Cayce—The Sleeping Prophet,* Bantam Books, Inc., 1967.

17. Sternbach, Richard, *Principles of Psychophysiology,* Academic Press, New York, 1966.

18. Wooley, D.W., *The Biochemical Bases of Psychoses,* John Wiley and Sons, Inc., New York, 1962.

MIGRAINE HEADACHES

We all know of people who have had sudden, violent attacks of headaches that may or may not be associated with visual or gastro-intestinal disturbances. What causes them is unknown. Some theories on cause include allergy, swelling of the pituitary or other endocrine disturbances, vasomotor disturbances, reflex irritations, duodenal stasis, cerebral edema, toxins. None has been supported by clinical studies. There is some evidence that symptoms are related `to functional disturbances of circulation in the cranium. Flashes of light, paresthesia, hemianopsia are due to vasoconstriction, vasodilation, head pain due to extra cranial arteries (dura, scalp).

Headache is usually the presenting symptom. It may be preceded by a short period of depression, irritability, restlessness, anorexia, scintillating scotomas, visual field defects, or paresthesias. These symptoms may disappear soon after the headache appears or may persist. Pain is usually generalized but frequently it is localized to one side of the head. Nausea, vomiting, and photophobia are common during the attack. The arms and legs are cold and cyanosed, and the patient is irritable and desires seclusion. Arteries on the head are prominent, and their pulsations increased. The headaches may last for hours or days. Frequency of attacks may vary from daily to once in several weeks, months, or years. (Cf. *Merck Manual*.)

I. Physiological Considerations

A basic etiologic relationship exists among all cases of migraine headaches. There are many kinds of headaches which may arise from many sources. Most of them, Cayce said, begin from congestion in the colon which causes pressures on the sympathetic nerve centers and the cerebrospinal system indicating distress somewhere in the body.

Each reading respresents an individual case, though there is a cause-and-effect similarity in all of them. In most instances, factors of a physiological nature are related to the migraine for which corrective suggestions were made.

In examining the readings, one finds statements such as these:

The blood supply. . .carries in same the effects of disturbances through the activity of the glands, making for disorders in the eliminations. . .[the blood lacks] sufficient oxygen to purify the whole bloodstream. . .to create the proper resistances. . .

As to the nervous system. . .incoordinations between the mental reaction and the physical forces of the body. . .

The organs of the body show their disturbances through the glands' activity. . .[through] the lung supply or blood activity and in the heart's action. . .also in the digestive system. . .Inability for the proper assimilations. . .   **739-1**

. . .in the nervous system which causes severe attacks of headaches. . .

The blood supply indicates a taxation in the nervous system as well as poor eliminations.

These. . .affect the digestive forces by the natural *abnormal* conditions of the stomach itself.

. . .pressures arising—through the pneumogastric and hypogastric nerve plexus, through the secondary cardiac plexus and combined with the vagus nervous system—that produce. . .disturbances through the temples, sometimes the eyes. . .top of the head. These are *severe* reactions. . .that are reflexed in the activity of the digestive and assimilating system.   1567-1

. . .in such a manner until the nervous forces of the body and the reactions of the digestive system do give disturbances to the body in many ways.

This as we find was primarily a glandular disturbance. . .

However, the primary cause lies in a subluxation. . .through the lumbar and sacral area.

Thus we have sick headaches. . .distress is caused both from the cerebrospinal and the nervous system.

There is a form of nervous indigestion. . .making for the slowness with which the digestive forces have acted or have emptied. . .

The blood supply indicates nervous strain. . .the catabolism. . .is naturally upset. . .through the digestive forces more than the metabolism of the body.

However, the metabolism is under stress. . .there has not been the correct coordination of the circulatory forces through the lungs, the heart, the liver and the kidneys.   **1651-1**

. . .the conditions to which the body becomes allergic in the digestive system should be looked for—that deal with all migraine headaches.
. . .it is in the digestive system, causing—through a state of circulation—an inflammation in the connections of the intestinal tract through which blood and nerve supply bring nutriment and activity to those portions of the body.
3326-1

After examining the readings, one realizes that the various organs and systems of the body are not functioning normally. These incoordinations include assimilation and elimination, sympathetic nerve centers and the central nervous system, blood supply, and spinal column. These disorders or imbalances may be precipitated by gastrointestinal allergies or subluxation in the lumbosacral spine. The results are the development of nervous indigestion, visual disturbances, altered assimilations and eliminations, irritability, restlessness which are signs that the body is upset and one has a migraine headache.

II. Rationale of Therapy

To Cayce, there was no incurable ailment—there were only "incurable" people: The patient had to be ready and the therapist knowledgeable. He was familiar with migraine headaches, and where many thought these the result of a nervous, tense disposition, the readings noted this was again only the symptom, not the cause. We should remember that the body has a capability of normal function.

. . .we would administer those activities which would bring a normal reaction through these portions, stimulating them to an activity from the body itself, rather than the body becoming dependent upon supplies that are robbing portions of the system to produce activity in other portions, or the system receiving elements or chemical reactions being supplied without arousing the activity of the system itself for a more normal condition.
1968-3

Thus these conditions taken in these beginnings may be eradicated entirely from the system; but the taking of sedatives of any form only adds fire to the condition. True, it may ease for the moment, but it requires continued excesses of same that involve the gastric flow even of other portions of the

system. However, if the correct applications are made, the causes of the condition may be removed.   3326-1

As we find, these may be builded back to near normal manner, if there is the consistent and persistent effort on the part of the body, but necessitating the applications—in a consistent and persistent manner—that may in the beginning appear to be aggravating rather than allaying.

But if there is the persistency, we will find we may be able to remove those inclinations for the lack of coordination in the nerve reflexes and the nerve impulses, and through same stimulate the circulation to a more normal activity.

And thus through the foods or the diets apply those necessary elements for the creating of a balance in the chemical reactions of the system as between the sodas, the potashes—or the alkalinity and the acidity—and the reactions for the body of the ability for replenishing itself.   1476-2

Therapy must be directed at restoring proper functioning of the body, through the following measures:

1. First, x-ray the colon and find areas in the ascending and transverse colon where fecal forces are as cakes.

2. Have colonic irrigations.

3. Use a radio-active appliance along with an hour of meditation for self-analysis.

4. Get osteopathic adjustments to relax the neck area, the sixth dorsal, the mid-back, and in the lower back, the lumbar axis.

5. Correct the diet.

The readings felt that patients needed more than physical advice—and they were counseled: Keep the mental attitude of a useful, purposeful life, using the abilities to be helpful to others. Stop complaining.

Migraine could be cured if the sufferer cleansed himself, got osteopathic adjustments of the spine, and improved general mental attitude; for that builded, that held in the mental image becomes the condition.

III. Suggested Therapeutic Regimen

In the manner of the diet: Beware of *any* character of food that even creates a great quantity of alcohol, or of *any* alcohol. . .Those drinks with a little charged water would be very well—as Coca-Cola or Orangeade or the

like, if taken once or twice a day; for their reaction upon the system as related to especially the hepatic or the kidney *and* liver circulation would be good.

Beware of starches or combinations of starches that produce the excesses.

Let this be rather as an outline, though not *just* these foods taken—but foods of these natures:

Mornings—citrus fruit juices, or whole wheat cereals—as Maltex or Crushed Wheat, that are well, *well* cooked (but do not combine cereals *and* citrus fruits at the same meal!). These may be altered at times also with stewed fruits; as figs, the pieplant, or tomato juice. . .all of these should be taken at one time or another. Coffee may be taken if it is desired, with brown toast at the meal—but *without* cream or milk in same!

Noons—preferably have as a portion of same only raw vegetables combined together. Vegetable juices may be taken at this time. The shellfish may be taken at this time, in their various forms.

Evenings—only the vegetables and meats that are well cooked and well balanced. No fried foods at any time. The meats should consist principally of fish, fowl or lamb. Have three vegetables above the ground to one below the ground.

1476-2

Here, with this body, it would require sufficient colonic irrigations, scientifically given, to keep the colon cleansed for a period sufficient for reaction of the body energies themselves in supplying nutriment to the folds in the colon itself.

This extends and becomes much more active in the jejunum (this is speaking universally now, not in this individual case) but its beginnings are in the area (as in this particular body) of the caecum—where the jejunum empties into the colon for further digestion and absorption by body forces.

Hence with this body, to be sure, throughout these periods keep away from excesses of sweets, especially chocolate and any sedimentary forces (such as brans or as raisins). Prunes will work just the opposite, for these carry another form of activity to the walls of the system itself. It would be well to include prunes in the diet, if they are cooked—or even fresh. Plums of all natures, then, are very well to be taken.

Certain forms of apples are well, but most of these for this body through these periods should be cooked.

Watercress, especially, should be taken—and these raw; including celery and lettuce; at times carrots. All of these grated and combined with the gelatin would be much better for the body.

Do drink plenty of water, at least six to eight glasses of water each day.

Do have sufficient enemas, scientifically given, to cleanse all mucus from the body. This may be done each time the colonic is given. So put them about ten days to two weeks apart, and there should be required at least four or five of these.

During that same period, relax the body osteopathically; with special reference to reducing a lesion that exists between the sixth and seventh dorsal.

Do these, being mindful of the diet, and we will correct conditions for this body. These are the sources of migraine headaches. 3326-1

Ray O. Bjork, M.D.

Edgar Cayce readings referenced:
739-1
1476-2
1567-1, 3
1651-1
1689-1
1807-1 through 6
1904-1
2078-1, 3
3047-1
3169-1
3326-1
3329-1
5052-1
5111-1
5200-1

MULTIPLE SCLEROSIS

In the Edgar Cayce material a total of 100 readings for 69 separate persons have been indexed to date as multiple sclerosis (see "Case Breakdown by Groups"). For the purpose of this study these 69 cases were divided into three groups on the basis of the readings themselves as well as resultant correspondence. Definite *post facto* diagnosis was made difficult in most cases by inadequate medical history, lack of description of disease symptoms, and sparsity of follow-up reports. In some readings multiple sclerosis or simply "a sclerosis condition" was mentioned by name as the basis of the condition, but in most cases a description of the etiology and treatments was the only information given.

Group I contains 34 cases in which the diagnosis was most certain and could be considered possible. In these readings the condition was named, a medical history with diagnosis was supplied in the correspondence (sometimes before and sometimes after the reading), or there was some detailed description of the symptoms, such as spotty motor and sensory loss, remissive course, evidence of multiple lesions, etc. Group II contains 22 cases in which the diagnosis was less certain and could only be considered possible because no description or diagnosis was given other than that there was some trouble with motor or sensory function. In other cases in Group II, the reading alone mentioned the diagnosis or an etiology suggestive of the condition without any external confirmatory evidence. Group III contains 13 cases in which the diagnosis did not seem to be multiple sclerosis as ascertained from the correspondence and/or readings. In many cases it was probably something else (in the majority of cases, as Parkinson's disease).

It should be noted, however, that even in Group I where a diagnosis of multiple sclerosis was assumed as probable, not enough information was available to make a satisfactory and certain medical decision in differential diagnosis. In no case was there an autopsy report to confirm the diagnosis. Therefore, a limitation which was imposed by the nature of the data must be acknowledged at the outset.

In addition to the 56 cases in Groups I and II (comprising 80 readings), one reading (907-1) was given on the etiology of multiple sclerosis at the request of Charles Goodman Taylor, M.D. Specific questions about etiology and treatment were answered. In consideration of the material, the data from reading 907-1 was weighted more heavily in constructing a theory of the disease as seen from the viewpoint of the Edgar Cayce readings than the material from the 56 cases of Groups I and II (not all of which can be presumed with certainty to have been multiple sclerosis).

I. Etiology and Pathology

In an attempt to construct a unified theory of etiological and pathological physiology of multiple sclerosis, reading 907-1 (as explained above) was used as a basis and supplemented by data found in the case readings. Both agreements and contradictions will be pointed out in the following discussion.

The basic mechanism stated was that multiple sclerosis was a result of a lack of gold which caused a glandular imbalance, in turn resulting in a hormonal deficiency or imbalance, disturbing proper functioning of the nerves.

Reading 907-1 indicated that the normal balance of metals in the system was out of equilibrium primarily due to a lack of gold. In 40 out of 56 cases in Groups I and II (71.5%) gold was mentioned as a factor which needed to be added to the system. Gold deficiency was tied to a defect in the assimilating system (by this was probably meant the digestive system) which in turn was kept in proper working order by hormones from the glands. Because the glands were in turn dependent upon the proper amount of gold in the system, this would apparently lead to a circular feedback relationship between gold, the glands, and the assimilating system. Though not explicitly stated, it could be assumed that the disease was not caused from simply a lack of gold in the diet, but perhaps from a lack of the capacity of the digestive system to assimilate gold or perhaps inability of the body to use the gold assimilated. In reading 907-1 a genetic factor was suggested as the underlying cause of the imbalance between these three factors: gold, glands, and assimilation.

In connection with the genetic factor, a lack of the normal balance of metals in the system may be discovered in the male by lack of sperm (i.e., some degree of sterility). However, it was not clear whether this was simply a decreased sperm count or a decreased potency due to a lack of metals, most notably gold, in the sperm. There is no medical data to confirm the theory that sterility is a result of multiple sclerosis. However, impotence, priapism, and/or increased sexual excitability have all been reported.

Some types of glandular disturbance was mentioned in 30 out of the 56 cases in Groups I and II (53.6%). However, a clear and consistent statement of the details is lacking. In reading 907-1 the question, "Which glands are involved?" was answered by, "Those about the liver and gall duct." The only glands in that anatomical neighborhood are the Islets of Langerhans, in the pancreas and possibly the adrenals. Perhaps the lymph nodes around the liver and gall duct are indicated, but no specific hormone-producing function is known for them. In some cases the liver, pancreas, and spleen were mentioned as if they were "glands." (1623, 1031) The liver was said to enable other glands to function normally, presumably by production of a substance which affected the glands. (3275) A thyroid and liver balance was described in case [1031]. The adrenals were mentioned in [2564] in regard to the effect of mental attitude.

However, the readings were not clear in their description of the exact relation of the liver to the pathologic process in multiple sclerosis. Reading 907-1 mentioned the excretory function of the liver as an aid in the assimilation of food in cooperation with the pancreas. (See also cases [1623] and [3907].) This presumably would be the production of bile which aids in the digestion of fats which are absorbed in the small intestine through the lacteals. Other readings mentioned the relation between the liver and the glands and also implied that there were glands within the liver itself. (2983, 3306) One lobe of the liver was said to have been softened (5238), and a whitening in the liver was described (2997). Thus the exact relationship of the liver, glands in the liver, and other glands remains unclear.

The glandular disturbance, which the readings indicated in a general way was caused by an imbalance between the digestive system, the amount of gold in the body, and the function of the liver, was repeatedly linked to malfunctioning of the nervous system. The lacking hormone was not named nor was this substance's action upon nervous tissues spelled out in a detailed way. This substance missing from the glands was supposed to be a nutrient to nerve tissue, and the nerves were repeatedly said to lack proper balance of energy or "stamina." (e.g., 1031, 1865, 2983)

Reading 907-1 stated that this lack of nervous energy caused a poison to form in certain nerve cells, and that other surrounding cells were then poisoned. A description was given of the pulling apart and elongation of originally round cells, whose location or name was not given. These could be presumed to be either neurons or microglial cells, but the latter is more probable because microglial cells when stimulated by degeneration myelin do become bipolar and migratory in their action as macrophages. Perhaps this was the same process referred to in case [1865] in which the hormonal lack was said to cause a breakdown of the cellular forces in the nerve walls leading to an inflammation and irritation via an action on the nerve plexuses and ganglia between the central and the autonomic nervous systems. This breakdown of nerve "walls," coupled with a description of wasting away or dissolving of the nerves [907] could be taken as a pathological loss of myelin sheath or white matter in multiple sclerosis, although such an explicit identification was not given in the readings. In fact, a lack of gray matter was mentioned in case [3626]. Pathologically there is damage to both the "white" myelin sheath and the "gray" axon in this disease, although demyelinization is usually commoner and occurs first. In the pathology of multiple sclerosis the loss of myelin is most obvious in the spinal cord and brain.

The location of the nerve plexuses and ganglia *between* the central and autonomic nervous systems is more difficult to speculate about. Again, it would be most reasonable to assume the anatomical location to be in the spinal cord and/or brain probably where the autonomic preganglionic fibers join the central nervous system.

In the readings some other etiological factors were mentioned. Reading 907-1 indicated that a genetic factor formed the basis for the development of the disease, but no more specific information was given. A genetic influence could possibly affect the process described above at many points (e.g., the assimilative system, the liver, the glands, the nervous system itself) and in many ways (biochemical processes, structural defects). The effect of mental attitude upon the functioning of the glands was mentioned in two cases, [2564] and [2994]. Some type of spinal injury was described in 11 out of the 56 cases in Groups I and II. However, no mention was made of this in 907-1. Therefore, the described faulty alignment of the vertebral column can be presumed to have been a coincidental occurrence etiologically unrelated to the disease itself.

An explicit denial was made that an infectious agent was responsible for multiple sclerosis. An infection in the gall duct area was described in case [1623], but it was stated that this was an effect and not the cause of the basic condition. The only other case which mentioned infection (in the glands) was [3306].

In summary, it must be said that equilibrium between organs and systems was emphasized. Some factors which are not part of current medical knowledge about the disease were mentioned: A glandular imbalance caused the lack of a hormonal substance which acted in cells in the nervous system to form a poison which was responsible for the pathological process in the spinal cord and brain. The glandular imbalance was caused both by a lack of gold and by lack of a substance produced by the liver. All three of these factors were said to be interdependent and associated with the assimilative system. A genetic factor was also mentioned, but a more exact description of where and how it came to bear on the disease process was not spelled out. An infectious agent was explicitly denied. It is apparent that the general nature of most of these suggestions raises more questions than they answer.

II. Discussion of Treatment

In an analysis of the various treatments recommended in the 56 cases of Groups I and II the most consistent and frequent emphasis was on three main types: addition of the atomic effect of gold through the use of the wet cell battery, massage, and diet.

The atomic effect of gold was said to be necessary for the glandular production of the hormone which maintained the proper structural condition and functioning of the nerves (see above). However, gold was not to be added directly to the system by ingestion or injection, but vibratorily through the use of the wet cell battery. Essentially, the wet cell was a weak battery composed of two poles (one copper and one nickel) suspended in a solution containing a specific mixture of copper sulfate, dilute sulphuric acid, zinc, and willow charcoal. A wire from the nickel pole was suspended in a solution of gold chloride and then attached to the body via a nickel plate three inches in diameter. The copper pole was wired to the body via a copper plate one inch in diameter. The readings indicated that the vibration given from the gold in solution would be electrically transmitted into the body and have the glandular effect described above. Reading 1800-6 (concerning the theory of the wet cell) suggested that the vibration did not act directly, but only enabled other elements (perhaps gold already in the body in an inactive form) to become active and have the desired effect.

In the multiple sclerosis readings other elements were suggested for use with the wet cell (e.g., iodine trichloride, silver nitrate, spirits of camphor), but gold chloride was by far the most frequent recommendation (the wet cell was given for 42 out of the 56 cases—75%—and gold chloride was to be used in 39 of these—69.6%). The percentage is even higher in Group I where the wet cell was recommended in 28 out of 34 cases—82.4%—and gold chloride in 26 out of 34—76.6%. However, in as many as 10 cases iodine trichloride was used on alternate days instead of the gold chloride in the solution jar. Spirits of camphor was advised in 13 cases in the same manner and sometimes all three solutions were to be used in a three-day series.

The nickel plate was to be placed on what the readings called the umbilical and lacteal duct center which was located on the right upper quadrant of the abdomen at a point over the distal end of the duct of the gall bladder. The position was individually specified in relation to the umbilicus (e.g., two to four finger breadths to the right and two to four finger breadths toward the right costal margin). Various locations along the spine were given for the copper plate but the most frequent were between the ninth and tenth thoracic vertebrae (18 out of 56 cases—32.2%) and at the level of the fourth lumbar (18 cases out of 56).

The wet cell was to be "recharged" (i.e., new solutions added) every 30 days and to be used each day for 30 to 60 minutes. The best time seemed to be before retiring at night, but this was not an absolute rule.

The use of the wet cell and more specifically with the gold solution was a fairly consistent recommendation in the readings. However, the details as to use were varied. The position of the umbilical and lacteal plexus seemed to vary from person to person as did the proper placement of the upper plate on the spine. The strength of the gold chloride solution varied between one and two grains per ounce of distilled water. The amount of concentrated sulphuric acid varied between one and one-and-a-half ounces. Sometimes willow charcoal was advised to be added to the wet cell and sometimes not. The length of treatment varied between 30 and 60 minutes per day. As has been shown above, sometimes iodine trichloride and/or spirits of camphor were also suggested for use in the solution jar. In 6 cases (5073, 5108, 5129, 5238, 5324, 5403) the wet cell without the solution jar was to be slow charged (not over three amperes input) before use as a lead storage battery would be, but in most cases "recharging" meant changing the solutions. These six readings (all given between May and August, 1944) also recommended that a glass-stoppered bottle containing two or three ounces of tincture of iodine was to be suspended in the wet cell acid solution while it was being electrically charged and remain there also when the appliance was being used.

The following quote is presented as a general example of the description of the use of the wet cell and also as a clarification for this seeming exception to the usual use (as described in the other multiple sclerosis readings).

In the applications, then: we would begin first by having prepared the low wet cell appliance that will carry to the body vibratorially certain elements and properties which are the basic influence in the activity of the gland and blood and nerve supply to the body, and taken through these means or channels may be assimilated by the body, with the activities of the digestive forces to either the sympathetic or cerebrospinal nervous systems or blood supply, or without creating a taxation to any of the central organs of the body.

We would prepare this with the two pounds of the copper sulphate and the rest of the ingredients in proportion.

We would make the chloride of gold solution one grain to one ounce of distilled water, using 3 ounces of the solution at a time. This would be changed (the solution), as would the recharging of the appliance, every 30 days. This also would be an appliance in which there would be the charging of the appliance with the solutions to charge; that is, making the appliance in the manner indicated, then suspend in the solution 3 ounces of the tincture of iodine. Preferably have the bottle with a glass stopper, this suspended and then put on a battery charge, slow battery charge, and let it be charged for one hour. Then the solutions would be given.

The larger plate would be attached always to the umbilical and lacteal duct plexus, which on this body would be the width of 4 fingers from the navel center to the right, and 2 fingers up from that point. And attach the larger plate which passes through the gold solution, see? The Atomidine or iodine solution is already in the appliance, so only the gold as a solution is to be given vibratorially to the body. For the rest goes with the gold solution.

The small plate should be attached to the lumbar axis, see? Fourth lumbar axis. This is to be taken each day for 30 minutes.   5108-1

Interestingly, in these six cases iodine trichloride was never suggested to be used in the solution jar alternately with the gold chloride as described above in ten cases. Thus, some form of iodine was suggested as part of the wet cell treatment in 16 out of the 56 cases. (28.6%) In other cases where neither of these iodine therapies was recommended, iodine trichloride by mouth was suggested in six cases and seafood as a source of iodine in the diet, in eight others. Thus, in 30 out of 56 cases (53.6%), some form of iodine was recommended in the treatment.

A thorough massage of the body especially the spine and extremities was suggested in 48 out of the 56 cases—85.6% (28 out of the 34 cases in Group I—82.4%)—and usually followed the daily use of the wet cell. In all but two of the cases the massage was to be done with a variety of mixtures of oils. These mixtures have been classified into two types: the simple (31 out of 56 cases—57.2%) and the complex (14 out of 56 cases—25.0%). The simple mixture was usually a combination of equal parts of olive oil and peanut oil plus melted lanolin in the following ratio: two ounces of olive oil, two ounces of peanut oil, one-quarter ounce of lanolin. The complex mixture usually used an olive oil base plus peanut oil, various combinations and amounts of Russian white oil, oil of cedarwood, oil of sassafras root, oil of pine needles, Nujol, lanolin, oil of wintergreen, tincture of benzoin, tincture of myrrh, witch hazel, spirits of camphor, spirits of turpentine, mutton suet, and/or oil of mustard. The most frequently used oils in the complex group were the first seven in the preceding list.

The directions for the massage were as varied as were the different combinations of oils. In the majority of cases it was suggested to massage from the spine to the distal portions of the extremities, but in some from the tips of the extremities to the spine. Although the spine and extremities were mentioned most, the chest and abdomen were also suggested. When it was specified, a circular motion for the massage was recommended.

The use of massage is one of the current medical treatments (as supportive therapy) for multiple sclerosis and certainly helps to maintain the tone of muscles which have lost their normal innervation. The advantage is that, when and if function returns (e.g., after one of the characteristic spontaneous remissions in the disease), the muscle will not have atrophied and shortened. The Cayce readings implied that the various oils used in massaging would be absorbed by the skin and somehow aid the healing process. From the standpoint of modern medical knowledge the oils would mainly perform a lubricative function and thus aid in making the massage more easy to perform. Certain of the oils might stimulate circulation in the skin. In the readings from 1941 to 1944 (during World War II) the simple mixture was almost always suggested. This may have been because certain of the ingredients used in the various complex mixtures may have been difficult to obtain. However, the simple mixture would probably serve the lubricative function as well as the complex.

Diet recommendations were given in 43 out of 56 cases. (76.8%) The diet in general was alkaline-reacting, non-constipating and low-fat in nature. Foods containing B vitamins were stressed and sometimes brewer's yeast or wheat germ was advised. Seafood, liver, wild game, and fowl were recommended as the meats to be eaten but broiled and not fried. The bones of chicken and fish were to be chewed. Fried foods were generally prohibited. Raw vegetables such as watercress, carrots, celery, beets, and salads with gelatin were stressed. Vegetables, fruits, and cereals were to be eaten much more than meat.

The relationship of the diet to the etiology of the disease is not too clear. None of the emphasized foods was designated as providing gold in any form. Seafood was explicitly mentioned as being especially important because of its iodine content. The Cayce readings elsewhere state that iodine has an effect on all the endocrine glands, not only the thyroid. The stress on the vitamin B complex was suggested as an aid to the proper functioning of the nervous system, but the relation of this to the pathologic physiology of multiple sclerosis was not spelled out.

Other treatments were recommended for a minority of the cases, such as iodine trichloride or gold chloride by mouth, the violet ray bulb applicator to the spine, or manipulation of the spine. However, these treatments occurred very infrequently in the readings compared to the three main types discussed above: wet cell with gold, massage with oils, diet.

The readings insisted many times that the treatment for multiple sclerosis had to be of long duration—three to seven years usually. The importance of completeness, continuity, and consistency as well as a hopeful mental attitude both by the patient and those who were to give the treatments were emphasized.

III. Recommendations

1. Readings about other diseases of the nervous system which resemble multiple sclerosis could be examined to see whether the etiological mechanisms or the treatments fall into any patterns similar to those suggested above. Perhaps a theory of the functioning of the nervous system as seen in the readings would emerge. These other diseases should include those considered in the differential diagnosis of multiple sclerosis, such as polio, Parkinson's disease, amyotrophic lateral sclerosis, the muscular dystrophies, pernicious anemia, Wilson's disease, and pseudosclerosis.

2. Autopsy reports in cases of multiple sclerosis could be checked for any gross or histological pathology in the liver, pancreas, or adrenals which are possible sites if the mechanisms of pathological physiology suggested by the readings are correct.

3. The action of the wet cell battery could be analyzed by biophysicists to discover whether any vibratory effect from gold chloride can be measured in the human body.

4. A controlled clinical trial of the three main types of treatment discussed above could be undertaken on a group of patients with a definitely established diagnosis of multiple sclerosis. The trial should be supervised by qualified physicians with a thorough system of record keeping and standardized methods for objective measurements of the condition of the patients at regular intervals. The normal course of the disease makes any clinical trial very difficult because of the occurrence of temporary, spontaneous remissions and the long duration of the disease—sometimes for 20 years with only slow progress. The study would have to be carried on for at least three to five years. The time required each day for the wet cell and massage (about two hours) to be given for three to five years to a large enough number of patients to make the trial statistically significant would involve considerable persistence and manpower. In this regard it might be noted that only an exceptional patient who got Cayce readings for multiple sclerosis consistently received the wet cell and massage treatment for more than six months and most of them for much less time before giving up (at least as can be judged from the reports received).

With the possibility of such a clinical trial in mind, the following treatment outline has been prepared. The treatment represents an attempt to abstract from the many readings given for individuals with their peculiar needs a general or average treatment. The broad outline of the treatment into three main types occurred repeatedly and fairly consistently. However, as pointed out in the "Discussion of Treatment" section above, the details of each type were varied to a greater or lesser degree for each case. For the purpose of an experimental clinical trial, a somewhat artificial "average" treatment has been abstracted.

IV. Treatment Outline

1. Wet cell appliance: The following ingredients should be added to one-and-a-half gallons of distilled water: two pounds of copper sulphate, one ounce of concentrated sulphuric acid, 30 grams of zinc, one-half pound of willow charcoal. The gold chloride solution should be made in the strength of one grain to one ounce of distilled water and three ounces of this solution should be used at a time in the solution jar through which the nickel pole lead passes before being attached to the nickel plate on the body. The solutions should be changed every 30 days.

The wet cell should be used for 45 minutes each day (preferably in the evening) in the following manner: The three-inch nickel plate should be lightly sandpapered and then taped to the right upper quadrant of the abdomen at a point which would correspond to the location of the distal end of the duct of the gall bladder. (This position would be somewhere between two to four finger breadths to the right of the umbilicus and two to four finger breadths toward the right costal margin.) The one-inch copper plate should be similarly placed on the spine between the ninth and tenth thoracic vertebrae one day and at the level of the fourth lumbar the next day.

2. Massage: Immediately after the wet cell treatment each day the body should receive a thorough massage with a mixture of oils in the following ration: two ounces of olive oil, two ounces of peanut oil, and one-fourth ounce of melted lanolin. The massage should start with the base of the skull and work down the spine and paravertebral areas to the distal ends of the extremities. The massage should be done with a circular motion. No more than an hour should be required for the massage.

3. Diet: The diet which was specifically emphasized is outlined in the "Discussion of Treatment" section above.

V. Conclusions

This report has been a preliminary step in the study of Edgar Cayce readings given for multiple sclerosis. An attempt has been made to organize the data, which appears in a somewhat confusing language and terminology, into an understandable pattern. With the reservation that all the cases classed in Groups I and II actually may not have been multiple sclerosis, the majority of the cases seemed to indicate a complex although only generally stated etiological theory. The majority fell into a tripartite scheme of treatment. Here again the broad outlines were consistent, but the details varied from case to case. No conclusions can be drawn about the validity of either the etiological theory or the treatment program from the results of this study. Many questions are raised on the one hand because of the generality and vagueness of many statements in the readings, and on the other because of specific mechanisms and treatments which are not substantiated by modern medical science. A study such as this can only hope to give hints and point the direction for further research which perhaps may help to unravel some of the present unknowns in the etiology and treatment of multiple sclerosis.

Walter N. Pahnke, M.D.

The Most Common Types of Etiology and Treatment

Classified According to Frequency of Occurrence in the 56 Cases of
Groups I and II

Items Specifically Mentioned in Readings:	Group I (34 cases)		Group II (22 cases)		Total Percent (56 cases)	
Etiology:		%		%		%
1. Glandular disturbance or hormonal imbalance	19	56.0	11	50.0	30	53.6
2. Lack of the effect of gold (mentioned directly or implied by treatments)	26	76.6	14	63.1	40	71.5
3. Liver misfunction	5	14.4	4	18.4	9	16.1
4. Assimilative problem	6	17.4	5	22.8	11	19.6
Treatment:						
1. Wet cell appliance	28	82.4	14	63.7	42	75.0
a. Using in the solution jar:						
1. Gold chloride........	26	76.6	13	59.1	39	69.6
2. Spirits of camphor ...	10	29.4	3	13.7	13	23.2
3. Iodine trichloride (Atomidine)	7	20.6	3	13.7	10	17.9
b. Slow charging with tincture of iodine in glass bottle suspended in the acid solution	5	14.4	1	4.6	6	10.7
c. Placement of electrodes on body						
1. Nickel—on umbilical and lacteal duct plexus	28	82.4	14	63.7	42	75.0
2. Copper—using lead passing through gold chloride solution						
a) Level of ninth to tenth thoracic vertebrae.........	13	38.2	5	22.8	18	32.2
b) Level of fourth lumbar vertebrae ..	13	38.2	5	22.8	18	32.2

2. Massage:	28	82.4	20	90.9	48	85.6
a. No oil	0		2	9.0	2	3.6
b. Simple mixture	20	58.8	12	54.6	32	57.2
c. Complex mixture	8	23.6	6	27.2	14	25.0
3. Diet	26	76.6	17	77.4	43	76.8
Cases in which a source of iodine by mouth was mentioned, but in which no iodine via wet cell was recommended.	8	23.6	6	27.2	14	25.0
a. Seafood	5	14.4	3	13.7	8	14.3
b. Iodine trichloride (Atomidine)	3	8.8	3	13.7	6	10.7

Edgar Cayce readings referenced by Groups:

Group I: 34 cases		*Group II:* 22 cases	*Group III:* 13 cases
1623	4048	464	1119
1865	5031	1031	1555
2159	5073	1199	1571
2453	5108	1545	1618
2983	5129	1676	1898
3041	5158	2053	1905
3093	5238	2499	3011
3118	5268	2564	3114
3124	5324	2619	3303
3151		2994	3310
3186		2997	3384
3218		3080	3491
3232		3095	5019
3275		3103	
3306		3367	
3382		3567	
3521		3602	
3612		4005	
3626		5107	
3695		5402	
3779		5403	
3907		5500	
4014			
4036			
4044			

MUSCULAR DYSTROPHY

The muscular dystrophies may be defined as a group of primary, degenerative diseases, characterized by progressive muscular wasting and weakness, and occurring usually in the first three decades of life. The muscular abnormalities are always associated with organic disturbances, varied and widespread.

Some of these myopathies are congenital in nature, the onset occurring at or shortly after birth. These appear to be genetically determined. Others are diseases of late onset. They are related to but not identical with the congenital type. The early childhood variety is associated with a pseudo-hypertrophic condition wherein the muscles apparently become larger, whereas the limb-girdle variety, usually of late onset, is more often associated with a wasting, even in the presence of myotonia.

More commonly, the muscular dystrophies are seen without the syndrome of myotonia (continuous muscular tension or contraction), but its occurrence leads to a sometimes separate classification as a myotonic disorder.

The etiology of these myopathies has remained quite obscure. Earlier studies had suggested that the muscular dystrophy patient could not regenerate his muscle cells. However, regeneration has now been demonstrated in nearly every form of muscular dystrophy. Its amount is usually dependent upon the rapidity of the disorder and the degree of inflammation. Thus, the more active the disease process, the more active the regeneration.

It becomes evident that these myopathies are not strictly diseases of the muscle tissue, if we look at the associated findings in the terms of non-muscular pathology.

A good example is dystrophia myotonica—a type of muscular dystrophy which is associated with tonicity of certain muscle groups, particularly the tongue and the thenar eminence of the hand. This condition is transmitted as an autosomal trait, thus is a chromosomal abnormality. Symptoms begin during adolescence or early adult life. Aside from the muscular involvement evidenced by disappearance of reflexes, involvement of cardiac musculature in 80% of the cases, loss of sternocleidomastoid and mastication muscle function, involvement of muscles of phonation, and the profound wasting of both upper and lower extremity musculature—a large group of other findings are indicative of the widespread nature of the disease process. These non-muscular findings are common: premature baldness, posterior capsular cataracts, testicular atrophy with decrease of seminiferous tubules, disturbance of the level of corticosteroids and 17-ketosteriods, diabetes mellitus, intellectual decline, elevated protein in cerebrospinal fluid with enlarged cerebral ventricles, and a thickening of the osseous structure of the skull or a small sella turcica.

I. Physiological Considerations

The muscular dystrophies would seem to be a group of diseases in which the primary pathology is found in the muscles and is in the nature of an abnormal development or a degeneration of the muscular tissue. Throughout the readings given by Edgar Cayce, however, this disease process is seen as a primary glandular malfunction with a secondary effect on the motor nerves to the muscles, and a tertiary result in the muscular tissue which demonstrates itself as a degenerative process. The body apparently can balance itself at any given point if the conditions are right, and the different manifestations are apparently caused by the variation of glandular function throughout the body in particular individuals, plus the nature or severity of glandular malfunction which exists.

Karma—the law of cause and effect—is a major etiological factor here. This would be understandable to those who have studied the readings at any length, for the glandular centers particularly are singled out as the bearers of karma and as the seat of soul memory. It was seen as purely karmic activity for [4014], a 27-year-old woman, while for a 10-year-old boy [5078], "this is karma for both the parents and the body." Occasionally karmic causes may be associated with chemical changes within the body; sometimes with birth presentations. One case, [5064], came about as the result of injuries to the spine and the structural portions of the body, while a 57-year-old woman found her disease brought into activity not from karmic or hereditary causes, "but [from] the use of those things that set the glands to react upon themselves, that supply to the nerve force itself the energies; as would be the tensile strength taken from a wire over which impulses of electrical force might move." (3099-1)

An interesting causative factor was discussed in the case of a 34-year-old woman whose sister was also afflicted with progressive muscular dystrophy. "In analyzing the conditions here, we find much of this prenatal, yet not that which might be called the sin of the fathers, nor of the entity itself, but rather that through which patience and consistency might be the lesson for the entity in this experience." (3681-1) From the standpoint of Cayce's unconscious mind, there were then those individuals who had chosen to learn patience and consistency in this rather difficult manner. At the same time, he could foresee methods by which they could overcome the bodily disease if they chose. In yet other readings he saw the disease process too far gone to offer any promise of recovery.

The glands throughout the body are those tissues which secrete substances needed for cells to reproduce themselves in all portions of the body. When this glandular activity breaks down at any point, the rest of the body is called upon in an abnormal manner if the substances are not supplied. This imbalance then brings about a lack of nourishment and what we know as a disease process. The following perhaps best explains this in the words of the readings:

> **One should consider, as in this body, that the physical body in its creation was and is given the ability to reproduce itself. Thus each organ, each portion of the body secretes, from the physical, the mental and the spiritual life, that needed to reproduce itself for a growth to better conditions—or the realm for which it prepares itself. When these activities break down, these have to be supplied or they call on other portions of the organism—and thus they become overcharged or undernourished. Then disintegration begins in one form or another.** 3337-1

The effect of this adjustment, the lack of proper glandular function, in the nerves and the muscle tissues is to deprive the nerves of energy and to create degeneration in the muscle tissues.

> **As we find, the disturbances here are of the progressive nature; that is, the condition has become constitutional, in that the body adjusts itself in many ways to the weaknesses and these continue to sap the vitality and strength**

from the nerves that control the tendons and muscles of the locomotories. This is indicated in the lower limbs as well as, now, beginning in the arms; and gradually, unless retarded, there will be the rolling up or folding up of the body-forces in *any* attempt to use the body muscular forces.   3099-1

For, the nerves are but the wires to the body forces themselves. And, through lack of generative power within the system, or the glands from which the secretions are taken for the continuing of strength in same, these become as burned wires, or cords, or threads through the body, and gradually fail to supply muscular forces, or the strength to the muscles and tendons through which these nerve energies pass.   3099-1

This condition is becoming quite progressive in that there is not the ability left in the nerves and muscular forces for the use of the limbs. Even the activities of organs are becoming involved so as not to be able to control them through the nerve energies.   3337-1

These three extracts point out that the real underlying pathology in these conditions which have been called muscular dystrophy is a malfunction of the glands of the body which create the energies and forces that pass through the nerve supply to the muscular tissue. The glands involved are those which secrete substances which allow reproduction and normal growth of nervous tissue, especially that nervous tissue dealing with locomotory activity. As the disease progresses, we see then "more of atrophy of the nerves which control the muscular forces of the body." (5078-1) Whereas the pathology becomes most noticeable and disabling in the muscles, yet we also recognize that a side effect of the primary disease process is a malfunctioning of organs throughout the body. These in turn finally break down under lack of proper nerve energies and the entire body thus becomes involved.

It is not clear from the readings what mechanism brings about the glandular malfunction, nor is it clear specifically where all these glands are located.

The nature of the affliction, however, has become clarified, as to the successive steps in the etiology of the muscular dystrophies.

II. Rationale of Therapy

In approaching therapy, we should remember that the body has a capability of normal function:

Thus, we would administer those activities which would bring a normal reaction through these portions, stimulating them to an activity from the body itself, rather than the body becoming dependent upon supplies that are robbing portions of the system to produce activity in other portions, or the system receiving elements or chemical reactions being supplied without arousing the activity of the system itself for a more normal condition.

1968-3

Therapy for the muscular dystrophies must be divided basically into two sections. The reason for this can be found in the preceding section, where karma seems to play such an important part in the causation. The difference between karmically induced illness and a disease on a different etiologic basis might be theorized as a difference in the degree of chromosomal changes or—if chromosomes are not deeply involved—the disease process in karmic conditions certainly involves the entity deeply at a physical, mental, and spiritual level. "Thus individuals must consider the whole entity when considering those things that would be helpful. Thus one must begin with the spiritual attitude of the entity toward life." (4014-1) This rather clearly points out the first area toward which therapy should be directed when this disease is karmic. We have no way of determining at the present time where karma is involved. Thus each case must be approached with this particular factor in mind. A prayerful attitude, as a constant activity, would be necessary for those who are responsible for the ill person.

At a physical level therapy should be directed at the three areas which have already been suggested as the site of pathology. The glands which control the rebuilding of the energies of the nervous system; the nerves themselves which probably suffer the most; and the muscle tissue which wastes away as a result of the other activities—all these need help. It is to be assumed that correction of the function of the first two named would lead to a restoration of normal function of the disturbed organs which may or may not be present in any particular case.

Keeping all these factors in mind, then, the following steps should be followed in arriving at a comprehensive therapeutic approach to the muscular dystrophies:

1. Begin with the spiritual attitude of the entity toward life.

Life itself is a manifestation of that called God in the earth. Give thanks for

the very fact that ye are conscious of yourself, even with the frailties of the body; that thy mind and thy purposes and thy hands may do much to show the appreciation in self of the opportunity in this experience to be a channel of blessings to others, in making known to others the love of the Christ for those who are weak in body, who are hindered from the activities of a normal physical world.

For He, thy God, thy Christ, is conscious of and hath need of thee; else thy individual self, as [5064], would not be aware of thy consciousness of being shut-in, would not be aware that there are material activities in which the entity might enter into—also that ye can, if ye will, be a witness for thy Maker.   5064-1

2. Bring added stimulation and strength to the muscle tissue. This will be done mostly with massage.

3. Direct therapy toward improving the glandular function.

4. Add that to the system which will assist the nerve tissue of the body in gaining strength and vitality.

5. Improve the assimilation so that the body will gradually regain its ability to take from the food those substances necessary and to distribute these throughout the system.

Cayce saw the massage doing many things. In addition to stimulating centers of spinal autonomic function to greater activity, he also saw massage of the abdominal areas as being an aid to assimilation. The abdominal lymphatic centers (the Peyer's patches), through massage, would distribute their energies through the system more efficiently: "Thus sufficient of the cellular forces may be enlivened, in the flow of the lymph as well as the corpuscle activity in the bloodstream, with these energies to revivify and build back the resistance and strength to the body." (3099-1) Even over distant parts of the body, the oils used act as food values which stimulate the lymph and emunctory circulation.

The wet cell is used in the majority of cases found in this file (six of eight), using at times camphor, silver, and Atomidine, but at all times gold, in the solution jars. Gold as it is used here performs a major function in this therapy in that it carries the vibration of gold to the central nervous system. This supplies a factor lacking in the nerves themselves and gradually builds toward a normal nervous system. The spirits of camphor supplies healing forces; while Atomidine brings about cleansing. (2514-1) In this same reading Cayce suggested that the Atomidine was given to aid in assimilating from the nerve forces. Elsewhere in the readings it is found that Atomidine "will not only be a curative property but a *preventative!* May be used internally and externally as well, and especially for any form of disorder in glands *or* tissue of body." (358-2) In another place it is described as a purifier and a cleanser for the glandular forces of the system.

Perhaps the attitude of the individuals who are concerned in the treatment is so important that it cannot be overemphasized. Treatment of any case must be approached cautiously, if the following extract can be thought of as applying to all:

The conditions may or may not respond. It will depned upon the determination of the body-mind of this entity to live, to supply, to call on those energies of the Divine within self to *unite* in the efforts to stay the energies in the body-force.

Then there would be supplied those elements that, if assimilated, may aid in supplying—through the mind forces and the body-energies—the physical reactions to the body.   **3099-1**

III. Suggested Therapeutic Regimen

Once the spiritual attitudes of the individual affected are considered and redirected, then the remainder of the therapy for the muscular dystrophies becomes somewhat simplified.

The four remaining goals of therapy can usually be achieved by the use of massage, which seems to be primarily used in every case; the wet cell appliance, with its gold chloride, silver nitrate, camphor and Atomidine used in the solution jars; and dietary adjustments which vary somewhat for the individual. There are several other suggestions—vitamins, beef juice, osteopathy (in one case), gold chloride and soda taken internally, and in one case a calcium additive—but these appear to be individualized and not essential to the outcome as a routine for all cases.

Massage should be given for a minimum of 30 minutes daily after the appliance has been used. It should be directed mainly at those areas of the spine that correspond with the extremities most afflicted. However, it should be continued down over the extremities and the joints, and even over the abdominal area. Plenty of oil should be used so that the skin absorbs as much as it can. Oils that have been suggested or combinations of oils are:

    1. Peanut oil, 2 ounces
       Olive oil, 2 ounces
       Melted lanolin, ½ ounce

2. Olive oil and peanut oil, equal parts.
3. Olive oil and tincture of myrrh, equal parts.
4. Peanut oil, 5 ounces
   Kerosene, 1 ounce
5. Peanut oil by itself. Add lanolin if a rash occurs.
6. Cocoa butter.

In case [3649], a massage with cocoa butter was to be given from the base of the skull to the soles of the feet with a rotary motion. The ones giving the therapy were instructed to use suggestions of a constructive nature while these treatments were being applied. The massage given to a 34-year-old woman, [3681], was to be given over the spine and the limbs, again using cocoa butter, and was to follow electrical-driven vibrator treatment to the spine daily. In all other cases the oils were suggested. It is important that these massages be given in a regular, consistent manner. Success in some cases was dependent upon the consistency and the persistence of "those about the body."

The wet cell appliance was suggested for use in six of the eight cases reviewed. In every instance the instructions were to use the wet cell 30 minutes daily. The large nickel plate was to be attached at the umbilical center, which was described as being three fingerbreadths to the right of the umbilicus and two or three fingerbreadths up from that point. The user was instructed rather carefully in nearly every instance to put the copper plate at the ninth dorsal vertebral area. This location varied with the type of solution carried in the solution jar. There was no clear pattern as to why the gold chloride solution would be alternated with sometimes silver nitrate, sometimes camphor, sometimes Atomidine. This apparently depended upon the needs of the body and the condition for which the reading was being given. On the other hand, the instructions were consistent and frequent to clean the plates before and after using; to keep all the parts disconnected when not in use; to take the tops off the solution jar and the wet cell battery when not in use and to keep these parts cleaned. If not kept meticulously clean, sometimes fever and perspiration would tend to clog the constant flow of energy from the vibrations present. The attachments should be removed after use and should be put together 20 minutes before being applied to the body each day. Different solution jars and connections should be used for the various solutions.

The battery is charged with one-and-a-half gallons of distilled water, one-and-a-half pounds of copper sulphate, one ounce of sulphuric acid, six drams of zinc, and one-half pound of willow charcoal. This is the usual charge. For most cases this solution and the materials in the solution jars should be changed after 30 applications. In some instances different strengths were used. For [4014], only three drams of zinc were recommended and no willow charcoal. For [3099], double strengths were advised—two gallons of distilled water, three pounds of copper sulphate, two ounces of sulphuric acid, one-half pound of willow charcoal and six drams of zinc. It is not clear why the different strengths were used.

The gold solution is made up to one grain of gold per ounce of solution, and three or four ounces is used in the solution jar. A silver solution was variable; in one instance—one ounce of 2% solution of silver nitrate was added to one ounce of distilled water and one ounce of ethyl alcohol. Atomidine was made up one ounce of the commercial strength to two ounces of water. A full strength of spirits of camphor was recommended.

A well-balanced diet should be used in all cases, varying at times according to the body needs. Consistent recommendations throughout the readings are to eat no fried foods, to avoid white flour and white sugar, and to take the fish, fowl, and lamb for meats.

Eliminations should be kept regular. Colonics should be utilized if necessary, and constipation certainly should be avoided. Good eliminations are always necessary to good assimilation.

Osteopathy was suggested weekly for six months for a seven-year-old boy, [2983], until he started on the wet cell appliance. The gold and soda were given orally in two instances. For [3099], one grain of gold chloride was added to one ounce of distilled water to make up the first solution. Then three grains of sodium bicarbonate were added to one ounce of distilled water to make up the second solution. Then each week, this woman was instructed to take one drop of solution number one, and two drops of solution number two, stir them in a glass of water and drink at once. They were not to be taken oftener than once a week. Beef juice was suggested to supply some of the vitamins, and Kaldak was suggested to be used in raw milk daily for one individual.

Therapy, then, consists primarily of massage of a thorough, yet gentle nature, directed primarily toward those areas most afflicted, and the use prior to the massage of the wet cell appliance, which brings into the system in a vibratory manner influences which apparently cannot be absorbed through the intestinal tract. These two modes of therapy bear the major portion of the load in restoring the glands of the body back toward normal, bringing a rejuvenation and resuscitation to the nerves which have been in a sense burned away, and revivifying and regenerating the muscular tissue. In the process, they reverse the changes in the internal organs which may have come about.

Do these, as we have indicated. . .Not as rote, but knowing that within self must be found that which may be awakened to the *building* of that necessary for the body, mentally and physically and spiritually, to carry *its* part in this experience. For the application of any influence must have that which is of the divine awakening of the activative forces in every atom, every cell of a living body.   726-1

William A. McGarey, M.D.

Edgar Cayce readings referenced:
2983-1, 2, 3	3649-1
3099-1	3681-1
3337-1	4014-1
3367-1	5064-1
3567-1	5078-1

References

1. Yudell, Alan. *Newly Defined Muscular Dystrophies,* Ariz. Med. 24:950-954, 1967.

2. Shy, G. Milton. *Diseases of Muscle; Textbook of Medicine,* W.B. Saunders Co., Philadelphia, 1967.

OBESITY

I. Physiological Considerations

The problem of obesity in the practice of medicine has remained a puzzle without adequate solution, in spite of the apparent simplicity found in the production of excess fat in the body from excess eating. The obese patient is usually dismissed with the advice to eat less food and he will lose weight. Endocrine abnormalities—notably thyroid and pituitary malfunctions—are currently recognized as etiologic agents in some cases of obesity, but this is understood to constitute a very small percentage of the total cases of excess body weight.

Clarity concerning this problem does not come readily from the Cayce readings, perhaps because of the fact that few readings were given only for the problem of obesity. Usually obesity was concomitant with other conditions and thus treatment and etiology were intermixed. It would probably be an accurate observation to state that the readings saw obesity as a side-product of other body changes that were in the process of causing what we know as disease.

In the cases reviewed in this Circulating File there are four major factors of a physiological nature which contribute in the greatest degree to the obesity for which corrective suggestions were offered.

The first and probably most important etiologic factor is what Cayce calls an "excess of starches in the diet," which we probably relate to the general problem of overeating. When these starches are in excess quantity they create drosses in the system, and these "make for a hardening upon the activity of the glandular system as related to the glands of the body." (1268-2) Apparently these changes in the glandular activity are not just in the endocrine glands of the body but also in those tissues in the small intestinal wall—probably Peyer's patches and other tissues which are active in the assimilatory process. Each of these has glandular tissue as part of its structure which directs and controls the reproduction and continuity of cellular structure unique to that tissue. Thus changes in the glands themselves might well alter the structure and nature of those cells which absorb and metabolize carbohydrates. Then we might find that "there has been produced in the glands—where the changes take place in the digestive system, just below the duodenum, that condition wherein *most* things turn to sugars, and these increase the avoirdupois of the system, especially about these portions of the body—the torso proper." (5603-1) We might say, then, that overeating starches is a prime cause of obesity and might create an abnormality in the assimilatory cells of the intestinal tract.

Improper or inadequate eliminations are the second cause of obesity. In [2455]'s case, lack and imbalance of eliminations were probably one of the prime causes of the woman's psoriasis as well as her obesity. In order to correct either, the eliminations had to be improved and the balance among the liver, kidneys, lung, and skin had to be restored.

Glandular imbalance was mentioned several times in those cases reviewed, and thus appears as a third major causative factor. The adrenals and the pineal particularly were mentioned as being faulty in performance, but we also see the production of obesity in an individual after [5240] had a thyroidectomy; almost immediately after [4030] had her tonsils out (obesity which existed 11 years after a reading was obtained); and almost immediately after [3386] had her uterus surgically removed. All of these are glandular tissues although the tonsils are not included among major glandular structures. In any event, glandular function or malfunction must be given its proper place in the etiology of obesity.

Incoordination between the cerebrospinal and the autonomic nervous systems apparently plays a fairly important role in creating conditions conducive to the production of excess body weight. As a fourth etiologic factor, these incoordinations arise from other causes and are not primary in themselves, but are found frequently enough to be considered as a physiological malfunction in understanding the process of obesity.

It is important to be aware that obesity *accompanies* the development of other diseases and thus we must question the theory that obesity *causes* other diseases. Perhaps it may be only that the changes in the physical body which occasion that which we call obesity might also bring about other disease processes as a matter of natural activity in a body that had adjusted itself to improper function.

II. Rationale of Therapy

In approaching therapy, we should remember that the body has a capability of *normal* function:

Thus, we would administer those activities which would bring a normal reaction through these portions, stimulating them to an activity from the body itself, rather than the body becoming dependent upon supplies that are robbing portions of the system to produce activity in other portions, or the system receiving elements or chemical reactions being supplied without arousing the activity of the system itself for a more normal condition.

1968-3

Any plan of therapy to produce a permanent alleviation of the condition which we know as obesity should properly be directed at entirely removing the causes of the excess weight. Thus, a program of fasting or strict regimentation of diet might bring a person down to normal weight where he would stay, in a small percentage of the cases, but most individuals following their normal diet would again return to the body weight they had originally, which is the state of obesity.

Recognizing that the body as a whole is the sum total of its functions or activities, it is easier to understand that each activity must be coordinated within itself, as well as with other physiological functions. We must then recognize that individual cells and groups of cells must be treated to restore their function to normal so that the organ or gland or system to which they belong might then be normalized.

In order to have a normal body weight, one should be eating a normal diet and should have adequate assimilations and eliminations with a balanced function of the circulatory, glandular, and nervous systems. This description certainly is one of good health, so correction of obesity often is producing a state of health wherein sickness was existing prior to that time.

Briefly, one might view the body as a site of constant construction of new cells to take the place of those that are dying. If assimilation is improper, not giving the bloodstream adequate nutritional substances, the rebuilding process becomes a disturbed, distorted, and incomplete thing. Likewise, if eliminations of dead cellular substances, of used energies and refused energies is not properly taken care of, again there is improper building because of the excessive amount of waste in the bloodstream. Lack of balance in the entire glandular system produces improper and insufficient amounts of those hormones necessary to combine with available energies to produce new cells. The blood and lymph circulation and the nervous system are intimately related to this whole process in such a manner that any malfunction here also produces lack of normal rebuilding. While it is understandable that the entire function of the body is not this simple, yet these characteristics of body function are undoubtedly valid. Thus when new cells are built properly, they function according to their nature which might be as cells of the retina, the skin, the hair, or perhaps even as cells of the adrenal cortex. Proper function gives balance and health in individual cells and in the entire body.

With this as a background, it seems then only reasonable to base therapy upon a restoration to normal of the cells which are abnormal in that particular body, keeping in mind the interdependence and the cooperation and coordination that are necessary among all functioning parts of the body.

III. Suggested Therapeutic Regimen

A program designed to accomplish the objectives just outlined in the second part of the commentary would necessarily begin with the most obvious point needing correction and proceed to those rather difficult complications that are often found in the obese patient. They might be enumerated as follows:

1. Rectify the diet;
2. Restore normal balance and efficiency of eliminations throughout the body—lymphatics and emunctories, liver, kidneys, lungs, and skin;
3. Bring about changes in the cells of the intestinal tract which will reverse the tendency of those cells to turn most things into sugar;
4. Balance the glandular system;
5. Correct other abnormalities which may be present: nervous system incoordination, circulatory system imbalance, etc.

The diet must be changed rather radically in order to begin therapy, and the major change brought about is the elimination of most starches. If starches are eliminated, fruits and vegetables must be added to take their place. No fried foods are allowed, and the meat intake is limited to fish, fowl, or lamb. Since eliminations are troublesome for most obese people, a diet including the factors just mentioned is extremely helpful. Such a diet taken from case [2096] is found appended to this commentary.

In obesity complicated by psoriasis, the problem of eliminations is more important. [2455] was advised to take occasional vapor baths with varying types of rubs afterwards to improve skin eliminations. Coca-Cola syrup without the carbonated water was suggested as a purifying agent for the kidneys; and as a purifier for the intestinal tract, a teaspoonful daily of a mixture of equal parts of sulphur, cream of tartar, and Rochelle salts was suggested. The importance of adequate liver function and production of bile cannot be over-emphasized. Attention is directed to the Circulating File on "Constipation" where this problem is discussed rather extensively.

The readings had a number of suggestions, all apparently designed to restore the liver and the eliminations through the intestinal tract to full activity. They suggested olive oil, one teaspoon with each meal, as one alternative. Zilatone tablets, one three times a day until bowels were moving actively and then cut down to twice a day or once a day over a period of 10 days, was another regimen for the bowels. Until the eliminatory organs are balanced and functioning adequately, the obesity problem cannot be completely overcome.

Over and over again in the readings grape juice—diluted two parts of grape juice with one part of water—was suggested as an additive to the diet, to be taken one-half hour before each meal and before retiring. This was to be done over a long period of time with persistence and consistency. Apparently this has a function of giving a type of sugar to the body tissues which does not promote weight gain. It was suggested that when the body was satisfied with this type of sugar, then those cells and glands in the intestinal tract that tend to change most foods to sugar would not be called upon to function in this abnormal manner. Only the passage of time and the replacement of these abnormal cells with those built in a normal manner would finally rectify the situation.

Glands throughout the body must be led into a normal function to rid the body of obesity. In the case of [5240] where the thyroid had been removed, suggestion was made to continue the thyroid extract by mouth. Stimulating existing glands toward normal function is often done with Atomidine given in series—one drop a day for five days, then left off for five days, and continued in this manner over a long period of time. It may alternately be given starting with two drops in a half glass of water the first day, three the second, and so on, up to a dosage of ten drops on the ninth day. At that point the dosage is decreased one drop per day until the original dose of two drops is achieved. Then there is a rest period of five to ten days and another series is begun.

In the difficult cases of obesity, the so-called radio-active appliance (which has been renamed the impedance device) is suggested for use. When it is used with the solution jar, in the case of obesity, Atomidine is used in the solution. In 5603-1 the impedance device was to be used every other day. Specifics can be seen in the individual readings. [4030] was a young woman who developed obesity after a tonsillectomy and who also was advised to use the impedance device. Apparently this battery brings into the body a therapy not readily obtained in other manners.

It would be proper to correct other abnormalities in function which may be present. Osteopathic treatments are frequently suggested in series of four or five up to 20 to 28 and also static electricity through the use of the violet ray bulb hand applicator for incoordination between the cerebrospinal and the autonomic nervous system. The use of this appliance is described in case 3386-1.

Disproportion of Body Parts

Eliminations seem to be a major factor in many disease processes. Obesity is no exception. In [2096]'s instance, the glandular function was not particularly a major factor in her obesity. It had begun to have an effect but, according to the reading, the eliminations were producing conditions in the body which would bring about trouble to the heart, principally through malfunction in the kidneys and through the sugars created in the system.

Perhaps more interesting to those who suffer with an overweight problem is that for [2096] faulty eliminations are the principal etiologic agent in producing disproportions of the body itself or the depositing of fat where one does not particularly want fat. Corrections were suggested (in addition to the diet which was primary)—for [2096] to take colonic irrigations once every ten days until four or five were taken, and sweat cabinet baths with massages afterwards. The following extract is interesting:

. . .eliminations are those that cause the disorders in the lower portions of

the system; feet, ankles and limbs, as well as those that produce a tendency for *portions* of the body, especially, to be out of proportion to the body as a whole.

The conditions. . .may be aided the most were the body to be more mindful of the diet; not as an extremist, no—but as one that would have the corrections made in the general eliminating system. . .

. . .this would be. . .an outline for the corrections of the physical conditions, that may later produce hindrances in the general physical health of the body.

We would begin first with those colonic irrigations—one every ten days until four or five are taken, which will overcome this tendency of constipation through the system. . .

We would also, at least twice each week, have those sweat cabinet baths, with a thorough rubdown afterwards with any of the eliminants—or prepare as this: Take Russian white oil, one pint; alcohol, one pint; witch hazel, one-half pint. Mix these together and massage the body with same following the baths, see? Well to occasionally leave off the oil rub and use the salt glow (that is, rub the body with salt).   2096-1

Since each individual case of obesity is different from the next, a routine of therapy must be designed for each person. Patience, persistence, and consistency certainly are necessities in bringing about a successful conclusion in this difficult physical condition. When one gets a bit discouraged, it might be well to keep in mind the following quotation:

Keep up what we have given. Be a little patient, but know that there is being brought about those conditions that will correct the disturbance *in* this body, and that the body's strength—the body-physical and the body-mental—*is* gaining. Set before self, mentally, that the body would attain. Make it *high,* and keep the mental *lifted* in that direction; for to heal the physical alone, and to have the mental still distorted—would only be the return of the conditions when *activities* would be renewed physically. But make the body physically fit, that the body-mental may act through same—and *make* the efforts to bring about that as *is* desired, in a mental *and* physical body—but make it high! Don't be satisfied with less!   5545-2

William A. McGarey, M.D.

Edgar Cayce readings referenced:

1268-2	2579-1	5240-1
2096-1	3386-1	5603-1 through 5
2455-1, 2, 3	4030-1	

Dietary Recommendations

Beware of sweets and of condiments. These are those [foods] that are flesh producing, or the weight producing for the body. 903-16

Q-11. Why is it hard to increase weight in portions [of the body] and decrease it in others?
A-11. The natural. . .trend in the development of the foetus forces in its inception, and then the general activities have been in these directions. This would go more into the psychological than in the pathological conditions to be sure, as we have indicated through these sources respecting the [activities and] associations throughout the sojourn of the entity and its bodily forces in the earth.   288-38

. . .there are tendencies that unless taken into consideration [they] may cause a great deal of trouble. These arise primarily from a condition which involves the glandular forces of the system, tending towards the creating of sugar in too great a quantity for the activity of the circulation between kidneys and liver and their effect upon the activities of the locomotion of the body. And this will increase the weight to such an extent that hindrances would arise in a form either of deterioration in the muscle and tendon forces of the body or in the activities that would affect the heart, the liver and the kidneys.

There is a subluxation. . .that exists in the 9th dorsal, the 6th and 7th dorsal. One is in one direction; the other in the [other direction]. This we would correct osteopathically.

Also we would keep better activities by the use of the Jerusalem artichoke as a part of the diet three times each week. Prepare this in a special way. . .Use one about the size of a hen egg, cooked in its own juices and served in its own juice—being prepared in Patapar paper. Boil in the Patapar paper, then mix the bulk of the artichoke with the juices (after taking off the peeling) and season with a little butter and salt, and a little pepper if so desired, and eat all of it.

Do not take this without having the osteopathic correction, for these are to work in unison.

If these are done, we should have better activities for this body.
3240-1

Q-2. Are there any exercises that I can take to keep my weight down that will not be detrimental to my back?

A-2. Take grape juice regularly four times each day, about half an hour before each meal and before retiring. Use three ounces of pure grape juice (such as Welch's) with one ounce of plain water, not carbonated water. This with the [recommended] sweats or baths will keep down the weight as well as remove poisons.   3413-2

Q-15. Why should the body take grape juice?
A-15. To supply the sugars without gaining or making for greater weight.   457-8

PROSTATITIS

Medicine today generally identifies problems of the prostate as encompassing acute infectious prostatitis (mostly in younger males), the more slowly developing prostatitis (in the middle or older aged individuals), those chronic infectious processes, and the benign prostatic hypertrophy (enlargement). In addition there is the prostatitis caused by gonorrhea and the cancerous prostate.

In the Edgar Cayce readings, the term "prostatitis" is used more loosely by those who asked for readings. Thus, most of the above conditions were dealt with, although not identified as such. In spite of this lack of specificity, there does emerge a pattern of causation and treatment which would imply—if these readings are to be taken as factual insight into the physiology of the human body—that differences in individuals and differences in age and resistance perhaps play the greater part in what kind of prostate condition is diagnosed. The real cause lies in the complexity and interrelationships of the body's functions and how they became unbalanced and/or incoordinate. The most effective permanent therapy restores a coordinated, balanced homeostasis of physiological functions and a greater oneness between the body, the mind, and the spirit.

To a 62-year-old medical doctor—who certainly never heard of holistic medicine and who stated he had lived an "honest and a spiritual life"—Cayce had much to say. The doctor was suffering intense pain from intercostal neuralgia, severe prostatitis, and arthritis centralized in the sacral and coccygeal area. Cayce was not easy on this man, and there was no response after the reading was sent, but the following extract from his reading sets the whole problem of prostatitis in perspective:

There is body, there is mind, there is soul. They each have their attributes,

they each have their limitations. The soul, in a material world, is controlled by mind and body. . .

The heart changes in its beat. Remember, the things you applied once—now you are meeting them! Live with this in mind (and every soul should take heed): *Ye shall pay every whit, that ye break of the law of the Lord.* For the law of the Lord is perfect, it converteth the soul. It doesn't always convert a hard-headed man nor a body that is beset with habits that have left their mark upon those portions of the body through which mind and soul may work. What are these?

Nerve and blood forces of the body!   3559-1

I. Physiological Considerations

Habits control most of our body movements and the great majority of our mental-emotional-physical reactions. At one point in time or another they are created by our own minds. And they act through the autonomic nervous system to the cerebrospinal nervous system, affecting all of the functions of the organs in the process of creating physical body activities in the outside world. It is a fact that the blood supply to various parts of our bodies is controlled by autonomic nerve fibers which, for the most part, travel on the arteries, arterioles and capillaries which bring blood with its life-giving food to those parts served.

Among those cases studied, prostatitis occurred rather frequently in conjunction with other problems: arthritis, neuritis, sciatica, diabetes, gastritis, and renal disease. At times, the only apparent diagnosis was simply prostatitis, but always there were causative factors in the manner in which the body's physiology was malfunctioning.

For instance, one 45-year-old man [763] had certain nervous system incoordinations which created problems in the kidney eliminations. This made for "seepages and poisons" in the bloodstream, which in turn seeded out in the prostate gland—and in other organs and structures. With [1501], however, an excess of uric acid in the bloodstream prevented proper coagulation in the system and an improper elimination through the kidney circulation as related to the liver and gall bladder circulation. On the other hand, with [3559], resentments in the past had had their influence from other experiences. (3559-1) For [4408], a problem with assimilation precipitated prostatitis; with [5074], the disturbance in assimilation affected the kidneys and seemed to predict an elevated blood pressure and a greater disorder in the kidney, bladder, and prostate areas of activity.

For [5376], poor assimilation and poor eliminations caused those tendencies toward an arthritis reaction, involving both the liver and the kidney—and the prostate, too.

The creating of symptoms and associated disease difficulties can be illustrated in the case of [763]'s nervous system problem:

As to the nervous system, here we find disturbances both in the cerebrospinal and the sympathetic nervous system; some—through those irritations that have been indicated—became more sympathetic reactions, and we have at others those where pressures are made, and we have an upsetting through the digestive area when nothing apparently tends to digest properly, while at others there is the tendency for the headaches, the dull heaviness that comes to the system, portions of the body where the skin becomes very dry and at others when there will be on the feet or hands or portions of the forehead or portions of the neck a cold, damp sweat. These are *nervous* reactions; the worriments that come from these pressures on various portions of the organism affecting the system and thus producing those distresses. These necessarily, through the sympathetic system, affect the organs of the sensory system, so that the ear, the speech, the hearing at times become involved (not always, but)—these become accentuated, or there may be buzzing, or there may be phlegm accumulations in the bronchials or in the vocal organs. These are *nerve* refractions and show disturbances through the circulation, as indicated, and where there is the constant use of any of these there is irritation produced to the organs themselves. For instead of carrying altogether replenishing forces and then carrying away drosses through the other portions of the cellular forces in the bloodstream itself, there are *deposits* at times in any used portions. Hence muscular forces, as well as portions of the extremities, become affected. Hence we have a neuritic effect over the whole system.   763-1

This man cleared up many of his symptoms by therapy directed at his general condition and obtained a check reading which then suggested specific treatments for his prostate (still enlarged and giving him some difficulty). The etiology of prostatitis is not simple.

II. Therapeutic Regimen

When conditions in the human body reach that point wherein the prostate is enlarged, tender, obviously inflamed or symptomatic with urination, the Cayce readings suggest several steps that might be taken toward resolution of the problem:

1. A diet should be adopted that is high in fresh green vegetables and low in fats, red meats, condiments, sugars and alcohol. Such a

diet would allow fish, fowl, or lamb (never fried), lots of fruits—the kind of diet that would be called alkaline-reacting.

2. Osteopathic treatments should be given to bring about a better alignment of the spine and a coordination between the cervical, the upper and mid-dorsal, and the sacrococcygeal outflow of nerves.

3. Full body massages should be added to the regimen of therapy, preceded by hydrotherapy—steam baths, Epsom salts baths, colonics, or sitz baths. And special massages to the sacrococcygeal area of the low back should be included.

4. Lacking availability of the Elliot machine to bring heat locally to the prostate gland, diathermy to the pubic-perineal-low back area could be a helpful application.

5. Packs, such as Glyco-Thymoline, Epsom salts, or hot salt, applied to the pubic or to the low back area, might be added.

The above therapy suggestions were the most frequently recommended in those readings studied for this report; however, numerous other suggestions were made, aimed more at correcting problems in the intestinal tract, kidney or bladder, or liver/gall bladder/spleen complex.

In any given condition Cayce consistently recommended therapy applied toward the causes rather than the noticeable effects. When a serum was given to [763] to control the irritation, Cayce had this to say: "...if the applications are continued for effects rather than causes we will eventually produce greater distresses and upsets in portions of the system." (763-1)

In the instance of a 28-year-old chiropractor whose prostatic irritation and enlargement was due to unequal eliminations affecting the kidneys as well as the prostate, an interesting combination of treatments was suggested. The doctor was already on an excellent diet (and probably was receiving adjustments with some degree of regularity). It was recommended that a saturated solution of sodium bicarbonate be applied over the sacrum and both sides of the gland in the groin and massaged in well. Then a hot pack of heavy sea salt was to be applied. The reading said that this would reduce the inflammation and cause correct functioning in the kidneys. (1447-3) Following each of those treatments, the man was to use the violet ray across the lower dorsal and entire lumbar and sacral region to strengthen the nerve centers and tissues in that area.

Proper eliminations depend sometimes upon better assimilation through the upper intestinal tract. The readings often suggested—in addition to a proper diet—an aid to correct the functioning of those cells in the stomach and small intestine. To [5376] was given this prescription:

> Fusion of wild ginseng, two ounces
> Fusion of wild ginger, ½ ounce
> Essence of lactated pepsin, enough to make four ounces (add enough alcohol to preserve mixture)
> Mix these and take one teaspoonful at bedtime.

In another instance [763] was told to take one teaspoonful of milk of bismuth, add six drops of essence of lactated pepsin, stir them together in a full glass of water, and take the mixture three or four times a week. This, he said, would increase the gastric flow and activate the mucous membranes through the lymph circulation and the jejunum, to help in healing and not irritate these portions. (763-1)

The massages recommended in the readings were invariably general massages, with specific reference to correcting incoordinations between the autonomic and cerebrospinal nervous systems, and locally in the lower back, the pubic, groin and prostate areas (the latter probably referring to the inner aspect of the thighs and perhaps the perineum). Massages were recommended more frequently than any other therapy.

Next in frequency were the osteopathic treatments. Then the Elliot machine (no longer available), in which hot water circulated through a rubber attachment inserted into the rectum, thus treating the prostate directly with heat. As mentioned earlier, diathermy may be used for the same purpose. Diet, of course, was always recommended or implied.

Packs were usually placed over the lower abdomen across the pubic area. Warm Glyco-Thymoline packs were suggested for a 44-year-old man [5180], repeated for 15-20 minutes as needed, for prostate disturbance. For [3559], a more complicated regimen was suggested: First, Epsom salts packs across the sacrum and hips, "an hour at a time, as hot as the body can stand them, changing them at least two or three times during the hour." (3559-1) This was to be applied daily for a period of time. Following the pack, the whole area was to be massaged with a mixture of olive oil, two ounces; peanut oil, two ounces; and lanolin (liquified), one-quarter ounce; as much as the body would absorb. Then a Glyco-Thymoline pack covered with a heated salt pack (one-inch thick, quilted) was to be applied. All of this was to be done every day.

Not to be neglected, however, are those steps that must be taken by the individual who is ill—the choices to correct attitude, to see life in a different light, to bring into the consciousness more of that which we know as the Christ Consciousness, and the awareness that we all are indeed spiritual beings who have a oneness with God, the Creator. And begin to make that consciousness active in relation to those about us.

Since attitudes, emotions, the soul's destiny and the activity of the Spirit are all a part of the problem we call prostatitis, then increased awareness—along with application of that awareness—is a necessity. Cayce pointed this out to the doctor:

But turn thy thoughts and thy mind more earnestly to the Divine that is within self. And know that He meant what He said, "If ye ask in my name, believing it will be done in your body." He meant it! Then *do* it!   3559-1

Working with a change of attitude, then, and adding an alkaline diet (as discussed earlier), osteopathic treatments, massages, packs, and diathermy—one can then forge for himself a program of therapy that promises aid and improvement. If one remembers to be patient, persistent, and consistent, changes come.

One gentleman, [5376], in all sincerity, wrote Mr. Cayce many years ago: "I have pains in my right shoulder and in the region of the prostate gland. My stomach is real bad and I am constipated. I hope the Lord will help me to regain my health. I am trying to be fair with Him." Let's be fair with ourselves, too, for the Lord helps those who help themselves.

William A. McGarey, M.D.

Edgar Cayce readings referenced:
763-1, 2
1447-3
1501-1
1539-3, 4
2392-1, 2
3369-1
3559-1
4408-1, 2
5074-1
5162-1
5180-1
5376-1

PSORIASIS

I. Physiological Considerations

Psoriasis is a chronic disease state manifested in the skin by red, dry, scaly lesions most frequently found on or about the knees, elbows and scalp, but may involve almost any area of the skin surface. The lesions are generally patchy in appearance, well demarcated, and may or may not be accompanied by itching. There can be acute flare-ups on occasion, or remissions, either partial or complete, for variable lengths of time. It is not unusual to find pitting and scarring of the nails as a result of psoriasis. A form of arthritis not unlike rheumatoid arthritis may also be present in some cases.

The readings have some rather specific things to say regarding the pathologic process that brings about the skin eruptions which are commonly known as psoriasis. In reading after reading it is mentioned that the diseased state of the skin and joint tissues is due to a thinning of the walls of the intestinal tract. In most cases the readings specify the jejunum as the site of the intestinal lesions although the lower portion of the duodenum is also quite often mentioned. This thinning of the intestinal walls then allows toxic products from the intestinal tract to leak into the circulatory system and find their way into the lymph flow of the skin. When the blood and lymph systems of the body are unable to eliminate these poisons then the inflammatory skin reaction known as psoriasis is produced.

There are disturbing conditions which prevent the better physical functioning in this body. These have to do primarily with an intestinal disorder and the lack of proper coordination in the eliminating systems. There are those conditions, then, in the duodenum and through the jejunum where there are the effects as if there were tiny thinned walls, as if the walls of the duodenum had been smoothed—rather than the folds that should exist with the gastric flow which should come through these areas at periods of

digestion. The results are a disturbance in the blood supply and an irritation in the superficial circulation, so that those areas in the epidermis show eliminations that should be carried through alimentary canal, for these are being eliminated through perspiratory system.   3373-1

This would indicate that, at least in case [3373], the thinning of the intestinal walls also included a loss of the villi normally present on the mucosal surface of the duodenum.

The smoothing of the mucosal surface and thinning of the intestinal walls is not always due to the same initial cause; however, it is stated that there is always involved a lack of lymph circulation through the alimentary canal.

Q-1. Is psoriasis always from the same cause?
A-1. No, but it is more often from the lack of proper coordination in the eliminating systems. At times the pressures may be in those areas disturbing the equilibrium between the heart and liver, or between heart and lungs. But it is always caused by a condition of lack of lymph circulation through alimentary canal and by absorption of such activities through the body.
          5016-1

Thus we see that while the initiating factor may vary, the disease process is always essentially the same.

In some times back we had a condition that existed from toxic forces, or by the accumulations through and to the stubborn condition in an *improper* elimination through the alimentary canal. This strain at the time from fecal forces in the system tended to make for a thinning of the walls of the intestines themselves, making a secretion that—having to be taken up by the lymph and emunctories, and the blood being impoverished—produces a rash on the exterior forces of the body at times.   622-1

First, in the blood supply there are the indications of poor eliminations. While the activities in the system would first indicate these are not of a great disturbance, the conditions are rather of an unseen or hidden nature; arising from the effects of a disturbance had some time ago, where the nature of congestion has affected the lymph circulation more specifically in the jejunum circulation. We have from same some perforations that are of such natures that in the circulation they produce blemishes and spots and conditions over various portions of the body. . .   745-1

In summary, it may be said that psoriasis is a disease state in which variable factors reduce the lymph circulation through portions of the gastrointestinal tract causing a thinning of the intestinal walls, usually in the jejunum and/or duodenum, and at times a loss of the villi which aid in selective absorption of intestinal contents. As the lesions in the intestines become more pronounced there occurs a seepage or leakage into the circulatory system of toxic substances from the intestinal tract. When the emunctory systems of the body are unable to eliminate these toxic products as fast as they are absorbed, the circulation becomes overburdened and they find their way into the lymph flow of the skin in sufficient quantity to produce congestion and the inflammatory reaction which is characteristic of the disease.

II. Rationale of Therapy

Treatment should be directed primarily toward ridding the body of the circulating poisons and bringing about a gradual healing of the offending intestinal lesions, while improving coordination between the organ systems. This would serve effectively to clear the skin permanently by eliminating the cause of the inflammatory reaction.

In nearly every case improvement in diet is one of the first treatments to be instituted. Since toxic accumulations in the circulation and tissues tends to be acid in nature, the general character of the diet is such as to promote alkalinity and thus bring about a better acid-alkaline balance to the entire system. The diet is much more specific in some cases than in others, but in all cases it tends to be alkaline in content. It also emphasizes fresh fruits and vegetables to promote better eliminations through the intestinal tract.

In the diet we would keep rather to the non-acid foods; that is, keeping rather the alkaline-reacting foods; letting one meal each day consist of raw vegetables wholly. With such there may be used an oil or salad dressing.

745-1

The matter of proper bowel evacuation is second only to diet in importance. Good eliminations are not only necessary to help the body rid itself of the toxic intestinal contents but also to improve the condition for the healing of the intestinal lesions. Proper adherence to diet is considered the best means of establishing good eliminations;

but enemas, colonics and laxatives are also used rather frequently to keep the bowels functioning efficiently.

In some cases a mixture of sulphur, Rochelle salts and cream of tartar is prescribed as a cathartic and to help purify the alimentary system. Since it is prescribed only in the more complex disease states and in conjunction with osteopathic adjustments, it is not recommended for routine administration, and not at all without first consulting a physician.

A variety of measures including physiotherapy, hydrotherapy, the violet ray and sunlight are used to stimulate and improve the circulation. Osteopathy is also designed to relieve pressures on related autonomic ganglia and their cerebrospinal connections and thus promote improved circulation to the impoverished tissues and organs of elimination.

Herbal remedies for healing the lesions in the intestinal wall are nearly always prescribed. These include yellow saffron, camomile, and mullein teas. Ground elm bark mixed with water or chewing slippery elm bark are also recommended to stimulate the flow of digestive secretions.

First, then, we would change the *character* of water taken by the body. There should be no water taken unless carrying elm bark or yellow saffron tea. While these may be in small quantities, the effect of these upon the gastric flow throughout the stomach, throughout the activity of the organs of the system, will so stimulate the walls of the organs themselves as to bring *healing* to those portions that are distressed.   745-1

We would keep to the taking, more often, the saffron tea as indicated; and we would change or alternate this at times with camomile tea. For these tend to form, in the regular activities of the body, the best in the gastric flows for the intestinal disorder.

The chewing of slippery elm would also be well. While it would be necessary that this be done in private, owing to the looks of it, we find that it will be most beneficial to the activity of the glands—the salivary glands as well as those in the pylorus, and in the duodenum also. Swallow the saliva that is indicated in the chewing of same; not the powder, but the bark itself, see?

Alternate, though, between the saffron and the camomile.   641-7

Little attention is given in the readings to treating the skin manifestations directly since these only reflect the diseased state of organs elsewhere in the body. Applications of Resinol or Cuticura ointment are at times prescribed as palliative procedures.

III. Suggested Therapeutic Regimen
Treatment is threefold in purpose: to restore balance and coordination between the various organs of assimilation and elimination; to clear the circulatory and alimentary systems of the accumulated toxic substances; and to promote healing of the intestinal lesions which allow the toxic substances to leak into the circulatory system.
1. *Diet:* The utmost importance must be placed on the proper diet since this aids substantially in accomplishing all three desired objectives. The diet, of course, will vary somewhat from case to case but generally emphasizes fresh fruits and raw and cooked vegetables with no meat other than fish, fowl and lamb.

. . .stress seafoods and fowl. Little of beef or other meats. Use at least three vegetables that grow above the ground to one that grows under the ground, and we will find better conditions for this body.   3373-1

Eliminate fats, sweets and pastries from the diet. Do have a great deal of fruits and vegetables.   5016-1

Q-2. Can the body take any kind of alcoholic beverages?
A-2. Wines; but not the stronger drinks—not rum or the like.   745-1

A rather detailed diet is outlined in reading 840-1 included in this report. The reader is referred to the readings in the Circulating File on "Psoriasis" for more specific information concerning diet.
2. *Eliminations:* Almost as much emphasis is placed on good eliminations as on diet.

Be sure there are the full eliminations through the alimentary canal each day; preferably use enemas instead of too great a quantity of cathartics or laxatives. But when laxatives are used, alternate with the various properties that have the senna base. These are better for the body.   641-5

Q-8. Should the use of enemas be continued to aid in eliminations?
A-8. Continue these until there is better peristaltic movement from the better flow of the lymph through intestinal system. In most of these use soda and salt. Do not take them with plain water.

Q-9. How often should an eliminant be used for general cleansing?
A-9. This depends upon the eliminations. Be sure there is one or two good evacuations each day. When there is not, take something—Castoria or those of the senna base are the better for the body, this body.   641-7

In some cases colonics are recommended early in the course of treatment. These should be professionally administered.

Within a week, but almost seven days apart, have two good colonic irrigations. Begin there first, so that there is no mucus. Two should be sufficient. Three may be better, dependent upon how thoroughly these are given.   3373-1

In more than one case a compound of sulphur, Rochelle salts and cream of tartar is recommended in conjunction with osteopathic adjustments. In one case the patient was cautioned against getting the feet wet or taking a cold following the administration of this compound. For further details the reader is referred to readings 2455-1 and 5016-1, both of which are included in this Circulating File.

3. *Herbal remedies:* Since yellow saffron tea is so frequently recommended as a part of the general treatment, it probably should be included along with diet; however, there are occasions when other herbs are used either in conjunction or alternately with the yellow saffron. Ground elm bark is recommended almost as frequently as yellow saffron tea and the two may be taken alternately.

Just before the drink is to be taken, we would have a pinch of ground elm bark stirred in a glass of water. Do not take this after it has stood for longer than twenty to thirty minutes. The saffron tea would be made in the proportion of three ounces to sixteen to twenty-four ounces of water, steeped as ordinary tea. Let the quantity or the strength be rather in accord with the taste of the body. These may be altered, or one taken one day and the other the next.   745-1

Also prepare mullein tea, which we would begin after the elm water has been taken for about ten days. Use the green mullein if it can be obtained; otherwise use the dried mullein. Crumble it, put a teaspoonful in a glass or crock container and pour a pint of boiling water over it. Allow this to stand for thirty minutes, strain, then cool and drink; not necessarily all of it at one time, but in the course of three to four hours after it has been prepared.   3373-1

4. *Stimulation of circulation:* To improve both the superficial and deep circulation, hydrotherapy and physiotherapy, including massage with olive oil and peanut oil, are recommended in 2455-1. The violet ray is advised in 2455-2 and 2455-3. The effects of sunlight are also recommended.

Keep in the sun more; not so much as to cause sunburn, but be in the sun often enough to work up a good perspiration—this would be good for the body. **641-7**

Osteopathic manipulations must, of course, vary with the condition found, but in general should be of such nature as to promote better coordination of the circulation through the kidneys and liver. Further information on osteopathic adjustments is found in readings 2455-1, 2455-3, and 5016-1 in the Circulating File.

5. *Palliatives:* Resinol and Cuticura ointment are suggested when needed to relieve itching.

In the evenings when the bath is taken, we would apply Cuticura ointment followed by Resinol—both applied, you see, one following the other. Apply these especially over the areas of the abrasions. Do not apply it in the hair, but around the edges—and on all other portions of the body where the skin is irritated. If we rid the condition from the system, then these disturbances should be eliminated. **2455-2**

As a final comment on treatment, the following is particularly worthy of mention:

Q-1. Is there an absolute cure for psoriasis?
A-1. Most of this is found in diet. There is a cure. It requires patience, persistence—and right thinking also. **2455-2**

Frederick D. Lansford, Jr., M.D.

Edgar Cayce readings referenced:
622-1   4461-1
641-5, 7   5016-1
745-1
840-1
2455-1 through 4
3373-1

Dietary Recommendations

Diet:
1. No carbonated water.
2. No meat other than fish, fowl, and lamb.
3. Eliminate fats, sweets, pastries.
4. Wine is permitted, but no other alcohol.
5. Emphasize yellow colored foods such as corn meal, carrots, and peaches. Peaches should be the only sweets eaten. Grape juice is also good.

Suggested Breakfast

Three mornings a week: Cereal consisting of rolled, crushed, or cracked whole wheat. Do not overcook. On other mornings: citrus fruit or juices, yolks of soft-boiled or poached eggs, whole wheat toast with butter. Beverage: milk or black coffee. Occasionally breakfast may consist of a baked apple with cream or stewed prunes or apricots or figs. *Do not eat citrus fruit and cereal at the same meal.*

Between breakfast and lunch: malted milk with a raw egg in it.

Lunch

Salad consisting entirely of fresh raw vegetables. Include tomatoes, lettuce, celery, spinach, beet tops, mustard, onions, or similar produce (except cucumbers). Salad oil or dressing permitted. Make the salad do for the entire meal.

Evening

Small cup of soup or broth. Cooked vegetables should make up the major portion of the meal. There may be small portions of lamb, fish, or fowl. No fried foods should be eaten.

Teas

Yellow saffron (American saffron or saffron). Drink one cup each evening at bedtime. Place the tea (start with a pinch) in a cup of boiling water and allow to steep for about 20 to 30 minutes. Use more tea if preferred.

Mullein tea may be taken on alternate days. Use 1 teaspoon of tea to a pint of boiling water. Steep for 30 minutes, strain, cool, and drink within three to four hours.

Eliminations

There should be a full bowel evacuation at least once a day. If not, a senna base cathartic or enema should be used. Enemas should be used not more than once or twice a week. Prepare the enema with a mixture of soda and salt, one teaspoon each to quart of water.

PYORRHEA

I. Physiological Considerations

The readings indicate that the causes of pyorrhea included both the invasive action of a particular bacillus upon the gums and teeth and certain predisposing conditions in the mouth, teeth, and gums which prepared the way for an attack by this bacillus. The action of this organism was described as first finding a site for growth and multiplication in the film which accumulated on the teeth. According to the readings, this film was caused from deposits left from soft and overcooked foods. The decay of such food particles on the teeth produced an acid condition whereas the normal condition of the mouth from the secretions of the glands of the mouth should have been alkaline. Such soft food also led to lack of proper exercise of the gums which lowered the resistance of the gums to attack from the bacilli which had found refuge in the film of the teeth. Eating and drinking of extremely hot or cold foods or drinks also lowers the resistance of both gums and teeth to attack.

The symptoms of the attack of the bacilli were said to be receding and bleeding gums and loosening teeth. Such symptoms are those of early pyorrhea. In this disease, if the process continues, the gums become infected and ooze pus and blood. The teeth themselves eventually become riddled with decay. The end result of the process is loss of teeth because they have to be extracted, or because they fall out.

The readings suggested that the microorganism responsible for phorrhea could be isolated and identified. The method suggested was to take pus and blood from the gums of a patient with advanced pyorrhea and to incubate this material in a medium composed of material from the teeth and saliva from the mouth of the same patient with pyorrhea. Both scrapings of the film and of the debris from accumulations of decayed food were to be used This mixture was to be incubated at 98.7° F. The organism was described in 1800-21 as having the same shape as a bedbug but with larger legs. Presumably it could be identified by microscopic examination of samples from the incubation mixture.

Another experiment suggested in the readings (1800-28) was that equal parts of blood and Ipsab be kept for nine days. Each day a smear was to be taken and examined microscopically. No other instructions were given. Presumably this mixture was to be incubated at body temperature and evaporation prevented.

II. Suggested Therapeutic Regimen

A. Treatment of early acute cases where infection is present, gums are bleeding and teeth are loose, but are not decayed beyond repair.

1. Massage gums thoroughly for five minutes twice a day with Ipsab. Repeatedly apply a liberal quantity of Ipsab to the tip of the finger and massage the gums vigorously on all surfaces. In extreme cases, take a small tuft of cotton which has been dipped in Ipsab and use a pair of tweezers to rub this saturated cotton between the gum and each tooth which is very loose. This maneuver will insure the contact of the Ipsab with the growing organisms. After the massage, rinse out the mouth with an undiluted solution of Glyco-Thymoline followed by tap water. Do not swallow any of these solutions.

2. Brush teeth once each day in the evening before retiring with a mixture composed of equal parts of common table salt and sodium bicarbonate. Brush teeth each morning after breakfast with any good dentifrice.

3. Eat a large raw vegetable salad each day.

4. Corrective dental work should be done on any carious teeth.

B. Prevention of pyorrhea in cases where the only symptoms are bleeding gums and perhaps early loosening of the teeth, but where no infection is present.

1. Massage the gums thoroughly with liberal quantities of Ipsab on the finger for five minutes three times per week.

2. Brush the teeth twice a day and for some of those brushings use the mixture of salt and soda solution mentioned above, at least once every other day.

3. Eat a large raw vegetable salad each day.

4. Corrective work should be done on any carious teeth.

The treatment outlined was not designed for bad breath or decayed teeth, but specifically for a disturbed condition in the gums which would soon develop into or had already become pyorrhea. The basic purpose of the treatment was to strengthen the gums and increase the resistance to infection. If this purpose were accomplished, presumably infection would be dispelled, loose teeth would become tight, and bleeding of the gums would stop.

Ipsab is a compound composed of prickly ash bark, sea water, calcium chloride, sodium chloride, iodine trichloride (trade name: Atomidine), and essence of peppermint. The ingredients of Ipsab were described in the readings as a specific for destroying the bacillus which was given as the causative factor in the infection of pyorrhea. The massage and the Ipsab itself were supposed to increase circulation which probably would aid the absorption of the chemical properties of Ipsab. This increased circulation would also increase resistance through the natural defense mechanisms of the body. The properties in Ipsab were also supposed to stimulate the glands both in the entire system and especially those in the mouth both directly and by reciprocal action with the other glands. Stimulation of secretion of glands in the mouth would help to bring about the normal alkaline condition. Brushing the teeth with the salt and soda mixture was supposed to remove the film from the teeth. Thus the readings gave the basic effects produced by the treatment as destruction of the organism which causes the destruction of tissue and enamel, stimulation of circulation to the gums, increase of natural resistance of the gums, restoration of proper secretions of the glands of the mouth, and cleansing of the teech. Because this treatment was not for restoration of decayed teeth, carious teeth must be dealt with by the procedures of modern dentistry. This treatment was given to combat pyorrhea and as a way to save only teeth not yet decayed irreparably.

Statements about the effectiveness of the treatment in the readings or which were given by persons who tried the treatment on a scattered individual basis cannot be used to prove definitely that this treatment will cure and prevent pyorrhea. Controlled clinical trials are needed under the supervision of qualified dentists. A summary of treatment has been presented for this purpose.

Walter N. Pahnke, M.D.

SCARS AND ADHESIONS

I. Physiological Considerations

Scars are such a common occurrence in everyone's experience that little attention is paid to them unless a large area is involved or a cosmetic or functional problem results from the location of the scar.

Scars are regarded as products of the natural repair of injured tissue. The healing of surgical incisions or lacerations which are closed by approximation with sutures differs from the healing of open wounds such as third-degree burns, stasis ulcers, or decubitus ulcers. Other types of scars may be produced by infections or certain inflammatory diseases.

The healing of surgical wounds begins with the body's outpouring of blood and serum into the defect, the formation of fibrin from fibrinogen, and the migration of fibroblasts and blood vessels into this matrix. New collagen is laid down by the fibroblasts, and a new epidermal surface forms from the migration of epidermal cells across the wound gap. At first the newly formed collagen is very cellular and richly supplied with blood vessels, but in time both the cellularity and blood vessels diminish. The bright red color of the new scar gradually fades to a pearly color in a year or so, and at this point the scar remains more or less stable.

In superficial wounds, where only a portion of the dermis is destroyed, epithelial cells may migrate from the remnants of sweat glands or hair follicles to form the new surface. The final healing might be a slightly depressed scar such as often is seen in acne or the deeper infections of impetigo or chicken pox. Large boils or papular or cystic acne may produce considerably deeper scars, sometimes of the "ice-pick" variety.

Large deep wounds—where the dermis is destroyed, such as in third-degree burns—pose a different problem for the body. In the absence of adnexal structures such as hair follicles, sebaceous and sweat glands, repair of the defect is by way of granulation tissue. Granulations are capillary buds extending upward to the surface and carrying with them fibroblasts and inflammatory cells. Once a good granulating surface is established, epidermal cells may migrate across to cover the healing surface, but if the wound is large, grafts may be required. Beneath the new thin epidermis new collagen is laid down. The resulting scar may be smooth, but often it presents an irregular, sometimes ropy surface. Shrinkage of the tissue may result in contractures and deformity.

Keloids and hypertrophic scars result from an abnormal growth of collagen tissue in a scar. They are elevated, swollen, tense, and sometimes painful. Usually keloids and hypertrophic scars develop in recently healed wounds. Keloids may be quite massive and deforming; excision frequently results in an even larger keloid. This type of growth is most commonly seen in the black race, and often they are found on the upper portions of the trunk, neck, or ears. Unlike keloids, hypertrophic scars may regress spontaneously after a few months, but at times the distinction between hypertrophic scars and keloids is impossible to make.

Of the 16 readings in the Circulating File on scars, only two touch on the physiology of scars, and thus comments necessarily will be brief. Do scars impair the normal functioning of the body?

Apparently some do, as in 487-17, "any scar tissue detracts from the general physical health of a body, for it requires a changing in the circulation continually." In contrast, in 440-3, when asked if apparently extensive scars on the abdomen and legs were detrimental, Cayce replied, "little or no hindrance." The same reading also gives a tantalizing hint on the origin and nature of scar tissue: ". . .where tissue has been in the nature of folds—or scar tissue, produced from superficial activity from the active forces in the body itself, in making for coagulation in any portion of the system, whether external or internal."

Just what is meant by "folds" is difficult to guess. Perhaps it refers to an as yet unappreciated feature of scar collagen. The term "coagulation" is used repeatedly in the readings. [2423] had a lack of it, and healing could not take place. [1377] had an abnormality of coagulation, and adhesions resulted, and in reading 440-3 it appeared to refer to a healing property. It seems to be a broader term than simple clotting of blood, and might be referring to complex biochemical processes involving fibrinogen and other serum proteins and numerous enzymes. (Further study of many more readings mentioning coagulation may be necessary to clarify Cayce's meaning. In Dr. William McGarey's commentary on "Leukopenia— Leukocytosis," coagulation is seen as the rebuilding of cells throughout the body.)

The essential, practical point in these readings is that scars are not necessarily the end point in the healing process. In some cases, at least, total eradication is possible; "remember the whole surface may be entirely changed if this is done persistently and consistently. . .in the course of two to two-and-a-half years, a new skin!" (440-3) Some scars, however, cannot be entirely eradicated. In 3167-1 regarding the scars from abscesses which had been lanced, "Can't pull out nail holes!. . .may pull out the nails, but we can't pull out the holes!" This would seem to indicate that incision and drainage of abscesses indiscriminately would be a poor practice, although Cayce did recommend at times lancing of boils.

II. Rationale of Therapy

The treatment of cutaneous scars is covered in all readings but two which deal with adhesions and chronic inflammation. These two will be discussed separately at the conclusion of this review.

In most of the readings on cutaneous scars, by which is meant healed wounds, camphorated oil was suggested, either alone, or alternated with olive oil and tincture of myrrh, or diluted with other oils. The best description of the effects of these prescribed medicines is given here:

> . . .*olive oil*—properly prepared (hence pure olive oil should always be used)—is one of the most effective agents for stimulating muscular activity, or mucous membrane activity, that may be applied to a body. . .*tincture of myrrh* acts with the pores of the skin in such a manner as to strike in, causing the circulation to be carried to affected parts [scars]. . .*camphorated oil* is merely the same basic force [olive oil?] to which has been added properties of camphor in more or less its raw or original state, than the spirits of same. Such activity in the epidermis is not only to produce soothing to affected areas but to stimulate the circulation in such effectual ways and manners as to combine with the other properties in bringing what will be determined, in the course of two to two-and-a-half years, a new skin!   440-3

The muscle activity stimulated by the olive oil may refer not only to striated skeletal muscle, but also to the smooth muscle in the intestinal walls, and in the walls of small arteries and arterioles. Perhaps such activity stimulates the circulation within the scar tissue leading toward that activity which is necessary to absorb the scar collagen. Both the camphor and tincture of myrrh were also described as stimulating the circulation. Camphor is also called a soothing force. Camphor is classified by Goodman and Gilman as a hydroaromatic gum obtained from the bark and wood of the tree, *Cinnamomum camphora,* which is grown in Taiwan and Japan. It is classed as a rubefacient, which means it produces capillary dilatation, in accordance with the Cayce information. If taken internally it causes nausea and vomiting, and large doses of solid camphor in children may cause convulsions. Therefore, camphor lotions should be kept out of the reach of children.

III. Suggested Therapeutic Regimen

Since camphorated oil appears to be the key to the treatment of cutaneous scars, it is important that it be accurately defined. Camphorated oil is no longer made commercially as it was in Cayce's day. At that time, it was made with natural gum camphor in olive oil. Presently available is a synthetic camphor in cottonseed oil; therefore, it may not be a satisfactory substitute for the camphorated oil referred to in the readings.

Case [440] was experiencing extensive scarring on the legs and abdomen. Massage was suggested alternating equal parts of tincture of myrrh and olive oil on one day followed the next day by camphorated oil. (The olive oil is to be heated before adding the tincture of myrrh, and only enough for the day's massage is to be prepared.) This sounds like an ideal program for extensive scars.

The successful removal of severe burn scars on [2015] was accomplished with a formula that has become a classic Cayce remedy:

> Camphorated oil, 2 ounces
> Lanolin, dissolved, ½ teaspoon
> Peanut oil, 1 ounce

Dr. James L. Rowland, D.O., Ph.D., of Kansas City, apparently has used this lotion successfully in wound scars and keloids. The lotion should be gently massaged into and around the scar with the fingertips once or twice a day.

For active acne in case [528], an interesting lotion was prescribed:

> Camphorated oil, 2 parts
> Witch hazel, 1 part
> Russian white oil, 1 part

This lotion must be shaken very well and massaged for several minutes into the acne areas twice a day. It was said to help clear the skin and treat and prevent scars as well. (Nujol is one form of Russian white oil.)

Note that the camphorated oil is diluted about in half in the last two formulas. A similar dilution was suggested in a burn scar case (487-17), but the diluent was sweet oil (olive oil).

Case [4003] had severe scarring, possibly with calification and contractures, which followed an injury. Treatment was aimed at removing the scar by absorption and excretion through the respiratory, perspiratory, and alimentary systems. Local therapy consisted of hot Epsom salts packs followed by massage using cocoa butter. Exercise, hydrotherapy, colonics, and diet were also part of the program.

Finally, in any healing, the spiritual status of the patient may be most important.

Let the scars be removed from the own mental, the *own mental and spiritual self*. Turn to those things of making application of the fruits of the spirit of truth, love, patience, gentleness, kindness, long-suffering, brotherly love, putting away those little tendencies for being "catty" at times or being selfish or expressing jealousy and such.

Let that mind be in thee as was in Him, who is the way and the truth and the light, and He will make the light of love so shine through thy countenance that few, if any, will ever see the scars made by self-indulgence in other experiences.   5092-1

A. Adhesions

Body cavities, such as the peritoneal cavity, are lined with serous membranes which extend around the organs in the cavity and allow them to slip over each other freely. Inflammation of the serous membrane may cause it to lose its slippery character and stick to itself forming an adhesion. The Cayce concept is much in accord with the traditional, but goes a bit further in defining the problem as system-wide.

As indicated by that as has been given, the *inflammation* as produced in system that caused irritation to the general *plasm* of the blood supply tends to make the scar tissue [inflamed serous membrane?] become adhesive in its nature.   1377-8

Treatment of adhesions was to be accomplished by vibratory applications to the back.

These will *keep* the conditions so that the adhesions will be broken entirely by the absorption that is created in the active forces of the blood supply circulation; circulation here meaning not *just* blood supply but the lymph and emunctory circulation, and nerve circulation as well. 1377-8

In addition, malt and codliver oil (in Pure Food tablets) were recommended for [1377] to "carry those vitamins in such quantities to assimilate best with the system." An improper coagulation in the blood apparently could be remedied by such vitamin forces.

B. Chronic Inflammation (Infection?)

The situation in [2423]'s case is difficult to diagnose from this distance. It may have represented a chronic paronychia or perhaps a granulating wound. The finger had been splinted, and this may have led to the diminished flexibility mentioned in a subsequent letter to Cayce. The reading virtually ignored the finger, instead getting to important systemic disturbances:

. . .first an unbalancing of the chemical system, until little reaction, or assimilation of values of vitamin B-1 is possible, or the coagulating elements; then poisons from hydrochloric acid, or excesses of same in the system, as combined with influences without.

Hence the inability for the coagulation, or for abrasions or injuries to heal. 2423-1

Treatment consisted of Atomidine and the "triple salt" combination:
     Rochelle salts, 1 level tablespoonful
     Sulfur, 1 level tablespoonful
     Cream of tartar, 1 level tablespoonful
These are to be mixed with a mortar and pestle. The use of precipitated sulfur rather than sulfur flowers is suggested. Precipitated sulfur is much finer grained, and thus presents a larger active surface for the same amount of sulfur. A level teaspoonful was to be taken first thing in the morning for five days.

The same prescription has been found in readings on acne, boils, and psoriasis. At times the warning was given to avoid chills or wet feet while taking the prescription, and in some cases osteopathic treatment was to follow. However, in [2423]'s case, the use of small doses of x-ray was to follow five days on the "salts." Local treatment was almost incidental. Cayce suggested "cocoa butter that is dissolved or rubbed in with olive oil; as this will aid in preventing scars, even upon the areas where old sores and injuries have been so disturbing to the body." In addition the apple diet for three days was suggested for cleansing the system. At the end of the three days a tablespoon of olive oil was to complete the purge.

This case is indexed under "scars" because of the advice on prevention of scars with cocoa butter and olive oil. Physiologically it may be more closely related to other cutaneous conditions such as boils or psoriasis.

Robert Forbis, Jr., M.D.

Edgar Cayce readings referenced:

440-3	1377-8	2423-1
475-1	1566-4	3167-1
487-17	1567-4	3334-1
528-2	1765-1	4003-1
1000-22	2015-6, 10	5092-1

SCLERODERMA

I. Physiological Considerations

Scleroderma is a disease process more technically known as progressive systemic sclerosis. It involves the collagenous connective tissues and may cause widespread, symmetrical, leathery induration of the skin, followed by atrophy and pigmentation. The cutaneous lesions are believed to be the external manifestation of a systemic disease, and the muscles, bones, mucous membranes, heart, lungs, intestinal tract and other internal organs may be involved by the same process, resulting in functional impairment such as heart failure or pulmonary insufficiency. The reader is invited to review this disease process in Cecil's *Textbook of Medicine* for a more thorough understanding of what modern medical opinions are at the present time concerning scleroderma.

Scleroderma, as it is seen in the readings, affects not only the skin but the blood-forming structural areas such as the bone and the lung tissue itself in a process which produces a hardening or a clotting of the blood, mainly as a result of the blood attempting to bring about what is called coagulation—that creative process within the body which is the building up of new tissue as old tissue normally dies. This is seen most graphically in the skin, wherein the superficial circulation to the various layers of the skin is involved in this process. Nerve endings in these areas become deadened, in turn resulting in acute pain as well as reflexing to the autonomic nervous system which then becomes involved itself. In this manner the organs become disturbed throughout the body.

Glands within the body—principally the thyroid, the adrenals, and the liver—become deficient in supplying elements which keep the epidermis normal. These glandular elements are necessary in the formation of structure out of energy, as Cayce has described many times in his readings. With these hormones absent, the effect of the influence of the glands is to produce, apparently, a tubercle bacillus or germ in the lymphatics of the skin itself as a direct result of the skin being destroyed and becoming hardened more rapidly than it can be rebuilt. This becomes a "consumptive" condition with an inflammation of the lymph in that area that *consumes* the circulation between the outer, the middle, and the innermost portions of the skin covering.

Another way to understand the process or course of events: The glandular deficiency creates a lack of nutrition in the circulation of the skin itself, which in turn checks the flow of the lymph circulation. As the disease progresses, conditions in the circulation become more disturbed and areas harden where the lymph or emunctory flow is destroyed. The nerves in these areas become involved as described earlier and then swelling reflects the body's attempt to better conditions. As the lymph flow is destroyed, the lymphatics themselves become inflamed, creating the germ or the tubercle bacillus, which consumes the circulation of the skin creating a malformation. In the more advanced cases of scleroderma, the perspiration becomes involved with the destroying of the sweat glands. Without this normal breathing of the skin, a gradual increase in acidosis within the body occurs. This makes the body more susceptible to colds and to intercurrent infections.

Far advanced cases, of course, have nearly all portions of the body involved. Thus little of the oxygen needs of the body can be met by a malfunctioning respiratory system, and the entire body is thus put under a greater strain. As these conditions progress, assimilation becomes more difficult, and the lack of reconstructive activities in the body grows progressively more acute.

Review of the above information points up the fact that the body's endocrine glands, in their disturbed functioning, become the primary cause of this disease process, with the collagenous changes being secondary to the inadequate restoration of circulatory structures within the skin itself.

II. Rationale of Therapy

In approaching therapy, we should remember that the body has a capability of normal function:

Thus, we would administer those activities which would bring a normal

reaction through these portions, stimulating them to an activity from the body itself, rather than the body becoming dependent upon supplies that are robbing portions of the system to produce activity in other portions, or the system receiving elements or chemical reactions being supplied without arousing the activity of the system itself for a more normal condition.

1968-3

A primary therapy in scleroderma certainly should be to eliminate the basic cause of the disease, which has already been described as a malfunction of the glands of the body. However, emphasis should be placed upon the need for persistence in gradually reestablishing a normal function throughout all those areas of the body which have been disturbed. Thus, the primary aim of therapy would be the gradual redirecting of the forces and energies of the body itself back toward what we know and consider to be a normal function.

Therapy should be directed at achieving certain goals which might be enumerated in order to establish a clear-cut direction. These goals should be kept in mind as attempts are made to restore the functioning of the body step by step. The following are self-explanatory:

1. Cleanse and purify the glandular system of the body. This will aid in the blood-building forces as well as bring more normal activity to the circulatory system of the skin and the other tissues which need rebuilding.

2. Promote a more adequate assimilation of food substances. Attention needs to be paid to the diet and to the functioning of the digestive organs and assimilative tissues.

3. Correct the functioning of the superficial circulation and the lymphatic circulation of the skin. Local therapy should be considered as well as those influences which are brought about through the other goals which are listed here.

4. Add to the system that which will purify the blood; set into motion those parts which have become disturbed; and build up the necessary forces to bring a nearer to normal reaction. This would imply the use of the wet cell appliance, which apparently reintroduces assimilative influences into the body that have been rejected in the establishing of scleroderma.

5. Improve the oxygen intake where needed and stimulate a more normal functioning of the lung tissues. Insure adequate eliminations and maintain a balance of the nervous systems of the body.

The use of any of the applications in a condition as chronic and deep-set as scleroderma requires a persistence that often taxes the patience of anyone faced with this particular disease, whether the sufferer or the therapist. The necessity of consistent application, however, exists, and Cayce emphasizes it in a variety of ways. One of the best examples is as follows:

Do not make the applications merely as a routine—either the rubs, the diets or the appliance. Let these be done with the continuous spiritual purpose to be healed of the disturbances *for* a definite purpose, that is to be constructive and helpful to others; to those about self and to others.

Keep optimistic. Pray often; seeing, feeling, asking, desiring, expecting help—from Him; who is the way, the truth, the light. He faileth not those who keep His purposes.   2514-1

III. Suggested Therapeutic Regimen

Therapy for scleroderma must be initiated according to the severity of the individual case. Among those cases in this Circulating File, [528] is obviously the most critically ill. Thus, the basic therapy used in all cases of scleroderma is closely joined to procedures designed to control and reverse some of the most distressing complications in her particular instance.

For this 28-year-old young woman, the Atomidine either by mouth or through the wet cell appliance is for cleansing and purifying the glandular system as well as "supplying to the system those forces or influences that will add to the bloodstream in such a way and manner as to give that resistance in the hemoglobin and the effluvia of the blood itself, those abilities to destroy or throw off the conditions." (528-3) These were not used at first. Rather [528] was kept at bed rest and given fresh air or allowed to breathe oil of pine or eucalyptus and benzoin burning in the room. Eliminations were insured through the use of enemas—not cathartics. Assimilations were improved with Ventriculin (see Appendix), beef juice taken frequently (see Appendix), and occasionally egg mixed with whiskey (which has been burned to remove the toxic portion of the alcohol), and a no-starch diet designed to bring an alkaline condition to the body. Castor oil packs daily over the abdomen and also the back, extending from the level of the diaphragm down to the sacrum, disseminate energies to the body. Packs should be followed by a thorough sponging off of the body with a saturated bicarbonate of soda solution. The soda removes substances from the skin that otherwise might be disseminated through the system and create unfavorable results. A review of readings 528-3, -4, and -5 would be instructive and helpful in understanding this particular case.

Later on, enemas were suggested with two tablespoons of Glyco-Thymoline added to one-and-a-half quarts of water at body temperature to prevent "reinfection from the tendency for the system to exhume this disturbed circulation through the alimentary canal." (528-5) Also, at this time, [528] was given instructions to inhale fumes from pure apple brandy in a charred oak keg. The keg was to be at least a gallon or a gallon-and-a-half in size, with one-half to one gallon of the brandy added. It should be kept close to the radiator or warmth of some sort, so gasses may be inhaled from the charred oak as well as from the brandy. [528] was instructed to inhale once a day at first, but when aching or feeling shaky, two or three times a day, "For this will assist the circulation in healing tissue that has been impaired by the effect of the condition as given." (528-6)

Red wine taken with some black bread or rye crisp in the late afternoon further strengthens the body. In other references through the readings this apparently strengthened the blood and corrected anemia to some extent. Alcohol rubs were also designated as a strengthening factor, if grain alcohol were used and not rubbing alcohol. These were especially to be used on the limbs and across the shoulders and "this will also tend to make for a better lymph circulation." (528-5)

Primary therapy, however, in all cases that have been reviewed, is directed at bringing iodine into the system in the form of Atomidine to improve the glandular system through a cleansing and purifying action. [2514] and [2526] took the Atomidine by mouth first and then the wet cell appliance was used thereafter. [528] did not use Atomidine by mouth until much later in her recovery period. Instead she was given the wet cell appliance at first.

Still another variation is seen in which [2526] was given Atomidine by mouth, one drop daily for five days and then off five days, then one drop daily for five days then off, etc. At the same time she used the wet cell appliance with only gold chloride in the solution jar. At the beginning of her therapy, however, she used Atomidine one drop daily for two days, then two drops daily for two days, and then three for two days, four, and then five. At the end of this 10-day period she stopped the Atomidine and then took an Epsom salts bath in 30 gallons of tepid water with 15 pounds of Epsom salts in it for 30 minutes, while massaging the body thoroughly over the lower limbs. Following this, a peanut oil massage was directed from the base of the head downward, especially around the thyroid, then down the spine and particularly over the lower part of the spinal system; the whole of the sacral area and down the limbs, both the underside and the "overside," as Cayce described it. As much oil was to be massaged in as the body would absorb. This procedure was to be repeated once with a slightly warmer bath, and then the wet cell was begun.

The wet cell battery and its application was part of the therapy in every instance. For [2514] a double charge was suggested, except for the willow charcoal. Thus, her battery was charged with one-and-a-half gallons of distilled water, three pounds of copper sulphate, two ounces of sulphuric acid, six drams of zinc, and one-half pound of willow charcoal. Separate solution jars were to be used for the three different substances that were recommended. The gold was suggested for supplying the nerve energies, the camphor for healing forces, and the Atomidine for cleansing. Four ounces of each solution was to be used—the Atomidine and spirits of camphor to be used as usually obtained, and the gold chloride to be one grain per ounce of water. The three solutions were to be alternated with the negative electrode attached over the lacteal center (three finger breadths to the right and three up from the umbilicus). The positive electrode or the small copper electrode, attached first, was for the gold to be attached at the fourth lumbar vertebra; the spirits of camphor next at the ninth dorsal vertebra; and the Atomidine solution at the second and third dorsal area, which would "aid in governing the assimilating forces from the nerve forces in the body." (2514-1) The solution jar is always attached to the negative lead.

The diet recommended was an alkaline-forming one with many leafy vegetables as the main portion. Fish, fowl, and lamb are all right, but fried foods should never be used. Vegetable soups and other foods easily assimilated are recommended, vegetables cooked with Patapar paper or the equivalent parchment paper which may be purchased in most health food stores. Meat should not be cooked with the vegetable soups.

Stimulation to the superficial circulation and the lymphatic circulation of the skin is brought about through massages and fume baths. The massage already described for [2526] is essentially the same as that used in the other cases. Apparently the sacral area, the legs and the hips, need more massage than other areas. This may have to do with reflex influences to the glands or to the nerve plexuses in those areas. A witch hazel fume bath (described in 2526-4), which could be done at home, was to be followed with peanut oil and olive oil massage.

Local areas of hardening are treated in various ways. Castor oil packs over hardened areas were suggested every other day over a long period of time for [2514]; Ichthyol over the sore places until the area was cleansed and then Cuticura after that. Unguentine was suggested to be massaged in the skin for soreness and pain through the shoulder. These seem to be palliative measures for the most part.

A rather comprehensive therapeutic regimen would include the Atomidine and the wet cell appliance to work on the glandular system, the nerves, and the bringing into the body those energies needed; a dietary regimen and care for the organs of assimilation to provide that which is needed through the alimentary canal; local therapy of the skin through massages and applications such as castor oil; and those other factors such as cleansing of the bowels with enemas and aiding in more extensive complications of the disease process. It is perhaps of most vital importance to emphasize that persistent, patient, consistent adherence to the applications be maintained.

Do these, as we have indicated. . .Not as rote, but knowing that within self must be found that which may be awakened to the *building* of that necessary for the body, mentally and physically and spiritually, to carry *its* part in this experience. For the application of any influence must have that which is of the divine awakening of the activative forces in every atom, every cell of a living body.   **726-1**

William A. McGarey, M.D.

Edgar Cayce readings referenced:
528-3 through 6
2514-1 through 15
2526-1 through 6

STUTTERING

Stuttering can be described as a disturbance in the flow or rhythm of connected speech. It is usually characterized by repetitions of syllables (e.g., buh-buh-balloon), prolongations of certain sounds (e.g., fffffeather), and occasional cessation of airflow (i.e., air ceases to flow through the vocal folds and the vocal folds cease vibrating; thus, no sound is produced). In advanced cases of stuttering certain secondary phenomena occur. Extreme tension in the musculature of the vocal folds, tongue, lips and face cause "struggle behavior"—grimaces, tics, head jerks, etc. Most stutterers develop fear of certain words or speaking situations as well, and try to avoid these.

For centuries the cause and treatment of stuttering has puzzled both stutterers themselves and those who have attempted to treat them. Of all the speech disorders, stuttering is both the most researched and the most baffling. In the last 50 years particularly, medical and paramedical journals have been filled with scientific studies and case histories. As a result, vast amounts of facts about the physical dimensions of stuttering have been collected. However, the knowledge gathered has not resulted in any consensus regarding the etiology or treatment of stuttering.

There are literally hundreds of theories about the cause of stuttering—each theory is supported by some research, and each has generated a specific treatment approach. However, these theories can be grouped into four major categories:

1. The organicity theory. This group of theories has been most prevalent throughout the ages. Basically it states that dysfluency is due to some physical defect in the stutterer. Since connected speech requires intricate timing and coordination of many simultaneous movements (including action of the lungs, vocal folds and surrounding musculature, soft palate, tongue, and lips), a breakdown in the

function of any one of these can disrupt the rhythm of speech. Virtually every organ involved in speech production has, at one time or another, been viewed as the defective one—including a "frozen" tongue, enlarged tonsils, specific nervous dysfunction and brain lesions. In light of the information contained in the readings of Edgar Cayce, one theory—that of Seeman (1934)—is particularly interesting. Seeman felt that the sympathetic part of the autonomic nervous system became hyperactive due to emotional stress or lack of inhibition from the cortex. This "oversupply" of energy produced a disturbance in all the fundamental processes upon which speech is based.

2. Neurosis theory. After Freud's time it became fashionable to view stuttering as the result of some deep-seated emotional or psychological problem. According to this specific school of thought, stutterers were felt to be "stuck" at the oral or anal level of emotional development, or experiencing deeply inadequate personal relationships. At present, many therapists still view stutterers as being basically neurotic.

3. Learning theory. Historically many observers have viewed stuttering as a bad habit. Research in the '60s showed that approximately 80% of all preschool children go through a brief period of "normal non-fluency," which can easily be confused with stuttering. According to learning theorists, this non-fluency can be turned into stuttering by the reactions of the child's parents, friends, teachers, etc. The child learns to fear speaking because of others' reactions, and this fear disrupts the intricate coordination pattern required for fluent speech, resulting in increased dysfluency.

4. Disturbed auditory feedback theory. We all rely on sensory feedback to monitor our speech. If a person is deprived of kinesthetic (sense of touch) feedback by local anesthesia of the palate, his speech becomes slurred. If auditory feedback is delayed (by use of a tape recorder with a delay built into it), normal speakers suffer fluency breaks very similar to those produced in stuttering. This has led to the theory that stuttering is due to some distortion in the auditory feedback system used to monitor speech.

Each school of thought has produced methods of treatment related to supposed etiology. Organicity theorists suggest treatment of the underlying physical defect—ranging from wine to unfreeze the tongue, to removal of the tonsils, to training the central nervous system through patterned exercise. Adherents of the neurosis school of thought use psychoanalysis, group therapy, and systematic desensitization to overcome non-fluency. Learning theorists try to change parental reactions to the young stutterer and extinguish specific stuttering behaviors. Other therapists try to mask disturbed auditory feedback with "white noise" or further delay the feedback. (When stutterers are placed on delayed feedback their fluency improves.)

Edgar Cayce gave readings for 10 individuals who regarded themselves, or were regarded by their parents, as stutterers. However, two of these individuals, [2705] and [2441], were told that their problem was not one of stuttering; rather it was a difficulty in choosing the appropriate words, or in putting thoughts into words. (These are language formulation problems, not the motor speech difficulty seen in stuttering.) A 21-year-old, [3245], was told in a life reading that his stammering—as indeed any situation—could be dealt with "if [the body] trusts in the ideal manner. Not in self. . .but in Him. . ." (3245-1)

These three readings have not been included in the Circulating File. Also excluded was a reading for a two-year-old, [402], in whom stuttering was secondary to a major illness. Very little information was given about the stuttering, other than a statement that her speech would improve as her general condition improved. A recommendation was given for spinal massage.

Of the remaining six cases, only three had stuttering as their primary problem—[605], [1788] and [2015]; of these, only [605] had follow-up readings about the stuttering. In the remaining three cases stuttering was a relatively minor problem of overall disturbed body function. A 33-year-old, [99], was presented with vertigo, imbalances in the blood, problems with the spleen and liver, a lesion of the cardiac plexus, and problems with the digestive system. A five-year-old, [1490], had a disfiguring skin condition due to disturbances in the glandular functions (specifically, the thyroid and adrenals), unbalanced body salts, nervous system incoordination due to subluxations of dorsal six and seven, and a lesion in the coccyx. For a nine-year-old, [1817], stuttering was secondary to blindness in one eye and a disturbance of kidney functioning. In these three cases treatments for the conditions must be separated from treatment specifically recommended for stuttering.

I. Physiological Considerations

According to the readings, the "sense of speech is the highest developed vibration in an organism," for it depends upon input from all the other senses and thus is heavily dependent upon the coordination forces in the body. These "coordinating forces" include the sympathetic nervous system (which is linked to the unconscious mind or imaginative body), the cerebrospinal nervous system, and the neurological connections, which "register impulse in [the] brain." (146-1) In other words, fluent clear speech depends upon coordination of impulses from both the sympathetic nervous system and the cerebrospinal nervous system.

When specifically asked what causes stuttering, Cayce responded: "The connections for the auditory as well as the vocal forces of the body derive their impulse from the 3rd cervical, as well as the 3rd, 4th and 5th dorsal.

"Hence it is necessary. . .to reduce. . .those tendencies of the body to oversupply energies to the vocal cords. . ." (1788-13) According to the reading, subluxations of these vertebrae, which produce pressure on the nerve, can cause nervous system incoordination, leading to disturbance in auditory functioning (ranging from a buzzing or humming in the ears to deafness) and vocal functioning (including stuttering, mutism and "unclear speech"). Other readings present disturbances in the spinal ganglia as causative factors in language disorders (some of which may resemble stuttering, but appear to be related more to word retrieval problems).

These six readings clearly implicate pressures and subluxations in the upper dorsal and cervical areas as the causes of stuttering. In five cases stuttering was specifically linked to a problem in the upper dorsal region. The third dorsal was always involved and the fourth and fifth dorsal were frequently involved. Problems with the second dorsal are mentioned in two readings. In a sixth case, [1490], no specific problem in the upper dorsal was pinpointed. However, an osteopathic coordination of the upper dorsal and cervical vertebrae was advised once the corrections suggested for specific lower dorsal vertebrae had been made. (The subluxations in the lower dorsal were related to the child's glandular deficiency, not stuttering.)

In three cases the readings specifically mentioned the third cervical vetebra as a causative factor. In a fourth case pressure along the cervicals was mentioned; and, of course, [1490] was told to have an osteopathic coordination of the cervical vertebrae along with the dorsal.

In two cases the overt stuttering was accompanied by a humming or buzzing in the ears. In another case the subluxations had caused an unspecified "deflection" in the auditory force; this was presented as a causative factor in the stuttering. In a fourth case an auditory perceptual problem was noted; the child had normally acute hearing, but there was a slowness in perceiving and reacting to auditory stimuli. Therefore, in a total of six cases, four had some specific problem with hearing.

In three cases the spinal problems had caused a hindering or slowing of blood circulation through the affected areas (throat, larynx, tonsils and adenoids)—and in one case blood had accumulated in these areas. Poor eliminations was a contributing factor in three cases.

In summary, then, the material in the readings falls primarily into two of the common theories on the etiology of stuttering. Clearly the speech problem is organically based, as it is caused by subluxations or pressures in the spinal column which "prevent[s] the normal flow, the normal impulse, the normal nerve activity through the bronchi, through the throat, through the vocal box, through the organs of the head and throat." (605-2) Another reading further defines the lack of normal flow as including an "oversupply [of] energies to the vocal cords. . ." (1788-13) In addition, the readings support the theory that disturbances in auditory perception are a causative factor. [1490] clearly had delayed auditory feedback, while [2015] had a "deflection in the auditory forces—which is indicated in the speaking voice." (2015-8) Two other cases had "head noises"— a humming or buzzing in the ears—which may have affected auditory perception. Concerning the learning theories, one set of parents was advised, "Do not curb or make the body aware, by anxiety, of too much difference of opinion." (1788-13) [605] was told to "be mindful that the body overcomes that tendency of becoming frustrated; and this lisping and stammering will disappear." (605-3) Clearly the readings indicated that anxiety and frustration cause stuttering to worsen.

II. Rationale of Therapy

The primary treatment, recommended in every case, was osteopathic or chiropractic adjustment of the affected portion of the spine. Most frequently a regular series of adjustments was advised; e.g., two or three a week for several weeks. [605] was advised to have more intensive treatments, as the dorsal subluxations were particularly difficult to correct. For the three youngest children (including [402], whose reading is not included in the file), spinal massage with peanut oil was also recommended—preferably on a daily basis. Massage throughout the dorsal and cervical areas was also recommended for [605]. (Please note that the type of massage recommended for [1490] was specifically related to her skin condition, not stuttering.)

In many readings, attitudinal factors were considered almost as important as physical corrections. [605] was told that "in meeting these [conditions], there must be made first in the mental body that determination that it will carry on in *normal* activity. . .that the hindrances will be removed. . .[for] without the activity of the mental body. . .even with the [osteopathic] changes, these would only make for partial corrections." She was also told to be "careful—painfully careful—in being mindful of the expression. . ." (605-1) Two years later, when she had a recurrence of stuttering (due to having an incomplete series of treatments), [605] was advised to be mindful of frustration. [1788]'s parents were told to foster an attitude of expectancy regarding the positive results of the therapy: "Do keep the body (though young as yet [4½]. . .) acquainted with that being done, and why, and the expectancy the body may have with the use of the treatments suggested." (1788-13)

Because the third and fourth dorsal have neurological connections to the digestive organs, three of the six cases had problems with overacidity or poor eliminations. For two of these cases an alkaline-reacting diet was recommended, with the further recommendation for one child of the use of Glyco-Thymoline to purify the alimentary canal. In two other cases a general body-building diet was recommended.

Other recommendations for treatment are to be found in these six readings. However, most of these are specifically related to a condition other than stuttering; e.g., Atomidine doses and use of the wet cell appliance were recommended for [1490] to overcome her glandular deficiencies. [99] was given a prescription to correct the imbalances between white and red blood cells; deep electrical vibration therapy was also suggested. Various other forms of electrical therapy were recommended, but only one appears to be related to the stuttering problems: [605] was advised to have diathermy to coordinate nerve impulses to improve blood circulation through the throat and head.

In summary, osteopathic or chiropractic adjustments sufficient to obtain a permanent realignment of the dorsal and cervical vertebrae were the primary recommendations. Attitude was also very important in achieving fluent speech. An alkaline-reacting diet was often recommended; the readings generally presented this diet as the optimal diet for good health as well. Other therapies appeared to be specific to other conditions and were not recommended for stutterers in general.

A word of caution: The readings for [605] warned against giving only partial adjustments (i.e., not having enough adjustments to ensure lasting spinal realignment). Apparently [605] did not have a sufficient number of adjustments and her stuttering symptoms recurred with greater severity two years later.

Lesley Laraby Boykin, DSPA, CCC-SP

Edgar Cayce readings referenced:
99-1
605-1 through 4
1490-1, 3
1788-13
1817-1, 2
2015-8

SYPHILIS

I. Physiological Considerations

Syphilis—commonly called lues, a word derived from Latin meaning pestilence (*Lues venerea,* venereal pestilence)—is caused by the spirochete organism *Treponema pallidum* which enters the human body through mucous membranes or skin abrasions, usually by sexual contact from an infected person harboring the organism. Upon entering an area of contact, a painless lesion called a chancre is formed. At this point the course of the disease is in the primary stage of syphilis. Before the lesion resolves itself, examination of the exudate of the chancre can sometimes show the presence of *T. pallidum* under the darkfield microscope. The presence of these organisms in the lesion at this point is diagnostic of syphilis.

One must be experienced to identify treponemes, since some spirochetes (such as *T. microdentium* in the mouth) can resemble the syphilis organism quite closely.

The chancre next resolves itself completely, and the course of the disease will progress to the secondary stage (two to ten weeks after the chancre heals) where cutaneous involvement occurs. A rash will appear in the ano-genital region, axillas, and the mouth. Secondary syphilis can also occur as meningitis, chorioretinitis, or periostitis. However, a goodly number of patients will pass through this stage without showing any symptoms.

The secondary lesions resolve themselves and the insidious spirochete will invade deeper into the surrounding tissue. This is then the tertiary stage of syphilis. Here granulomatous lesions (gummas) occur in the skin, liver, bones, and degenerative changes come about in the central nervous system. In some cases, syphilitic cardiovascular lesions occur causing aneurysms. Recently treponemes have been demonstrated in the gummas, and the tissue response must be attributed to a hypersensitivity to the organisms at this stage.

These various stages described are not absolute. Some people have no outward symptoms in the primary or secondary state, but these individuals may have profound involvement in the tertiary stage or may not show any involvement at all. It is interesting, too, that 25% of the cases of early syphilis will seemingly resolve themselves completely. The other 25% of the cases will go into a latent stage and remain so while the remainder will progress to full blown cases of tertiary syphilis. The time of appearance of late syphilitic manifestations will vary from patient to patient. In the latent stages, an arbitrary time of two years is selected. Under two years is called early latent, and the possibility of infection of a partner remains. After that time, the late latent stage is entered, and infection of another is unlikely although the possibility of tertiary syphilis appearing remains even for these persons.

Congenital syphilis can occur in the fetus since the treponeme can cross the placental barrier after the 18th week of pregnancy. The time of initial infection and the duration thereof during gestation will decide if the child will be stillborn, have fulminating syphilis, or be uninfected. If the mother has primary or secondary syphilis, the chances are quite high that the fetus will be infected. In late latent syphilis of the mother chances are somewhat better that the child will be well. These children that are affected and are born alive may have signs of congenital lues: interstitial keratitis, Hutchinson's teeth, Charcot's joints, saddle nose, periostitis, and a variety of central nervous system anomalies. Early congenital lesions may be shown in the neonate under two years of age. (These lesions may resemble the secondary stage in the adult.) After two years the secondary lesions will resolve as well as all the manifesting congenital signs. Sometimes the central nervous system symptoms may manifest themselves as late as the late teens. As in regular syphilis, no definite timetable can be given when late congenital lues will erupt as well as how it will show up.

There are two schools of thought concerning the origins of syphilis. One claims that its origin was in the New World when Columbus' men brought it to Europe from the Haitian Indians. The men passed it on to the prostitutes, who passed it on to the local population and the Spanish soldiers, who bore it to the religious wars that were to plague Europe along with syphilis—which was called then the "Great Pox." The second group maintains that the disease was always present in a benign form until the 1490s. Some scholars believe that evidences for late syphilis are noted in early records such as the Books of Leviticus and Job where late syphilis symptoms are described in Job's sores that covered him from head to foot and in the Levite's function to look for "leprosy" signs. The disease in Renaissance times was quite virulent until it evolved into the more mild, chronic form that it is today. While the disease is milder and usually not fatal in the secondary form, its fatality can result from complications of late syphilis nowadays.

The diagnosis of syphilis presently is made not only with clinical evidences but also with treponemal and serological tests. As mentioned before, the darkfield test is run to see the presence of spirochetes. Also an improvement in this technique is shown by the fluorescent darkfield test (FADF). In this test, the serum from the lesion containing spirochetes is put on a glass slide and allowed to dry. Then a fluorescent antibody is put on, rinsed off, and the slide is put under an ultraviolet microscope to see if the organisms are present. The microbes fluoresce if present. If they are not present, no fluorescence is seen. This test is convenient for physicians who do not have a darkfield microscope (the dried slide can be sent to the laboratory by mail).

Of course, many cases of syphilis do not show in lesions where the organism can be observed (especially after the lesions resolve), so serological tests must be made. When the treponemes attack body tissue, two reactions occur. One is the antibody response against the treponeme itself. The other is the formation of the antibody complex, reagin, which is formed by release from tissue debris of a hapten that in turn joins a protein to be attacked by an antibody. The ease and the ability to quantitate the reagin which is equivalent to the amount of treponemal involvement make the reagin test the test of choice for screening and to follow treatment. The effectiveness of treatment can be noted by the drop in titer. The rise in titer of reagin increases through primary and secondary syphilis and may drop in the latent stages, although the titer can sometimes rise in tertiary involvement.

The easiest reagin test is the flocculation test where lipiodial or cardiolipid antigen is added to the serum to form a visible aggregate. If no reagin, then no reaction. The VDRL slide test is usually done nowadays to test for reagin due to convenience and accuracy. The fact that it is a slide test (read with a microscope) and a fairly rapid one lends it to common use in the laboratory. During the early days since the discovery of a practical flocculation test in 1910, many other tests were developed such as the Kahn, Kline, VDRL, Hinton, and

Mazzini. The complement fixation test developed by Wasserman in 1906 (first practical serological test for syphilis developed) has been improved many times since then. (Kolmer in 1922 refined the complement fixation test to such a point that it remained a test of choice until the advent of a practical treponemal antibody test. It was more specific than the flocculation tests.) The principle is that complement is drawn away by the antigen and reagin from the sheep red blood cells and hemolysin which must have complement to complete the reaction and lyse the blood cells. If reagin is present, there is no lysis; if not, the lysis occurs. While a positive reagin test will be indicative of syphilis, reagin will also be formed by the following disease processes:

Malaria	Leprosy
Yaws	Pinta
Relapsing fever	Vaccina
Mononucleosis	Febrile diseases
Pregnancy	Lupus erythematosis

Immunological disorders (usually of genetic disorder)

In these cases, careful screening is needed by the physician. Reagin tests are not limited to serum alone. Some, such as the rapid plasma reagin test (RPR), have developed quite recently for fast screening. (This test has been automated to do reagin tests on a mass scale.) The reaction is essentially the same as the flocculation test with the addition of carbon to indicate flocculation. But the problem still remains to have a specific and sensitive test for treponemial antigen, especially in doubtful cases where the patient gives a negative history.

The test of preference is the treponemal immobilization test (TPI) developed in 1949. If the person's serum is reactive, then the live organism (in the presence of complement) is immobilized; if not, then it will remain mobile. While in theory this test is simple, technically it is very complex, sensitive, and expensive. The fact that live rabbits must be used to culture the organism (it can't be cultured *in vitro*) and the factors that can affect the serum to give a false positive (such as rubber stoppers on the serum tube which give off toxic material into the serum) make this test impractical for routine use. Rather it is used to be a reference to the fluorescent treponemal antibody—absorbed test (FTA-ABS), or "FTA" for short, developed in 1964 for general use.

II. Rationale of Therapy

Treatment in the 19th and previous centuries consisted of iodates, mercury, and bismuth. While these heavy metals were questionable in their bacterial activity in the body, they did seem to resolve the syphilitic lesions and provide a barrier to prevent further involvement of the organisms. The first good antitreponemal compound came about 1906 with Ehrlich's salvarsan "606" arsenic compound that could be injected into the bloodstream without undue toxicity to the patient. While it could lower the titer, its staying power, unlike the other heavy metals, was not long, and some persons had reactions to it. Treatment was long, and arsenicals had to be used with other heavy metals to have a lasting effect. In secondary or late syphilis, treatment sometimes had to be repeated as relapses would occur.

It should be noted that while iodine was thought to be non-antitreponemal, it did help to resolve granulomatous tissue and was less toxic than all the metals used. Iodine was used with arsenic therapy in central nervous system lues to avoid the allergic reaction (Herxheimer) to arsenic. The iodates were used since 1836 for treatment of central nervous system syphilis since the French discovered their use. Mercury (quite toxic to the kidneys) was used since medieval times. Bismuth was used preferentially to mercury since the 1870s. It could produce reaction when overused. Fever therapy (induced malarial infection—cleared up by quinine) was used with arsenic in 1918 (arsenic does not affect the malarial parasite) since the spirochete is sensitive to temperature change. A modification of this was steam cabinet therapy with arsenic—much to the discomfort of the patient. The treatments (all modifications) were long, uncomfortable, repeatable, dangerous, and sometimes painful; many patients decided that the cure was worse than the disease.

But the advent of penicillin therapy in 1943 with improvements in early 1946 (oil instead of water base) proved to be a godsend. Even to this day, it remains a drug of choice since the spirochetes have not developed resistance to the drug. Unless there is an allergic reaction to penicillin, the drug is non-toxic, spirocidal and can be applied in one course of treatment. In late syphilis, several injections may be needed to kill the hidden, widely scattered organisms. If the patient is allergic to penicillin, other antibiotics are needed. The course of treatment here is longer, as these drugs are not as effective.

As for epidemiology, sexual contact is the fomite—not the poor maligned toilet seat, dirty washrags, or other such nonsense. The spirochete is fragile, sensitive to temperature and drying (the spirochete will perish in 30 to 45 seconds when removed from the body and exposed to the hostile environment), and is sensitive to disinfectants. The organism forms no spores and must be spread by sexual contact from one partner to another to survive the generations. If mankind could refrain from pre- and extramarital intercourse and only have intercourse with uninfected or treated partners, the disease would eventually die out.

Accidental infection can occur if one touches an open wound or mucous membrane to an active lesion. Reinfection can occur, as a case of syphilis confers no immunity. What the doctor and the health department expect from the patient is cooperation in finding contacts to help stop the spread of disease. It is cruelty to the contact not to be reported. In this case, the disease is spread and the untreated person may be doomed to eventual death from late syphilis as well as to spreading the disease further.

III. The Cayce Readings on Syphilis

Several Cayce readings on syphilis in the male were given. In reading 862-2, the patient comes to him with a reactive blood test. All tests made in 1935 were of a reagin nature and thus did not confirm a case of syphilis. If you note reading 862-1, Cayce warned the patient of toxemia if normal hepatic circulation were not restored. With a positive reagin present, Cayce's diagnosis of an infectious force that produced a humor is borne out; but with the negative history, an irresolution of the toxemia had seemingly produced this biologic false positive (BFP) as far as syphilis is concerned. In readings 862-2 and 862-3, a low-acid diet and electrical stimulation by a low-voltage wet cell appliance are given to bring about coordination in the circulatory forces. Serum injections are suggested in the readings but were not considered necessary. However, in reading 862-3, it is mentioned that the patient might well be infected with late syphilis, though the information only hints at it and gets on with the treatment. In 862-4, the infection begins to resolve. A comment is given that the disease is infectious but not contagious, as is usual with late lues. Reading 862-5 is but a check reading. After this reading, [862] had injections (probably arsenicals) which activated the immunological system to reject a sac that contained shrapnel—synovitis. The treatment prescribed by the information is unusual, but it seemed to work in this person's case until the patient went against the information. (Surgery was suggested in 862-6 to remove the sac.)

Case [1289] is a sad one, of a child doomed by congenital late syphilis. The involvement is so profound as to cause Edgar Cayce to sign off with no absolute diagnosis of syphilis although he made the syphilitic nature clear in 1289-2. The readings gave forgiveness and benediction to the foster parents of the stricken child for whom he made a prophecy of death. The lack of a question period seemed to add finality to the first reading. But in 1289-2, hope is offered to the parents to meet their sin of poor attitude by administration of hot castor oil packs along with a diet to aid the child. While the readings did not offer conventional therapy, it did offer hope in the changes of heart and a possibility of a miracle.

Case [1854] is an accurate diagnosis of a gumma in the lung which was mistakenly thought to be tubercular in origin. Here apple brandy inhalations are suggested for relief. Calcidin (calcium iodate) was taken orally which would supply iodine to resolve the syphilitic tissue. Atomidine and electrical appliances were used for the stimulation of the lacteal ducts to throw off the infection. If you note the letters of follow-up, the young man had been diagnosed as a syphilitic and had been treated with arsenic and steam cabinet therapy. His reaction to the drug was taking its toll on him. The selection of Calcidin seems in line with traditional therapy to resolve the lesion.

Case [5061] is an example of paresis. Only hypnotic sedation is prescribed for the patient. So far gone was he that any therapy known to us or to Cayce's source of information would not have resulted in a cure.

In readings 5067-1 and 5067-2 we find a case of a malignant form of advanced tertiary syphilis throughout the body of the patient. The disease was so advanced that no treatment known at that time could have helped the person. An ultraviolet light filtered through a green glass was to be held over the area of the spine along with the application of a shortwave oscillator. This was probably for the encouragement of the immunological and cell forces throughout the body. Penicillin was a rare and expensive drug (rationed during World War II) and was in an aqueous state but had not proved to be reliable to clear up lues, especially in late cases. Injections had to be given over a long time, since an oil carrier had not yet been found (discovered in 1946) to provide staying power for the drug. Arsenic and bismuth were not used by the physican since it may have been too late to utilize these drugs with the patient in such a weakened condition. Even if the microbes were killed off, it would not have resolved the gummas present that were affecting the patient. We do not know if the treatment would have worked since not all the steps were carried out as prescribed. As is usual with severe late syphilis, the patient died.

In the cases of syphilis in the female we have an example of an early case of lues in [3120]. Not only is the disease diagnosed correctly, but also congenital malformation and possible death for the fetus was predicted. (The infant did die soon after birth.) Adjustments were given to the spine in preparation for childbirth. Internal and external applications of iodine were given in the form of Atomidine (taken orally and by douches). Shots given by a medical doctor previously (no mention of drug given) had not cured the infection. The follow-up reading, 3120-2, indicated no central nervous system lues and urged the patient to keep up the treatment, along with a pep talk. Here a good follow-up was done; and it indicates that the patient was still living in 1962 with no apparent relapse of symptoms. Since the reading took place in 1943, the time period with no evidence of a relapse is a good prognosis.

The patient in reading 4418-1 had pain and discomfort with the formation of a gumma. A codeine medication was given to ease pain and to prepare her for a following reading. Reading 4418-2 prescribes an herbal tonic, steam cabinet therapy with iodine, followed by oil of wintergreen (stimulates the pores) and a salt massage. This does sound like the steam cabinet treatment with iodine substituted for arsenic. There is no follow-up on this case.

Admittedly, the information by Cayce did not always agree with medical advice for syphilis at that time or even in our era. However, when his advice was followed, it did work (such as in [3120]). The treatments went into areas neglected by present medical science because of the advent of penicillin. Late and congenital syphilitic cases are rarely seen today due to early diagnostic techniques with routine screenings of people (premaritals, prenatals, and new hospital patients have their blood drawn nowadays for reagin tests as well as possible contacts) and eradications of treponemes by penicillin in one treatment. One can conclude from the readings the following:

1. Therapy consisted of iodine and the iodates—these being less toxic than arsenic and bismuth. Penicillin may not have been suggested since there was no practical treatment by it during the psychic's lifetime.

2. Where the system was overtaxed by the spirochete, stimulation was given to the lacteal ducts by ultraviolet light, wet cell application with noble metals and iodine. Electrical oscillation was used for severe cases.

3. Prescriptions were individual and could call for any of the combinations of the above.

4. Psychological and spiritual counsel was given as an adjunct to the treatment where applicable. Treatment was not limited to the body alone.

5. Applications of other drugs (the herbal tonic) were sometimes prescribed.

6. Treatments could be applied as long as the body and the mind were still capable of responding. Severe late syphilis lies beyond any help (such as cases [5067], [1289], and [5061]).

7. When treatments were applied, remission of symptoms occurred with no relapses.

Today's science has a long way to go to explain completely why these treatments worked. Such explanation would call for a complete understanding of the immunological, cellular, and organ systems. Some of the medications that were suggested should be studied for their effects upon the human body. The source of cellular resistance stemming from the lymphatic system are yet to be proven. The record remains open. As one physician said: "He who understands syphilis, understands medicine."

Richard M. Wright

References:

Bernet, C.W. *Clinical Serology.* Springfield, Ill., Charles C. Thomas Co., 1968.

Brown, et. al. *Syphilis and Other Venereal Diseases.* Cambridge, Massachusetts, Harvard University Press, 1970.

Stokes. J. *Modern Clinical Syphology.* Philadelphia, W.B. Saunders Co., 1926.

Syphilis, Synopsis. U.S. Department of Health and Welfare: Washington, D.C., U.S. Printing Office, 1967.

Jawetz, et. al. *Review of Medical Microbiology.* Los Altos, California, Lange Medical Publications, 1966.

Eagle, H. *The Laboratory Diagnosis of Syphilis.* St. Louis, Missouri: The C.V. Mosely Co., 1937.

TONSILLITIS

I. Physiological Considerations

Tonsils have a creative purpose and function within the body. They are not superficial in their function, and when the tonsils are removed the whole activity is never again present in that particular physical body. In talking about tonsils and adenoids, the reading for [759] declared "These are for a normal healthy development in body and mind, as we find, *necessary* to a body. These removed may or may not be harmful to the better conditions of a body, for they are as scavengers of portions of conditions for the system; they are as the activities for the relief of tension and strain in system." (759-7)

On occasion a tonsillectomy was suggested in the readings, this coming about when the body had not been cared for according to previous directions; or in those cases where other serious diseases intervened, and it became necessary to remove the tonsils which were adding toxins and poisons to the circulation, thus preventing more normal functioning of the body otherwise. This was seen in a case of rheumatic fever. (25-2)

The etiology of tonsillitis is the impairment of circulation either generally throughout the body or locally as the throat and head seek to bring about a local equilibrium. Tonsillitis results from the drosses (wastes and toxins) carried in the circulation. Eliminations— inadequate as a general measure of the body or as a local problem— underlie virtually every condition of inflamed tonsils and adenoids. Associated with this and often causative are lesions or subluxations in the cervical or upper dorsal vertebrae, these again producing a lack of proper function of the circulation in the throat and head.

As a portion of the total lymphatic system, the tonsils and adenoids act as local resistance to infection and find themselves related to the other lymphatic centers such as the Peyer's patch area in the upper intestinal tract. Most of the readings given for tonsillitis were to individuals who were quite young, this being the age in which the disease is most commonly found.

II. Rationale of Therapy
In approaching therapy, we should remember that the body has a capability of *normal* function:

Thus, we would administer those activities which would bring a normal reaction through these portions, stimulating them to an activity from the body itself, rather than the body becoming dependent upon supplies that are robbing portions of the system to produce activity in other portions, or the system receiving elements or chemical reactions being supplied without arousing the activity of the system itself for a more normal condition.

1968-3

Tonsillitis as such should be approached as a therapeutic problem with the whole individual in view. Other conditions, when present, need to be treated or brought into focus as part of the whole picture of the disease process.

The aim in therapy is to bring about adequate eliminations through all channels; to purify or clarify the blood and the intestinal tract; and to correct pressures and lesions which may be present in the upper vertebrae of the body. Corrections in diet should be made, and a period of time should be allowed without strain on the throat or on the entire organism.

In this manner eliminations will be brought into a high state of efficiency—even more so than during a state of normal health—and the system will be relieved of drosses and toxins which have accumulated. Through osteopathic adjustments the neurological impulses to the throat and the adjacent areas will be normalized, and the circulation will become more efficient and more balanced in its functioning. The dietary adjustments and the correction of the possible abnormalities of acid-base balance in the intestinal tract then produces a more normal assimilation—allowing the body to rebuild and resolving the inflammation and abnormalities of the tonsils.

III. Suggested Therapeutic Regimen
Tonsillectomy as such should be reserved for those cases which are refractory in their nature or which create a dangerous level of toxins within the system.

Osteopathic adjustments and manipulations should be begun immediately to correct abnormal impulses from lesions and subluxations and to bring about more adequate lymph drainage to the area of the tonsils and surrounding tissue.

Cleansing of the body should be instituted, using enemas or colonics where possible, or cathartics such as BiSoDol, phosphate soda, or syrup of pepsin (such as is found later in this commentary).

For those conditions in which drainage from inflamed nasal tissue and tonsillar tissue creates an acid condition in the stomach, Glyco-Thymoline in small doses is helpful. Most commonly an alkaline-reacting diet would be advisable.

Rest without straining of the body or throat or eyes is important in this condition. Persistence and consistency in carrying out the recommendations always seem to be a portion of the suggestions given in the readings.

It is important that the adjustments and the cleansing of the intestinal tract be done in cycles until the throat is completely normal and that a proper diet be maintained during this time.

Tonsillitis Tonic

If we would take a tonic such as Codiron, three tablets each day—these taken at mealtimes—we will find that we will make for greater improvement in the general health of the body.   815-4

This 35-year-old man was advised by his doctor to have a tonsillectomy. The reading stated it was not best to have his tonsils removed; that he would have difficulty; that his blood was not in a condition to have this done. Preferably, he should have osteopathic treatments.

Tonsillitis—Sinusitis

If there is trouble with the face and throat, we would wrap about same a cotton cloth (two or three thicknesses) well saturated with the Glyco-Thymoline, and keep it on for an hour and a half to two hours. This will aid in reducing the inflammation.   1788-12

Tonsillitis—Eliminant

...Caldwell's syrup of pepsin as an antiseptic and an eliminant. Give about

half to three-quarters of a teaspoonful two or three times a day, or about three hours apart, until there are good eliminations from the alimentary canal. Leave off two or three days (keeping the intestinal antiseptic and the massages, which we will indicate), then take again—until there are good eliminations.   1788-12

Upset Intestinal Tract

Now to give ease and to supply to the system those properties necessary to rebuild within the body those things necessary to rejuvenate those portions of the body, break up conditions as exist in the stomach and intestinal tract, reaction of forces as applied to the body, we would add to the system those properties that are necessary to produce a balance or an equilibrium to the body. We would first take this into the system:
In one half gallon water there would be added 16 ounces of common garden sage (dried); this would be reduced by boiling to one quart, strain, and while warm there would be added 6 ounces beet sugar (not cane sugar), 15 grains amber grey [ambergris] (black) dissolved in one ounce of alcohol (or six ounces of gin); 3 drams cinnamon stick or bark, rather than dried or ground. Dose would be a tablespoonful three times a day.   4499-1

In this case, the stomach, pancreas, liver, kidneys, and lacteal forces were all in a state of high disturbance. The tonsillitis came as a result of these imbalances.

Tonsillitis—Intestinal Antiseptic

. . .a few drops of Glyco-Thymoline; not more than six drops at a time, twice a day should be sufficient, in water. Keep this up until the odor of same may be detected in the stool. Leave off a few days and then take again.
                                          1788-12

Should we not attempt to awaken the inner forces to God's presence? "For, all healing comes from the one souce. And whether there is the application of foods, exercise, medicine, or even the knife, it is to bring the consciousness of the forces within the body that aid in reproducing themselves the awareness of creative or God forces." (2696-1)

William A. McGarey, M.D.

Edgar Cayce readings referenced:
24-1
25-2
341-5
759-7
815-4
1208-16, 17
1788-12
1968-3
4499-1

ULCERS

I. Physiological Considerations

Ulcerations of the gastrointestinal tract, particularly the stomach and duodenum, is a relatively common disorder which in most cases is associated with hyperacidity (at least in benign lesions). Increased acidity is brought about by a variety of mechanisms which again can be translated into disturbed function in the nervous, circulatory, and digestive systems.

It is now commonly accepted that people under high stress situations—e.g., tension jobs, the critically ill patient, etc.—have a greater tendency to develop ulcers. It is also known that there is ulcer diathesis with increased levels of steroid, whether endogenous (as in Cushon's disease) or exogenous (as in people on steroid therapy for various reasons). Yet another variation is found in the Zollinger-Ellison Syndrome, a condition associated with a gastrin- (a hormone) secreting tumor of the pancreas which in turn stimulates excessive acid production leading to ulcerations.

Malignant ulcers are more often associated with normal or low acid level, which probably reflects a process of degeneration (from chronic irritation) from an initially benign lesion. The rapidity of such a degeneration would depend on the presence and intensity of a multitude of carcinogenic stimuli and inherent weaknesses (predisposition).

Stomach ulcers

Turning now to the readings on stomach ulcers, we find that in reading 39-1, the inciting agent was excessive mental stress which brought about changes in the nervous and muscular activity leading to impairment in organ function. First the spleen, heart, and solar plexus were affected and then the stomach. The exact role of the spleen in the process of digestion is not well defined but seems to have to do with enhancement of digestive juices.

Malpositioning of the stomach then occurred with disturbances in pyloric sphincter activity, regurgitation of food (and thus digestive pancreatic enzymes) into the stomach, leading to lacerations and ulcerations.

The disturbed activity in the nervous system with attendant circulatory changes (these always go hand in hand) were responsible for a variety of symptoms and signs reflecting other organ system dysfunction, described in the reading.

In the majority of cases disturbances in assimilation and elimination were seen to be the underlying problem. The organs commonly involved are the stomach, pancreas, spleen, liver, kidneys, but other organs may also be reflexly involved.

Representative is case [732], in which there was deficiency in the secretions from the liver and gall bladder leading to overacidity and ulceration in the stomach, regurgitation of food into the stomach, impaired circulation, and poor eliminations through the blood, lymphatics, and gut. Pyloric sphincter disturbance and regurgitation into the stomach seem to be fairly common features, either causing the ulceration or being an associated condition.

In case [3570] this disturbance in the digestion/assimilation was brought about by an "overloading of the system" (overeating?) and that the resulting abnormalities were being perpetuated by an inadequate diet consisting of just fruits and vegetables (more on this under "Rationale of Therapy").

A somewhat different mechanism in the pathogenesis of ulcers has its origin in lesions in the spine (of traumatic origin or otherwise) usually in the third to fifth dorsal centers. (4786-1, 5641-1) Impaired nervous impulses result in malpositioning of the stomach, over-acidity, sphincteric disturbances and ulcerations in the stomach. In reading 5641-1, this patient had even undergone corrective stomach surgery but continued to have problems because the problem in the spine had been overlooked.

Ulcers more often occurred at the lower end of the stomach, though in one instance (4786-1) the cardiac position (i.e., the upper portion) was involved and even the intake of water was quite painful. Widespread inflammation along the digestive tract may be seen as a complication.

Other mechanisms mentioned include deficiencies in the quality of

the blood with functional abnormalities eventually leading to
ulcerations (3768-1, 5440-1); cold and congestion settling in areas of
weakness in the stomach thus producing ulcers. (5421-2)

In summary, ulcerations are brought about primarly by disturbances in the processes of digestion, assimilation and elimination.
Other causes include spinal lesions, mental stress, circulatory
disturbances, etc., which again reduce to the basic triad seen in all the
readings—the digestive, nervous and circulatory systems. What
affects one of these systems eventually affects the others if
compensatory mechanisms are inadequate.

The importance of the digestive system in this whole process is
reflected by the following passage:

**The vibratory forces of a body are made up of the cellular units of that as is
created by the digestive forces of the body, as they carry to the various
portions of the system that necessary to resuscitate the living organisms of
the body, that must reproduce themselves in the living organism. When these
impulses are such (as is here) as to bring more of acids, or more of those
impulses that bring those of distresses to a body, acting through the
sympathetic, acting through the hypogastric, acting through the forces of the
normal activity of brain itself, the impulses can be none other than that.**
5641-1

Duodenal ulcers

The factors leading to the formation of duodenal ulcers are similar
to those described under stomach ulcers. It is therefore not surprising
that both conditions quite often coexist in the same individual. For
this reason, it is recommended that the reader also consult the
Circulating File on stomach ulcers for additional details and read the
section on stomach ulcers above.

In brief, the causative factors described in the readings include
stress, described as overtaxation and general debilitation in the
digestive system in the case of a 29-year-old person. (137-94) The
stress may be primary as in the case of attitudes (negative), nervous
personality, or secondary to some other disease process which creates
anxieties. (1724-1, 5426-1) Also noted were disturbances in digestion,
assimilation and elimination which may in turn be caused by other
conditions; for example, intestinal flu (1724-1), adhesions (5021-1),
abnormalities in the liver and gall bladder (4885-1, 5426-1), blood
deficiencies leading to an overacid condition (5487-1), to name a few.

In the case of [1724] (ulcer caused by intestinal flu), the reading was given in 1938 and the patient only recalled a mild case of flu in 1918 with no gastrointestinal symptoms!

Common to all the conditions cited above are congestive changes which bring pressure to bear on nerve ganglia, producing a wide variety of effects (symptoms). In reading 137-95, for example, congestion in the gastric and hypogastric regions led to impaired ability to eliminate, which then threw toxins into the upper circulation, creating pressures in the head and neck region. This point is further illustrated:

Also reflexes are produced, of course, upon all the activities of the system through the digestive forces. Hence *all* the organs of assimilation become involved at times—as the activity of the liver, the spleen, the pancreas; as well as the eliminating forces and the excess condition for the activity of the kidneys, of course, in carrying off the disturbing forces.   1724-1

Again the majority of cases seem to fall into the category of disturbed function in digestion, assimilation and elimination which arise from other causes.

II. Rationale of Therapy

The main thrust of the treatments should be directed at correcting the underlying problem in addition to treating distressing symptoms. In some cases it may not even be possible to address one's full attention to the underlying problem until distressing symptoms are under control. Thus therapy may be approached in the following manner:

1. *Treating distressing symptoms.* This is what often brings the patient to the physician, e.g., treatment of pain, nausea, excessive gas, etc. Other symptoms of reflex origin may include headaches, dizziness, weakness, even pain and heaviness in the extremities, reflecting circulatory disturbance. Not all these symptoms need be treated individually since by correcting the underlying problem these usually resolve themselves.

2. *Correcting the underlying problem.* This is sometimes difficult to do since the original cause may be far removed in time and space (place) from the existing problem. In this instance when a simple approach proves ineffective, one has to rely on one's intuition (or seek

the help of a reliable psychic) or try a "shotgun" approach consisting of using all or most of the modalities under the section on treatments (this would be rather infrequent).

These would be aimed at:

a) Correction of digestive disturbances through proper diet, digestive aids, etc. One needs to be careful here, for a completely natural diet, when too restricted and carried on for long periods, is not necessarily beneficial, as reflected in reading 3570-1.

b) Avoidance of excessive strain on the nervous system through proper mental and emotional attitudes.

c) Correction of spinal lesions.

d) Correction of circulatory disturbances.

III. Suggested Therapeutic Regimen

This should be as simple as possible to promote patient compliance. In more severe cases or where the underlying problem is obscure, one may need to use all or most of the therapeutic modalities outlined below.

1. *Symptomatic Treatment*

a) Castor oil packs over the stomach, duodenal, and liver areas to improve lymphatic drainage, reduce inflammation, and relieve pain.

b) Grape poultice over the stomach and duodenal areas to relieve pain due to excessive gas formation. This could be used daily for two hours at a time. (1970-1) This may be alternated with Glyco-Thymoline or Lavoris packs. (5216-1)

c) Reducing intestinal acidity through charcoal prepared with honey (no directions on preparation). This would carry six times its weight in acid out of the system. (5641-1)

d) Others

1) Use of Glyco-Thymoline to soothe intestinal irritation, five to ten drops per glass of water twice daily; two to three drops may also be taken with elm water twice daily. (4148-1, 4464-1)

2) Taking olive oil by mouth one to two teaspoons two to three times daily to promote healing.

3) Combination of cinnamon and lime water helps to relieve nausea. (See 5641-4 for directions on preparation.) May be taken in sips every few minutes.

4) Massages once or twice a week using various oils. One suggestion was a combination of olive oil and myrrh.

2. *Diet*

This is of paramount importance since ulcerations and lacerations are invariably associated with inflammation and congestion, thus leading to digestive, assimilative and eliminative difficulties. The food intake should therefore be one that is easily digested and assimilated, leaving very little in the way of wastes to eliminate. Examples:

Vegetables and fruits. All types of vegetables, but tuberous ones should be avoided in plethoric conditions; all fruits except raw apples, bananas, and acid-producing fruits.

Liquids. Natural juices as tolerated, including citrus juices. Beef juice, two teaspoons three to four times daily. Herb teas, such as yellow saffron, elm tea or elm water (pinch of elm in a glass of water). In one instance only these two drinks (saffron, elm) were prescribed exclusively as liquids. (3763-1) Milk and crackers could also be used initially as well as jelly, gelatin, beef juice, liver and liver extracts in small doses, etc. In one instance (5226-1) egg enemas were prescribed for nutrition since oral intake was difficult. Carbonated waters should be avoided in general but may be helpful in moderate amounts in some cases. The diet may then gradually be increased after about 10 days.

Solids. Whole grain cereals, bread, fish, fowl, raw egg in malted milk are very good. Avoid fried foods, starches and other meats.

Digestive aids. The teas mentioned above would stimulate better function and thus aid digestion. The following prescription may also be used: 10 drops of essence of lactated pepsin in one teaspoon of milk of bismuth or Milk of Magnesia in a glass of water twice daily. This may be alternated, and would stimulate better digestive juice flow. (556-2)

3. *Maintaining proper eliminations*

This is especially important if this is the basis of the disorder. Step 1 will already aid in this, but in addition, regular colonics should be used. The frequency would be somewhere from three within a 10-day period to four to five at 10-day intervals.

Olive and white oils may also be used as enemas. (5440-1)

Castor oil packs to stimulate lymphatic drainage generally over the liver, stomach, and duodenal areas. The castor oil packs may be used five days in a row.

Begin Eno salts each morning after the first castor oil pack (one teaspoon in a glass of water). After the fifth castor oil pack, take a whole bottle of Castoria, one-quarter to one-half teaspoon every 30 minutes. (3570-1)

4. *Mechanical aids*

    a) Elastic stomach brace to correct malpositioning of the stomach. Manipulations would also be helpful, especially when spinal lesions are at the root of the problem;

    b) Electrically driven vibrator over the spine (556-2);

    c) Ultraviolet light treatment;

    d) Light, color and sun treatment;

    e) Radium appliance (no longer available);

    f) Radio-active appliance to balance the circulation.

5. *Others*

For adhesions: Castor oil packs five days on, five days off. Follow with olive oil, at least one tablespoon after the fifth day (night or morning). Massage area after each castor oil pack (not too vigorously) with olive oil (heated) two ounces, peanut oil two ounces, and lanolin (melted) 14 ounces.

Prescriptions

    a) For cleansing the blood in case of poor eliminations: To 16 ounces of water (distilled water), add six ounces wild cherry bark. Reduce by simmering (not boiling) to one-half the quantity. Add to this, when strained, two ounces of cane sugar, dissolved in one ounce of hot water. Reduce to six ounces, then add:

    Elixia calisaya, 1 ounce
    Elixia Peruvian bark, ½ ounce
    Tincture valerian, ½ ounce
    Fluid extract burdock root, ½ ounce
    Fluid extract poke root, 20 minims
    Podophyllum (dry), 3 grains

Cut in two ounces of grain alcohol, three drams balsam of tolu. Add all this to the solution. The dose of this would be a teaspoonful three times each day, taken before meals. (3968-1)

    b) A variation would be:

    Dogwood bark, 2 ounces
    Prickly ash bark, 2 ounces
    Buchu leaves, ½ ounce
    Black root, 2 ounces

Elder flower, 4 ounces
This should be put into one gallon of water, reduced by simmering, not boiling, to one quart. Strain; and add one-half pint
spiritus frumenti, eight years old, with six ounces of sugar (beet
sugar preferred). A dose of this would be one tablespoon four
times each day. (3968-1)

c) For coordinating the nervous system and eliminations:
To two ounces of simple syrup, add:
Compound syrup of sarsaparilla, ½ ounce
Tincture valerian, ¼ ounce
10% solution iodide of potassium, 20 minims
10% solution bromide of potassium, 10 mimins
Elixir calisaya, ¼ ounce
Then add to these solutions—when they are combined—one-
half ounce grain alcohol. Shake solution together before the
dose is taken. Take a dose about three times each day, one-half
to three-quarters teaspoonful, either plain or in water. (137-101)
6. Finally, one should have a proper mental and emotional
outlook, avoid stress, and have adequate rest during the acute phase
of the illness.

Hezekiah Chinwah, M.D.

Edgar Cayce readings referenced:

Ulcers: 39-1   *Duodenal Ulcers:* 137-94, 95, 96, 101
       556-2   481-4
       732-1   1724-1, 2, 3
       1834-1   3968-1
       1970-1   4885-1
       3570-1   5021-1
       3768-1, 2   5216-1
       4148-1   5426-1, 2
       4464-1   5487-1
       4786-1
       5216-1
       5226-1
       5421-1, 2, 3
       5440-1
       5618-1
       5641-1 through 5

VARICOSE VEINS

I. Physiological Considerations

When a person is standing, the force of gravity greatly opposes the return flow of blood and lymph from the lower extremities. Hence in the diseased state varicose veins most often occur in this area. While the body is in this position, efficient superficial circulation in the extremities depends not only on the pumping action of the heart to overcome gravity but also on the muscular activity within the extremities themselves. The normal flow of blood and lymph is further aided by and dependent upon smoothly functioning channels through which they may flow. A thinned out and sacculated vascular wall causes an unequal pressure in the system, thus allowing for stasis and even leakage into the surrounding tissues. This unequal pressure in the tissues impairs the lymph flow in that area, allowing an accumulation of toxic waste products from the cells which may further suppress or even inhibit the normal activity of the tissues supporting the vascular walls. This contributes further to the disease state.

The readings imply that the tendency toward varicose veins usually develops as a result of mechanical trauma or systemic toxicity, both of which tend to impair the drainage from the area affected. Mechanical trauma may exert its effect either through pressures on the autonomic ganglia and their connections with the cerebrospinal system as a result of spinal subluxations or through pressures exerted directly on the venous return from the lower extremities. In reading 1093-1, a 23-year-old maid sustained an injury to the end of the spine years before which brought about a gradual slowing of the circulation, resulting in varicose veins of the legs at an early age. In another case, trauma occurred more directly to the affected area as a result of standing after overexposure to the sun.

The present condition as we find arises from too much of the attempt to create or help the internal circulation from the sun heat, and standing too much on the feet has tended to increase the circulation *to* the portions and not sufficient of that as indicated to take the circulation *from* same.

Thus there became the tendencies for the swelling, as well as the spreading of the conditions through the system.   **1541-6**

Childbirth frequently causes varicose veins as indicated in 5037-1, which is included in the Circulating File on "Varicose Veins." Other cases are as follows:

Now as we find, there are conditions that are gradually causing distresses through this body. We find that these have to do with what may be called after-effects in childbearing, and thus are rather specific in their nature; but are producing pressures that cause a disturbance that is gradually cutting off the circulation through the lower limbs. This will also gradually cause a greater disturbance, and of a more definite nature, unless some measures are taken to correct same.

From those conditions or positions that developed during the periods while carrying the child, there are misplacements. This also has caused deflected circulation from the pressures in the lumbar and sacral segments, so that the return of circulation from the lower extremities is causing the enlarging of the veins.   **2867-1**

Q-22. Does the soreness along legs come from overweight, or poor circulation?

A-22. As just given, a pressure in the lumbar axis.

Q-23. Could this be a forerunner of varicose veins?

A-23. It could be, unless corrections are made—or unless there is the relieving of the pressure by equalizing the circulation.

Q-24. Why does childbirth cause varicose veins sometimes?

A-24. Owing to the pressure as indicated, or as created in the area just given, by the natural position of the child through the period of gestation.
                         457-9

A second cause of varicose veins is a slowing of the return circulation to the lower limbs brought about through toxic conditions originating elsewhere in the body. As the organs that aid in digestion become unbalanced in their function, subluxations are produced in the related areas of the spinal column and the resulting pressure on the autonomic and spinal nerves tends to bring about a slowing of the venous return from the lower extremities.

The blood supply indicates that there has long been a disturbance in the liver and gall duct area. Hence toxic conditions exist that have tended to add to the weight of the body or there is a glandular reaction from the sources or natures of the suppressions and subluxations existent in the lumbar, the sacral, as well as the upper portion of the dorsals.

These slow up the actions, and we have sediments in the gall duct areas rather than so much of a gall bladder disturbance. Thus we have also, from the same pressures, a slowing of the return circulation in the lower limbs. This has tended to produce an engorging of the veins, or varicose veins along on the inside and on portions of the limbs. 3523-1

In another case we find that acidity in the system brought about by improper eliminations plus dietary indiscretions and excessive strong drink exerted such an influence on the entire digestive and eliminative systems as to create lesions throughout the spine. Varicose veins was one of the results of this type of imbalance.

There is irregularity with the eliminations from the kidneys and bladder, and some distress in this area at times—which is also indicated by pressures in the lumbar and sacral axis, especially that produces a slowing of the circulation through the lower limbs and the dilation in the veins in portions of the limbs themselves.

We find that these are the effects, then, of this toxic force that is produced by the pressure existing in the distribution of energies and circulation in the lower extremities, from the 9th dorsal downward—as well as from that which has been and is a part of the condition by an excess of carbonated forces upon the system itself, combined at times with a toxic condition produced by strong drink.

These we find are the *sources* of this condition. . .

The acidity is producing disturbances more and more through the digestive system, as well as those influences upon the liver itself. This is causing a lesion in the upper dorsals and lower cervicals that is a part of the whole general condition.

The affectation is to the organs as indicated—the liver, the assimilating system, the colon, the activity of the kidneys, and those conditions in the superficial circulation; or the plethora in the veins—or varicose veins are showing their effect, which tends to make for slowing of activities through the body. 2461-1

II. Rationale of Therapy

Any system of therapy designed to restore and maintain normal function to the circulatory systems in the area of the varicose veins must concern itself with relieving the localized congestion as soon as possible, reestablishing and maintaining adequate venous and lymph drainage, and instituting measures designed to correct the underlying causes and resultant mechanical defects. In general, it may be said that patience and persistence are the key factors in application of treatment to assist the body in its correction of the diseased state.

Reestablishment of the normal circulation is assisted through frequent elevation of the affected part and applications of local medication; to relieve congestion of the tissues, massaging of the area using stimulating oils and supporting the weakened vessels through elastic stockings or bandages while standing or walking. Caution is given that prolonged standing or sitting is harmful, whereas walking is in general beneficial to the circulation. Of course, any complications such as infection, thrombosis, hemorrhage or ulceration must first be dealt with adequately. Caution must be used in making a concerted effort to deal with the underlying problem if such treatment might have an adverse effect on the presenting complications. In case [1956], surgery is advised if the patient cannot stay off his feet for adequate lengths of time or if rupture of the veins occurs.

Osteopathic manipulations designed to relieve pressures on the involved nerve pathways is considered to be one of the first treatments necessary in most cases. Likewise, any direct pressures obstructing the circulation should be alleviated as soon as possible. Any systemic toxicity that might have a bearing on retarding venous return must be dealt with. Usually this therapy consists of improving eliminations through the bowels and kidneys and improving the diet so as to reestablish the acid-alkaline balance. Mullein tea is often prescribed as a means of promoting better eliminations and improving the coordinations between the organ systems.

Take internally mullein tea not more than three times a week, but make it fresh each time it is taken. Prepare a tea made from mullein. For uniformity, preferably use the dry mullein, a pinch between thumb and forefinger. Put into a teacup and pour boiling water on same. Let this stand for 30 minutes, strain, cool and drink. This is a reaction to the liver, the lungs, the heart and the kidneys, as to produce coordinating activity in circulation. It works with

each of these and also makes a better condition through the alimentary canal.   **5148-1**

(In the 1960 edition of *The Herbalist,** by Joseph E. Meyer, under "Mullein" the properties and uses of mullein are listed as demulcent, diuretic, anodyne, and antispasmodic.)

III. Suggested Therapeutic Regimen

Therapy is directed toward correcting the underlying causes of the condition while relieving congestion in the affected area and restoring adequate circulation. Rest, with the feet propped higher than the head, is necessary to promote better drainage from the legs.

Keep off of the limb as much as possible. Keep off of the feet as much as possible, and when reclining keep the limb elevated a little above the normal, so that the circulation is tended *toward* the body-forces themselves.

1541-6

It is frequently advised that elastic stockings or bandages be worn when walking or standing. Walking is prescribed as an excellent exercise, especially if there is a tendency toward varicose veins while pregnant.

As we find, in the main, conditions are developing nominally. However, the body should take those precautions about being on the feet so much and not using them. Standing is hard on the body, as is being indicated by the swelling in the limbs—which will tend to make very bad circulation, and produce varicose veins unless there *are* some activities taken to prevent same. Either *walk* or *don't stand on the feet so much!* Walking is the best form of exercise for the body.

If there will be the walking, and not merely standing or resting, and the taking of a small quantity of mullein tea every other day, these will disappear—and this disturbance will disappear. The therapeutic reaction is to better circulation—through the kidneys, especially as related to the lower limbs.   **457-13**

The site for osteopathic adjustments to relieve pressure on the involved nerves varies from case to case and depends on correction of the lesions found. In general, lesions are found most often in the lower dorsal, lumbar, sacral and coccygeal areas, although in more than one

*Sterling Publishing Company, Inc., New York City, N.Y.

case lesions occurred as high as the lower cervical and upper dorsal areas. Treatments are usually given in a series and often in cyclic fashion with periods of rest in between. At times deep osteopathic manipulations are stressed.

Q-1. How often should the osteopathic treatments be given?
A-1. During this particular siege or period, as we find about twice a week—and four *should* be sufficient; and then they may be much farther apart—for the general correction.

This will require *deep* osteopathic manipulations in lumbar and sacral area, and with special reference to the locomotions for the sciatic centers.
1541-2

Mullein stupes or poultices are used either directly over the affected area or above the area of swelling if obstruction due to edema is present. The amount of congestion present determines the frequency with which the mullein stupes are applied. To prepare the stupes:

Gather the mullein leaves, bruise these and pour boiling water over them (in an enamel pan or glass container, not aluminum or tin). Then place over the affected areas.   **5037-1**

We would apply the mullein stupes now more to those areas that are the *sources* from which the limbs receive their circulatory activity, and those portions about the limb to reduce the swelling. Apply these about once a day, and for about an hour. . .
Q-1. Should the mullein at any time be applied to the back?
A-1. As has been given, apply it from the sources! or apply it to the sources from which the limbs obtain their circulatory activity! Does this mean from the toes or from the hips?   **1541-6**

Mullein tea is also to be taken internally from two ounces to one cupful daily. (Instructions for preparation have already been given under "Rationale of Therapy" in this commentary.)

Massaging the limbs and at times the entire body assists the circulation and prevents swelling. Various oils are frequently prescribed for this purpose. This should be done with caution or not at all in those cases where massage might have a deleterious effect on such complicating factors as thrombosis, phlebitis, or severe cardiac disease. These cases need individual professional evaluation. A mixture of olive oil, tincture of myrrh and compound tincture of benzoin is used in one instance (reading 1093-1). In another olive oil and myrrh are used (reading 1956-4); and in still another, peanut oil.

For the local condition—that is, in the veins, where the larger or varicose veins are indicated—we would massage same at least each day, *toward* the body, with peanut oil.

If these still cause distresses, then we would use—if it becomes necessary—the elastic stocking for the preventing of the filling of the veins. But these should gradually disappear entirely, with these corrections being made as indicated.   2867-1

Do use an equal combination of olive oil (heated) and tincture of myrrh to massage in knees, limbs and feet, right after these have been bathed in hot water. Massage these oils well into them.

Do these and we will find improvements for this body.   3523-1

Importance is also placed on eliminations. In many instances it is stated that the bowels should be kept moving a little above normal. Enemas, as well as a variety of laxatives, are prescribed in various readings.

Occasionally the enemas are preferable to *too* much of cathartics of *any* kind. And even when cathartics are taken, the enemas are well so that there is not the inclination for such to become reabsorbed in the system. Remember, poisons are accumulated by the infectious condition, and when there is swelling or inflammation these need to be eliminated.   1541-6

Senna tea or compounds containing senna are one of the more frequently prescribed laxatives. For more complicated conditions various laxatives in the form of both salts and oils are prescribed on some occasions. If it is felt that a more harsh laxative in a particular case is indicated, the prescriptions for same as well as some precautions may be found in the Appendix of this book. Strong purgatives are to be taken frequently only when individual evaluation of the particular case so indicates.

A balanced diet as well as certain foods are also advised to help maintain the eliminations.

Just a regular diet for this body would be well. Keep the well-balanced diet. While not too much fats nor yet too much of starches, but a well-balanced diet here will keep the body in the better conditions.

Do use plenty of those that are of the bulky nature, or that tend to be laxatives—that is, plenty of figs, plenty of prunes, plenty of pieplant and of such natures as portions of the diet. But a well-balanced diet for this body. For, those combinations, so far as the chemical forces are concerned, are very good in the body; else we would have had—with this particular sort of disturbance—a great deal more distress through portions of the system.

2867-1

Again it should be emphasized that persistence of treatment is of foremost importance in effecting improvement of this condition.

Frederick D. Lansford, Jr., M.D.

Edgar Cayce readings referenced:
457-9, 13
1093-1
1541-2, 3, 6
1956-5
2461-1
2714-1
2867-1
3523-1
5037-1
5148-1

APPENDIX

ACIDITY—ALKALINITY

The acid-alkaline balance achieved within the body is a product of the consciousness of the body's cells themselves in their various locations and in their various conditions of health or dis-ease, or disease. It is difficult to visualize how the body responds to the foods which are assimilated and the forces of life within the body itself to maintain a balanced acidity within the bloodstream and all the body tissues. Some organs or tissues normally have an acid pH while others are found in the state of health to be alkaline. (Medically it is known the body maintains a pH of 7.4 in the bloodstream, this being slightly above the neutral reaction, thus alkaline.)

The normal diet will have 80% alkaline-forming foods and 20% acid-forming foods, which, in the normally balanced stomach and intestines will be absorbed and produce the proper balance of acidity-alkalinity within the body itself. It can be seen in case [1959] that nervous indigestion caused a lack of balance between the acid and alkaline forces in the stomach proper or the hydrochloric and the lactic forces. The lactic forces would be those which are absorbed through the lymphatics of the intestinal tract, mainly the Peyer's patches found in the upper portion of the small intestine. With the inflammation in the pyloric and the lower portion of the duodenum, as in this individual, the lymph is not properly absorbed and the acid in the stomach is excessive. Thus, if the lymphatics produce the alkaline reaction or substances within the body—or if their activity is equivalent to the degree of alkalinity maintained within the body—then, in this case, a general tendency toward acidity or an imbalance would occur within the blood and the tissues proper.

On the other hand, in case [5009] there was constipation with a decreased flow of the gastric juices resulting in poor assimilation and certain deficiencies which were then described as producing a rather complex reaction and resulting in excess alkalinity within the system. Whereas the excess acidity in the system caused in [1959] a tiredness and languidness and a heaviness in his limbs, in addition to other disturbances, the alkalosis found in [5009] produced a type of irritation—"reaction existing between the circulation in liver and kidneys is gradually, through this alkalinity, causing irritation to the bladder and the tubes through which the urine passes."

It must always be kept in mind that the body strives very carefully as a unit to maintain a specific acid-base balance within its structure. Thus symptoms and some conditions of dis-ease might well be considered the response of the body as a whole trying to counteract an imbalance which may be found in the organs of assimilation—the stomach and upper intestines proper. These may swing either way, toward the acid or toward the alkaline, and thus the lymph as it becomes part of the blood—even to the nature of the lymphocytes themselves—in various ways then influences the body itself.

The balance of the body as a whole might better be understood if we see the various ways in which a woman's system was out of balance in addition to the acid-alkaline disturbance which was present. In [1254] the following additional incoordinations were mentioned as being part of the entire disease process:

1. Glandular (adrenal, thyroid, liver, thymus, pineal) incoordination.
2. Deep and superficial circulation incoordination.
3. Metabolism (anabolic-catabolic) incoordination.
4. Autonomic-cerebrospinal nervous system incoordination.
5. The ileum plexus reflexes to the lower portion of the cerebrospinal are not coordinated with those above the diaphragm area.
6. Assimilation-elimination incoordination.
7. Even the upper and lower part of the digestive tract (stomach and small intestines) are incoordinated.

From the above it can be readily seen that the acid-alkaline balance is only one of a portion of many coordinate activities which are carried out within the body. A rather fascinating concept was suggested in this particular reading (1254-1) that had to do with hormones and activities. Because of the glandular incoordination, there was a lack of hormones which coagulate the energy produced by the bloodstream into form and tissue throughout the physical body.

In various readings coagulation is mentioned without an explanation—this perhaps referring to the activities of hormones within the bodies.

More explicit treatment for these conditions can be found where more specific diagnosis is made. All types of disturbances play a part in producing this one incoordination within the body and thus specific therapy must be aimed at these various types of malfunction as they exist within the body. For this reason, further and more specific diagnosis is indicated.

Diet cannot be emphasized too strongly. The reader is encouraged to study material related to this topic.

In approaching therapy, we should remember that the body has a capability of normal function:

Thus, we would administer those activities which would bring a normal reaction through these portions, stimulating them to an activity from the body itself, rather than the body becoming dependent upon supplies that are robbing portions of the system to produce activity in other portions, or the system receiving elements or chemical reactions being supplied without arousing the activity of the system itself for a more normal condition.

1968-3

William A. McGarey, M.D.

Edgar Cayce readings referenced:
1120-2	1959-1
1254-1	2091-3
1749-1	5009-1
1866-6	

ALMONDS

Almonds are mentioned somewhat infrequently in the Cayce readings, yet, according to his rather definite statements, apparently have a very important job to do in the metabolism of the human body.

Cayce makes no statements about the physiology of the action of the almonds, although in one reading he did state that within the almond was a substance that he called a vitamin. He stated that taking two or three almonds a day would prevent a tendency toward cancer. Nowhere, apparently, does he mention almonds as a treatment for cancer. He did suggest the use of them to several people after they had a cancerous growth removed and likewise in several places to prevent the tendency for it ever occurring.

The almond, *Prunus amygdalus,* is closely related to the peach, *Prunus persica* (also called *Amygdalus persica),* and likewise to the apricot, *Prunus armeniaca.* The almond nut is of two distinct types, the bitter and the sweet. The bitter almond contains a ferment, emulsin, which in the presence of water acts on the glucoside, amygdalin, and yields glucose, benzaldehyde and hydrocyanic acid. Amygdalin, of course, is present in the sweet almond, but not the ferment, emulsin. It is interesting to note that a cancer therapy, Laetrile, which has been discredited and banned by government authorities, is described as an extract from the apricot kernel, and is for the most part hydrocyanic acid. It has been hypothesized by the discoverer that this acid is destroyed in the body by normal cellular oxidative metabolism, but cancer cells, functioning without oxidative mechanisms, are unable to destroy the acid; thus they absorb it and are destroyed themselves. Cayce mentioned none of these mechanisms in his readings. He suggested sweet almonds rather than the bitter, advised they be used in the prevention rather than the cure of cancer, and ascribed their value to a vitamin-type substance rather than an acid. Perhaps this followed his general philosophy of doing things gently and gradually rather than sharply and abruptly. However, it is interesting to note the relationships between these substances that have both been used now in human beings in relationship to the disease called cancer.

William A. McGarey, M.D.

Edgar Cayce readings referenced:
1158-30   3128-1   3515-1
1206-13   3180-3   5009-1

Readings Extracts on Almonds

Q-21. Shall I resume peanut oil rubs?
A-21. There is nothing better. . .they do supply energies to the body. And. . .those who would eat two or three almonds each day need never fear cancer. Those who would take a peanut oil rub each week need never fear arthritis.   1158-31

Q-5. What can I do to improve skin condition of face and back, and of scalp and hair?
A-5. At least once a week, after a good, thorough workout of body in exercise—following the bath afterward, massage the back, the face, the body, the limbs with pure peanut oil. Then this will add to the beauty. And know, if ye would take each day, through thy experience, two almonds, ye will never have skin blemishes, ye will never be tempted even in body towards cancer nor towards those things that make blemishes in the body-forces themselves. And the oil rubs once a week, ye will never have rheumatism nor those concurrent conditions from stalemate in liver and kidney activities.
                                        1206-13

. . .and if an almond is taken each day, and kept up, you'll never have accumulations of tumors or such conditions through the body. An almond a day is much more in accord with keeping the doctor away, especially certain types of doctors, than apples. For the apple was the fall, not the almond—the almond blossomed when everything else died. Remember, this is life!
                                        3180-3

[Background: This woman had been told that she had all the symptoms of cancer in her right breast and thus should have it removed. The reading advised removal of the breast, the taking internally of plantain tea, proper diet, etc., following surgery.]

Eat an almond each day—one almond—the body will have no more trouble or recurrence of this nature through the system.   3515-1

"Recently in reading *Psychology of the Unconscious* by Carl Jung, I came upon an interesting reference in ancient myths to the almond tree as having life-giving qualities. This reference is on page 557, #32." (3128-1 Supplement, from a letter following her life reading)

Letter Regarding [5009]

Ever since we left Virginia Beach, I have had in mind putting down on paper, as you requested—the story of my mother [5009], and the polyps and the almonds, so here goes:

In July 1957, my mother was operated on for a malignant mass in the intestines. The surgeon removed a segment of bowel to which was attached a polyp, as well as the mass. He told my brother and me that he would have liked to have removed also a further segment on which two or three more polyps (benign, of course) were located but he feared she could not have stood that much nerve shock. He said he wished to watch closely by x-ray the polyps every three months. Subsequently, I urged Mother—as soon as she was out of the hospital—to eat several raw almonds a day—whether she believed in them or not (and although she tends to discount and negate a lot she was scared enough to heed me!). In three months the x-ray pictures showed the remaining polyps "somewhat smaller"—the doctor reported. In another three months the doctor said he couldn't discern *any* polyps at all in the x-ray pictures and was so pleased that he changed her periodic x-ray pictures from every three months to every six months. In another year—he changed to x-ray photos only once yearly. It has almost been 3½ years now since her surgery and there has been no return of any trouble or of any polyps (and her last x-ray photos were of her entire body—torso as well as abdominal region). So, this is a good report for "the almond."

ATOMIDINE

A prevalent concept in the readings is that eliminations from the skin come about when eliminations through the enteric tract slow down or are inadequate. The skin is an eliminatory organ and suffers when the bowels are improperly functioning.

The glandular system apparently has a great deal to do with bringing together the normal functioning of the autonomic nervous system, especially as it relates to specific functions. If the glands are not coordinated, then various functions of the body apparently become incoordinate. The following reading is instructive in this regard:

Q-3. What should be done to clear the skin?
A-3. The combination of things as we have indicated. First the Atomidine will tend to make for the coordinating of the channels of elimination. The skin condition is rather from the improper coordinating of the activities through the peristaltic movement, or absorption in the torso of the body. Thus it produces a condition wherein the irritations are being produced from the poisons being eliminated through the perspiratory system rather than through the alimentary canal.   2579-1

BEEF JUICE

The body derives several benefits from regular use of beef juice. It apparently could bring about a strengthening of the body without irritating the cells in the intestinal tract which might bring about a change in the nature of the lymph and the lymphatic functioning that might in turn disturb the body, causing sleeplessness and general irritation. The following readings are commentaries on it plus descriptions of how to prepare it.

The combinations that have been indicated for the body as to diet are very good; yet we would add the greater strengthening influence without the addition of weight or of heavy foods—which would materially aid, and would not irritate those tendencies for the accumulations or separations in the active forces of mucus that has produced and does produce in the lymph those segregations and accumulations about which the body becomes so disturbed at times.

These as we find may be had in the Pure Beef Juice; not broth, but prepared in this manner:

Take a pound to a pound and a half preferably of the round steak. No fat, no portions other than that which is of the muscle or tendon or strength; no fatty or skin portions. Dice this into half inch cubes, as it were, or practically so. Put same in a glass jar without water in same. Put the jar then into a boiler or container with the water coming about half or three-fourths toward the top of the jar, you see. Preferably put a cloth in the container to prevent the jar from cracking. Do not seal the jar tight, but cover the top. Let this boil (the water, with the jar in same) for three to four hours. Then strain off the juice, and the refuse may be pressed somewhat. It will be found that the meat or flesh itself will be worthless. Place the juice in a cool place, but do not keep too long; never longer than three days, see? Hence the quantity made up at the time depends upon how much or how often the body will take this. It should be taken two to three times a day, but not more than a tablespoonful at the time—and this sipped very slowly. Of course, this is to be seasoned to suit the taste of the body.

Well, too, that whole wheat or Ry-Krisp crackers be taken with same to make it more palatable.   1343-2

Also once a day it will be most beneficial to take beef juice as a tonic; not so much the beef itself but beef juice; followed with red wine. Do not mix these, but take both about the same time. Take about a teaspoonful of the beef juice, but spend about five minutes in sipping that much. Then take an ounce of the red wine, with a whole wheat cracker.   2535-1

Q-5. What quantity of beef juice to be taken daily?
A-5. At least two tablespoonsful, but no fat in same. A tablespoonful is almost equal to a pound of meat or two pounds of meat a day; and that's right smart for a man that isn't active!   1424-2

Beef juice should be taken regularly as medicine, a teaspoonful four times a day at least, but when taken it should be sipped, not just taken as a gulp.
                                    5374-1

As we find, we would use small quantities at a time—but take almost as medicine—of the beef juices. . .This is easily assimilated, gives strength and vitality, and is needed with the vital forces of the body in the present. Take at least a tablespoonful during the day, or two tablespoonsful. But not as spoonsful; rather sips of same. This, sipped in this manner, will work towards producing the gastric flow through the intestinal system, first in the salivary reactions to the very nature of the properties themselves, second with the gastric flow from the upper portion of the stomach or through the cardiac reaction at the end of the esophagus that produces the first of the lacteals' reaction to the gastric flows in the stomach or digestive forces themselves; thirdly making for an activity through the pylorus and the duodenum that becomes stimulating to the activity of the flows without producing the tendencies for accumulation of gases.   1100-10

Beef juice is not a broth but a juice extracted from the meat through heat. It is prepared as follows:

Take about one pound of round steak preferably. Cut off the fat, leaving the muscle and pieces of tendon. Cut this then into half inch cubes, and put it into a glass jar without water in it. The jar should be covered but not tightly. Then put the jar into a pan with water in it, the water coming about one-half or three-fourths of the way toward the top of the jar. Put a cloth on the bottom of the pan to prevent the jar from cracking. Let the water then simmer for three to four hours. Then strain off the juice which has accumulated in the jar and the remaining meat may be pressed somewhat to extract the remainder of the juice. The meat will then be worthless. Place the juice in a refrigerator, but never keep it longer than three days. The quantity made, then, depends upon how much and how often the juice is taken. It should be taken two to three times a day, but not more than a tablespoon at the time—and this should be sipped very slowly taking perhaps five or ten minutes to use the whole amount.

It may be seasoned to suit the taste of the individual. It would be well also to use a whole wheat or Ry-Krisp cracker at the same time to make it more palatable. (See 1343-2 above.)

CASTOR OIL PACK

Prepare first a soft flannel cloth (preferably wool flannel, but cotton flannel is all right if wool is not available) which is two or three thicknesses when folded, and which measures about eight inches in width and 10 to 12 inches in length after it is folded. This is the size needed for abdominal application; other areas may need a different size pack, as would seem to be applicable. Pour some castor oil into a pan and soak the cloth in the oil. Then wring it out so that the cloth is wet but not drippy with the castor oil. Then apply the cloth to the area which needs treatment.

Protect the bed clothing from soiling by putting a plastic sheet underneath the body. Then a plastic covering should be applied over the soaked flannel cloth. On top of that, place a heating pad and turn it up to "medium" to begin with, then to "high" if the body can tolerate it. Then perhaps it will help to wrap a towel around the entire area. The pack should remain in place between one and one-and-a-half hours.

The skin should be cleansed afterwards by using a quart of water to which is added two teaspoons of baking soda. Keep the flannel pack in a pan for future use. It need not be discarded after one application.

Frequency: See recommendations in Circulating File on specific ailment.

Note: Take olive oil by mouth after every third treatment, if directed, in amount tolerated.

378

COUGH AND HICCOUGH THERAPY

As a cough medicine, an expectorant, and for a healing through the whole system, prepare:

Put 2 ounces of strained pure honey in 2 ounces of water and let come to a boil. Skim off the refuse, then add 1 ounce of grain alcohol. To this as the carrier, then add—in the order named:

> Syrup of wild cherry bark, 1 ounce
> Syrup of horehound, ½ ounce
> Syrup of rhubarb, ½ ounce
> Elixir of wild ginger, ½ ounce

Shake well the solution before the dose is taken, which would be about a teaspoonful—and this may be taken as close together as every hour. It will allay the cough, *heal* those disturbing forces through the bronchi and larynx, and make for better conditions through the eliminations.   243-29

In making applications for the body in the present, we would make this as an aid for the cold and for assistance in expectoration; this to be taken about three to four times a day, or at night when there is the tendency for spasms of coughing.

Dissolve 1 ounce of rock candy, as a syrup, in a pint of good rye whiskey. Then add, in the order named:

> Syrup of horehound, ½ ounce
> Glycerine, 10 drops
> Elixir of lactated pepsin, 10 drops

Shake these together before the dose is taken.   303-25

For the cough, for the activities to the *general* bodily forces, we would have at least three to five osteopathic corrections; these specifically in the dorsal and the cervical areas.

Do not attempt to treat the nerves of the face and neck in making these osteopathic adjustments.

Prepare an inhalant in this manner:

To 4 ounces of pure grain alcohol, add—in the order named (and in an 8-ounce bottle):

    Oil of eucalyptus, 20 minims

    Compound tincture of benzoin, 15 minims

    Rectified oil of turpentine, 5 minims

    Balsam of tolu in solution, 20 minims

Shake the solution together, inhale through the nostril and through the mouth, two or three times through each, and two or three times a day. This will aid in purifying, in clarifying the membranes in the nasal passages and in the throat.   2600-1

Q-2. What causes the severe headaches and cough?

A-2. The cough is caused by the pressures upon the bronchi, by this backing up of impulse. The headaches arise from the congestion in the liver.   1745-5

Q-5. What causes the small cough even without any cold?

A-5. This is rather a reflex condition. Nothing to be alarmed at. If there will be the use of Minit-Rub around the throat, at the trachea, we find that this would be allayed. Put this on every night or two for several nights and it will allay the condition.   3079-2

Q-1. What is the cause of the cough and what treatment will relieve it?

A-1. This is an effect of the deterioration and a drooping or dropping of the palate. Tie up a piece of hair in the center of the head. Keep it tied up, like a wig. Tie this tighter each day. Every three days make it a little bit tighter, a little bit tighter; it'll soon stop the cough and raise the palate.   3632-1

Q-4. What causes hiccoughs when she laughs? Please advise corrective measures.

A-4. Do this massaging as indicated over the liver and gall duct area. You see, a hiccough is the convulsion in the diaphragm where the esophagus enters the upper portion of the stomach. And as this rash is caused from incoordination of the elimination, you will kill two birds with one little pebble.   2752-3

Yes we have the body here. It is rather a serious condition as we have in this body. The body has grown rather weak. His coughing spells and hiccough spells are bad for him. Not very much to be done for this body for a cure. May be some things done to bring relief. May be some extension made to the life of the body. . .

Q-3. What causes him to cough and hiccough so much?

A-3. Condition of the eliminated elements in liver and hepatic circulation.

These are choked. The application will localize the condition, then we will be able to operate successfully. As it is distributed over the system, the blood is not capable of taking care of it. Do as we have given if we would bring the best to this body.   50-1

Q-1. What should be done to relieve hiccoughs which he has had for 6 days?
A-1. Let this be done by suggestion, through such as Kuhn.   1839-1

INHALANT BOTTLE

This bottle should be prepared with small stoppers, or else use the big plain stopper when not inhaling.

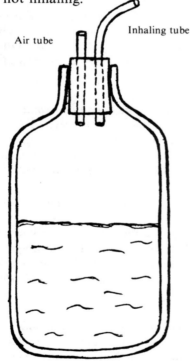

Air tube

Inhaling tube

Bottle: 6 to 8 ounces
Liquid: 4 to 6 ounces

Plain rubber or cork stopper to be used in bottle when not inhaling.

Keep all openings tightly corked when not in use, so as to prevent loss of strength of inhalant by evaporation.

Suggested Inhalants

Pure grain alcohol, 4 ounces
Oil of eucalyptus, 30 minims
Rectified oil of turpentine, 10 minims
Compound tincture of benzoin, 20 minims
Oil of pine needles, 5 minims
Tolu in solution, 15 minims

Grain alcohol, 4 ounces
Oil of eucalyptus, 20 minims
Rectified oil of turpentine, 5 minims
Compound tincture of benzoin, 15 minims
Oil of pine needles, 10 minims

Oil of eucalyptus, 20 minims
Rectified oil of turpentine, 5 minims
Compound tincture of benzoin, 15 minims

This type of bottle may be prepared by a drug supply house or a high school chemistry laboratory. When ready to be used, remove small corks from the tubes (after shaking the solution well), and then inhale through the nostril, each side, some three to four times—not the liquid itself, but the fumes that naturally arise if the ingredients are combined properly. Use the inhalant three to four times a day, or especially if, in the morning or evening, there is the tendency for sneezing, for cold, or irritation.

DIET: ACID AND ALKALINE

Acid

Q-5. What foods are acid-forming for this body?
A-5. All of those that are combining fats with sugars. Starches naturally are inclined for acid reaction. But a normal diet is about twenty percent acid to eighty percent alkaline-producing.   1523-3

Do not take in the system, then, especially any of those foods that produce an overacidity in the lower end of the stomach—such as pickles, or any food carrying overamount of acid or vinegar, or acetic acid, and never any canned goods having benzoate of soda. This includes relishes and things of that nature.   340-5

. . .necessary that occasionally the body be put wholly on that of the citrus fruit diet, that the body abstain from too much of the sweets—especially that of the cane sugar variety, though those that are of the grape, or that are fermentation forming, and sweets as come from chocolates or of fruits that do not carry potash—*these* will be helpful to the general system. Well that the fruit salts at times be taken for the condition in the system, or in the bowel itself. This will produce better clarification. Also well that the antiseptic for the intestinal tract [Glyco-Thymoline] so that those tendencies of exciting the mucous membranes throughout the system do not become infectious from the acidity as has existed there and has been thrown much through the system; else we may form conditions that either will be resultant in the destructive forces for kidneys' circulation or lungs, or both; for rarely (this would be well for *all* to remember) has there ever been a case of tuberculosis without *first* the kidneys going bad.   340-12

Alkaline

The diet should be more body-building; that is, less acid foods and more of the alkaline-reacting will be the better in these directions. Milk and all its products should be a portion of the body's diet now; also those food values carrying an easy assimilation of iron, silicon, and those elements or chemicals—as all forms of berries, most all forms of vegetables that grow under the ground, most of the vegetables of a leafy nature. Fruits and vegetables, nuts and the like, should form a greater part of the regular diet in the present—and in the preparations for those activities to come later, whether in relationships in the physical manner or those in the mental forces that are necessary in such activities. 480-19

Keep closer to the alkaline diets: using fruits, berries, vegetables particularly that carry iron, silicon, phosphorous and the like—and these as we have indicated. . .

Q-2. Can immunization against [contagious diseases] be set up in any other manner than by inoculations?

A-2. As indicated, if an alkalinity is maintained in the system—especially with lettuce, carrots and celery, these in the blood supply will maintain such a condition as to immunize a person. 480-19

As indicated, keep a tendency for alkalinity in the diet. This does not necessitate that there should *never* be any of the acid-forming foods included in the diet; for an overalkalinity is much more harmful than a little tendency occasionally for acidity. But remember there are those tendencies in the system for cold and congestion to affect the body, and cold *cannot—does not*—exist in alkalines. Hence the diet would be as indicated. Citrus fruits; or the smaller fruits occasionally with the cereals that are dry (but do not have citrus fruits and cereals at the same meal). Green raw vegetables should be a portion of the diet occasionally. The meats should be such as lamb, fowl, fish, or the like. Occasionally the *broiled* steak or liver, or tripe, would be well. A well-balance between the starches and proteins is the more preferable, with sufficient of the carbohydrates. And especially keep a well-balance (but not an excess) in the calciums necessary with the iodines, that produce the better body, especially through those periods of conception and gestation. 808-3

As to the diets: We would use not too much sweets, but preferably raw vegetables—at least have one portion of one meal each day consist of a combination of raw vegetables in a salad; such as celery, lettuce, tomatoes, peppers, radishes, carrots, beets, spinach, mustard, onions, lentils and the like. There is the need of such stamina that may be supplied by the combinations of the *green* vegetable forces with the activities in the system. Watercress, especially, is well for the body, and may be included in the salad. This should be eaten at least during one meal each day. And the rest of the diet should consist of the more alkaline-reacting foods. For, in all bodies, the less activities there are in physical exercise or manual activity, the greater should be the alkaline-reacting foods taken. *Energies* or activities may burn acids, but those who lead the sedentary life or the non-active life can't go on sweets or too much starches—but these should be well-balanced.

Keep an attitude of helpfulness, cheerfulness, hopefulness. *Be optimistic!* At least make three people each day laugh heartily, by something the body says! It'll not only help the body; it'll help others!   798-1

The diet also should be considered—in that there is not an excess of acids or sweets, or even an excess of alkalinity, that may produce such a drawing upon some portion of the system (in attempting to prepare the assimilating system for such activity in the body) as to weaken any organ or any activity or any functioning as to produce greater susceptibility.

Hence there should be kept a normal, well-balanced diet that has proven to be right for the individual body, if precautionary measures are to be taken through such periods.   902-1

DIET FOR DIABETES

Outstanding Factors

Use: Jerusalem artichoke, three to six times every week.

Avoid: Foods creating sugar, such as: pastries, candies, ice cream, sugar; spices. White breads, white potatoes, fried foods, fats—such as beef or hog fats. (Butter fats may be used in moderation.)

May use: Honey, honeycomb or saccharin for sugar substitutes.

Fruits: Plenty of fruits, especially apples. These fruits may be either raw, fresh or stewed. Citrus fruits (used in proper combinations).

Grains: Corn (corn bread) or cereal, gruel, barley, oats, brown bread, whole grain cereal (no white bread).

Vegetables: Lots of leafy vegetables (above ground); spinach, endive, cabbage, celery, green vegetables, tomatoes; not too many pod or tuberous variety. Exceptions: May use Jerusalem artichoke; beets and tops, onions, carrots, oyster plant.

Protein: Lots of fish and seafoods; moderate amount of fowl, meat stock. Nuts in moderation. Egg yolk but not the white; occasionally coddled egg. Milk, in moderation (Bulgarian type recommended).

Important suggestion from the readings

Rather those of the vegetable forces that will create for the system those of the *building* to the nerve, to the blood, and to the general strength of the body. Calcium foods, phosphates, sodiums. These will aid the system in *correcting* the conditions. **119-1**

Calcium: Spinach, steel cut oats, whole wheat, whole rye, halibut, cheese, onions, garlic, rhubarb, milk, raw cabbage.

Sodium: Okra, celery, spinach, strawberries, carrots, salt, apples, gooseberries, prunes, raw turnips, peaches, lentils, cheese, oats, beets, cucumbers, string beans, asparagus, figs, lamb.

Drinks: Little coffee or tea; no cream or sugar; cereal drinks all right; Postum, etc.; no carbonated drinks; no alcohol.

The Jerusalem Artichoke

The Jerusalem artichoke is an edible tuber also known as the gerasole. In the United States it is called the American artichoke. It is a species of sunflower and is unique in that it stores its carbohydrates as inulin or inulides, which yield levulose on hydrolysis rather than starch, and the levulose on hydrolysis yields glucose. The levulose is not as harmful to the body in diabetes as is glucose. Medical opinion has been divided on its use in diabetes. Some plants contain a substance called glucokinin, but apparently this has not been demonstrated yet in this type of artichoke. For sake of reference and information, it is noted that: Insulin is a protein hormone, inulin is a plant-derived fructose polysaccharide, while glucokinin is a hormone-like substance obtained from plants which will produce hypoglycemia in animals and will act on depancreatized dogs in a manner similar to insulin.

The tuber has a high thiamine and pantothenic acid content in addition to containing inulin. Inulin is not converted into useable sugar as are the common starches of potatoes and other tuberous vegetables, and the readings state that it is a type of insulin material for the body which helps restore normal function of the pancreas. For this reason, the Jerusalem artichoke is useful in the diabetic diet where sugars must be restricted. It is recommended in every reading given for a diabetic. Even prior to the discovery of insulin, the Jerusalem artichoke was used in diabetic diets.

The readings indicated the following directions for its use: Keep the artichokes in a flower pot or imbedded in the ground to preserve them. They will not keep on ice. Eat one about the size of an egg, twice a week, once raw and once cooked. Cook in Patapar paper [a paper of vegetable parchment] to preserve the juice; mix the juice with the bulk of the artichoke when it is eaten, after seasoning it. Eat it along with a regular meal; i.e., do not make a meal of just the artichoke or eat it between meals. The readings state that this kind of artichoke carries sufficient insulin to be easily assimilated and yet it is not habit-forming.

The following two quotations from the readings are interesting and informative:

Also we would have the stimulation that may be had through taking each day the Jerusalem artichoke as part of the meal—one day raw, the next day cooked. These properties are to aid in reducing this constitutional disturbance in the glandular force. They may also aid in reducing *materially,* in the present, the doses of the insulin; for taking the artichoke—especially this Jerusalem variety—is using insulin but in a manner that is *not* habit-forming, and is much more preferable—if it is governed properly—with the rest of the diet.   1878-1

Instead of using so much insulin; this can be gradually diminished and eventually eliminated entirely if there is used in the diet one Jerusalem artichoke every other day. This should be cooked only in Patapar paper, preserving the juices and mixing with the bulk of the artichoke, seasoning this to suit the taste. The taking of the insulin is habit-forming. The artichoke is not habit-forming, not sedative-producing in the body as to cause accumulations of poisons as do sedatives, though it will be necessary to take a sedative when there are the attacks, but take a hypnotic rather than a narcotic—only under the direction, however, of a physician.   4023-1

Although the readings recommended cooking the Jerusalem artichoke only in Patapar paper, the following recipes are given to allow some variation in the diet:

Jerusalem Artichokes with Almonds
1 lb. cooked Jerusalem artichokes   ⅛ tsp. nutmeg
¼ cup butter   salt, pepper
¼ cup almonds   2 tbsp. lemon juice

Mash the cooked artichokes. Sauce: Into the melted butter, add the peeled almonds and sauté slowly. Add the salt, lemon juice, nutmeg and stir well. Serve the cooked, mashed artichokes hot, and pour over them the almond sauce and almonds.

Variations: If desired, slice the almonds, or use cashew nuts, or peanuts, crushed. Or serve cooked asparagus tips, or green peas or string beans mixed with the artichokes.

Baked Jerusalem Artichokes
2 lbs. Jerusalem artichokes   1 tbsp. orange juice

(scrubbed, trimmed, cooked)   6 small pieces orange peel
2 tbsp. butter   1 tbsp. brown sugar or
½ tsp. nutmeg   molasses or honey

Cook the artichokes until only slightly tender; cool slightly, then cut into halves the long way. Lay on aluminum baking sheet, dot with butter, sprinkle with sugar and orange juice, lay on each a small piece of orange peel. Bake in moderate oven (or covered electric skillet) at 350 degrees for 10 to 15 minutes.

Broiled Jerusalem Artichokes

1½ or 2 lbs. Jerusalem artichokes (well-scrubbed, trimmed, cut into "finger" lengths)
2 tbsp. salad oil
salt, pepper
paprika

Dip the artichoke pieces in the oil, then lay them on an oiled baking sheet or heavy aluminum foil. Place under preheated broiler at high heat, until somewhat brown (about 2 minutes). Then turn, brown the other side; lower the heat and broil for 6 to 8 minutes.

DIET FOR ECZEMA

1. No fried foods. This includes potato chips, Fritos, and the like.
2. No carbonated drinks. This includes diet drinks, beer and ale.
3. No candy, sugar, pastry, pie, ice cream. Honey may be used occasionally on buckwheat pancakes.
4. No potatoes, white bread. Limit starches to 20% of diet.
5. No pork, beef, or ham. For meats use lamb, fish, and fowl prepared by baking, broiling, or stewing.
6. No butter, greases, fats. No oily salad dressings.
7. Vegetables should be a substantial part of diet. Carrots, okra, squash, and the like are especially recommended. Also fresh green salads (but without oily salad dressings!). Avoid peas, dried and baked beans, however.
8. Fruits: Eat only sparingly. Avoid raw apples and bananas.
9. Mullein tea: Every evening at bedtime drink a cup or more of mullein tea. This may be obtained at a health food store. Prepare by placing about one-half teaspoon in a cup and pour boiling water over it. Allow to steep for 30 minutes, strain, and drink.
10. Avoid heavy seasoning in foods.
11. Milk, eggs (yolks only), and cheese are all right.
12. It is suggested that you do not combine citrus fruits and cereal at the same meal.

ELIMINANTS

Here we may give for the body a very good eliminant, from which might be gathered that as would be good for children, babies, and grown-ups.

Make a fusion of senna; that is, in the proportions of six to eight senna pods to a pint of water. Boil this, and steep, but reduce to three times less the quantity. That is, if the first quantity is a gallon, reduce it down to at least one quart, see? Let it not boil then, but just simmer, so as to be strained off. Then, to this quart, add two ounces of strained honey.

Then make a fusion of pumpkin seed, these crushed, and prepared in the same proportions as the above, though only one-third of the quantity would be used, see? To this add (to the third of a quart, you see) one-half ounce of Rochelle salts.

Then add, for this same quart quantity that was used, one-half pint of alcohol.

You'll have a good eliminant! This may be used by anyone. The dosage, for an average adult, would be a teaspoonful or for this individual, you see. For babies, use from one minim up to fifteen drops, depending on the age, you see.
$\hfill$ 3053-1

General Concepts of Elimination

These [disturbances]. . .have to do with the assimilations and eliminations of the body. There should be a warning to *all*. . .as to such conditions; for would the assimilations and the eliminations be kept nearer *normal* in the human family, the days [of life] might be extended to whatever period. . . desired; for the system is *builded* by the assimilations of that [which] it takes within, and it is able to bring resuscitation so long as the eliminations do not hinder.
$\hfill$ 311-4

Q-4. Should anything be taken for eliminations?

A-4. Correct [your eliminations] better by diet than by taking eliminants, when possible. If not possible to correct otherwise, take an eliminant, but [alternate] between one time a vegetable laxative and the next time a mineral eliminant. But these [elimination problems] will be bettered if a great deal of the raw vegetables are used and not so much of meat, but do eat fish, fowl and lamb occasionally—but don't fry it!   3381-1

A vegetable as well as a mineral laxative should be alternated in the use of alkalizers, or of agents taken for increasing eliminations through the alimentary canal. It is well for those requiring any laxative to change about. Have a mineral and again the vegetable compound, so there is the better balance kept, and neither will become so necessary or it will not destroy entirely the sphincter activities of the muscular forces of the alimentary canal.   849-76

Q-2. What is the condition of my intestines. . .should I continue taking Castoria?
A-2. Rather than so much of the Castoria [vegetable base] in the present— for this *can* become irritating, of course—we would occasionally change to other eliminants. As we have indicated for other bodies, it is well to alternate these rather than continuing to take just one type of eliminant.
Occasionally, then, we would take the milk of bismuth—a teaspoonful, with a few drops of elixir of lactated pepsin in same—stirred in half a glass of water. This is to cleanse the system, or to absorb the poisons. Then afterward it would be necessary to take small doses of Eno salts or Sal Hepatica. The Sal Hepatica, of course, is partially mineral, while the Eno salts is practically all vegetable or fruit salts, see?   264-56

Set up better eliminations by the use of those foods that tend to produce better drainages. . .laxative foods such as. . .a great deal. . .of the black figs and the white and purple also, and the prunes and prune preparations.
                    3336-1

Mineral

First, we would use a saline laxative to make for better alkalization of the whole system, and to increase circulation in such a manner as to eliminate much of the poisons from the system, especially in the alimentary canal. Take a heaping teaspoonful of Sal Hepatica in half a glass of water, dissolved and then filling the glass—using a large glass, tea glass or the like. Do this each morning for three to five days—each morning before breakfast, see? Using a large glass and putting the dose in the glass half full of water at first will keep the properties from overflowing, when the solution effervesces.
Leave off this after the third or fifth day, provided there have been good

eliminations and the cold has been allayed, also the stiffness overcome. But continue to keep an alkalized condition for the body, and to keep up good eliminations.

2526-2

Then we would increase the eliminations so as to carry away more of the poisons and toxins from the system. For this body in the present, and with the activities, we would use the mineral rather than vegetable eliminants; especially such as may be found in Upjohn's Citrocarbonates. This we would take a heaping teaspoonful each morning before any meal is taken. Let it effervesce and drink a full glass of water with the spoonful dissolved in same, and then another glass of water afterwards.

Do drink more water.

2051-7

And keep occasionally a dose of Upjohn's Citrocarbonate and Milk of Magnesia; not both on the same day, no, but once or twice a week take each of these, or one or the other of these.

618-2

We would take at times the alkaline properties that may be had from the Upjohn's Citrocarbonates, taken in periods of one to two days. These will change the effects of the circulatory system as to allow better eliminations.

678-2

Oil

Then leave off the Atomidine, and begin with the use of castor oil packs; an hour each day for three days. Use at least three thicknesses of flannel, lightly wrung out of the castor oil, as hot as the body can stand it, and applied over the liver and the whole of the abdomen, especially upon the right side of same. Keep the pack warm by using an electric pad.

After the third day of using the packs, take a high enema to relieve the tensions throughout the colon and lower portion of jejunum; using a colon tube for same. Have the water body-temperature, and to each quart of water used (and use as much as three quarts) we would put a level teaspoonful of table salt and half a teaspoonful of baking soda, thoroughly dissolved.

2434-1

As we find, the acute conditions arise from the effects of a poison—pyrene.

From this activity the acute indigestion as produced through the alimentary canal has caused an expansion of, and a blocking in, the colon areas.

As we find in the present, we would apply hot castor oil packs continuously for two-and-a-half to three hours.

Then have an enema, gently given. It would be well that some oil be in the first enema; that is, the oil alone given first, see? Olive oil would be the better for this; about half a pint; so that there may be the relaxing.

And then give the enema with the body-temperature water, using a heaping teaspoonful of salt and a level teaspoonful of baking soda to the quart-and-a-half of water. Give this gently at first, but eventually—that is, after the period when there has been the ability for a movement—use the colon tube.

Then we would take internally—after the oil packs and the enema—a tablespoonful of olive oil.

This, as we find, should relieve the tensions and relax the body sufficiently to remove the disturbing conditions.   1523-9

Q-5. Would yeast be good for me to take?

A-5. Yeast is very well, but if the apple diet is used for the cleansing forces as indicated—about once a month—this would be preferable to the creating of greater disturbances in an already fagged condition in the system.

If there is the insistent non-activity of eliminations as well as should be, then, as we find, the small quantities of olive oil—with the activities of the system—would be preferable to the yeast or cathartics or the like. We would take about half a teaspoonful of the olive oil about three to four times each day, when it is taken. This will not only supply nutriment to the digestive tract but will aid in the eliminations, and is an intestinal food.   1622-1

Olive Oil

Q-1. What treatment to stimulate eliminations?

A-1. These are best stimulated by the diet and exercise. As has been in those given, these in the diet should be that as is a mild *laxative,* rather than *cathartics,* see? and when there is the tendency of this condition to become sluggish, those of oils—*preferably* much more of olive than just plain mineral oil, for olive oil—*properly* taken—is a food for the intestinal tract. This would be well to be considered by many: That, that may be *assimilated* by the system—of olive oil—pure—is food value for the system itself, and tends to stimulate peristaltic movements, see? Taken, then, in very small quantities—but rather often; and when found to disagree—or a tendency, from the foods or the character of drinks taken—discontinue; for nothing is more severe than rancid, or oil that has become overacted on by the hydrochlorics in the system. Only that as will assimilate. So olive oil or mineral oil—in moderation; but diet and exercise the best.   5603-5

Vegetable

Q-7. Are colonics also of value to body when not pregnant, and if so how often?

A-7. Value to the body when not pregnant, or when pregnant, if necessary. For a laxative take senna leaf tea, using four or five of the leaves placed in an empty cup and then pour hot water on it and let stand for thirty minutes to forty-five minutes, strain and drink it. Do this about once a week and it will be good for the body, as it does not become habit-forming and is a correct laxative for most individuals; though not everyone.   457-14

For the eliminations generally, we would use Zilatone as an activity upon the eliminating system; that the organs of the system may be cleansed throughout. Half an hour after the morning meal take one Zilatone tablet; half an hour to an hour after the noon meal take another; then in the evening about two hours after the meal take *two* tablets. And then leave off for at least two or three days, before this may be repeated again.   1523-1

It would be well, as we find, to use the Zilatone as an activative force for stirring the liver and its activities for the general eliminations. For this will also purify and clarify the gall duct area, stimulating the activities for the general system. We would take two tablets of morning and two of evening, the first day. The next day take only two in the evening. The next day take only one. Then skip two days. Then repeat these.

We would preferably use the Zilatone tablets as indicated, with the effective activities from same upon the liver and kidneys, the gall duct, the spleen and pancreas; *with* the combination of the White's Codliver Oil Tablets.   357-7

Q-6. What is a good laxative for this body?

A-6. Eno salts is the best laxative for this body, for this is of the fruit nature and not mineral, that would cause disturbance or hardening activities through the conditions in the stomach, as well as through those activities in the liver and the kidneys. This also should be taken in just small doses, almost every day, for periods of a week at a time, and will be most beneficial.   462-13

Castoria

The extracts which follow are all recommendations of Fletcher's Castoria, the laxative most often suggested by the Cayce readings. In the extracts, chosen at random, it is not only possible to compare the dosages given to individuals whose ages vary from four days to 62 years, but to discover yet another way in which the psychic readings of Edgar Cayce show their capacity for detail. During the years from 1936 to 1944, which these references cover in chronological order, it is a matter of record that the formula of Castoria was changed, and then changed back again. Note how the readings adjusted for the changes, even prescribing combinations of laxatives when necessary.

Take a laxative such as found in Fletcher's Castoria combined with syrup of figs. Take from a small bottle (of 900 drops) a teaspoonful, and add in its place a teaspoonful of the syrup of figs. Give half a teaspoonful every half hour (shaking well each time before pouring out the dosage), until there is a full reaction from the alimentary canal. 773-4

Do not take too much food in the system until there is a thorough cleansing of the alimentary canal. This would be well to be done with an alternation between the Fletcher's Castoria and the syrup of figs. These should be taken about every half an hour, or an hour apart, until there is the *thorough* evacuation. The dose would be half a teaspoonful, at one time of the Castoria and the next of the syrup of figs. 379-4

Q-1. *What dosage and how often should the Castoria be given?*
A-1. This only if it becomes necessary, you see; and then, of course, only one to two drops at each dose, three to six hours apart, until it has made the correction through the alimentary canal, which will be detected, of course, in the stool.
This would have nothing to do, of course, with the frequency of the Glyco-Thymoline—as these will work together, and the Glyco-Thymoline is for one thing—the correcting in the colon, while the Castoria is for the digestive system. 2015-1

Keep up, or increase, the eliminations. Use Castoria with syrup of figs as an eliminant; not leaving off the others, but this to decrease the elimination of poisons through the system and start the activity of the eliminating system through those channels which will be most beneficial. Better conditions are brought about by taking this in small quantities and often, you see; about half a teaspoonful every half hour. These—the Castoria and figs—may be mixed or alternated. 1541-9

Take internally a combination of syrup of figs *and* Fletcher's Castoria, in small or broken doses; half a teaspoonful every half-hour, even if it requires

more than nine hundred drops (or a small bottle of the Castoria). Take until there is *complete* evacuation, with an activity of the liver and of the kidneys *from* the taking of these broken doses.

The next morning after these properties have reacted, take two heaping teaspoonsful of Sal Hepatica in a glass of water to flush the system.2516-1

Begin with small doses every half hour of Castoria and syrup of figs. On one half-hour take half a teaspoonful of Castoria, then the next half-hour take half a teaspoonful of syrup of figs. Continue these, first one and then the other, you see, either one or the other every half-hour, until there are *full* eliminations from the alimentary canal. The basis of both of these compounds is senna, you see, yet there are active principles in each that will affect the hepatic circulation in quite a different manner—and their combinations are needed.   573-6

Begin with broken doses of Castoria or with Caldwell's syrup of pepsin (senna or fig base); half a teaspoonful every hour until good eliminations are set up. The Castoria formula has been changed and is not as complete as the syrup of pepsin; hence the suggestion for the pepsin as a substitute.

2824-5

Now to cleanse the system, we would set up the eliminations with Castoria. Taken as it is in the present, it is very good.   2752-3

We would give the Castoria in broken doses—ten to twelve drops every half hour until there are thorough, thorough eliminations.   2824-6

As we find, there are the aftereffects of the acute conditions in the body— arising from the lack of proper eliminations of the poisons which were caused from the poisoning as was indicated from an acid.

These, as combined then with the aftereffects of "flu," with so much of a vegetable laxative, have caused a contraction of the mucous membranes in portions of the colon, as well as jejunum.   1523-10

EPSOM SALTS PACK

Add as much Epsom salts as will dissolve in the amount of water necessary to saturate a bath towel. Apply as hot as possible over the area indicated. Keep repeating the hot applications for two or three hours at each treatment.

Instead of repeating the hot applications, one may place a piece of plastic over the packs to prevent soiling, and then use an electric pad to keep the pack warm until the Epsom salts have completely dried or have become caked in the pack.

FASTING

I. What Is Fasting?

Fasting has been looked upon throughout the ages as a means of spiritual growth in the practices of many religions; as a protest against civil injustices or as a means of protesting against the alleged or real injustices of the law of the land; as a means of binding an oath to seek revenge; in defending one's honor; and as a means of preparation for surgical procedures in more recent years. Fasting involves complete abstinence from food or more lenient diets partially excluding certain food substances.

Fasting as it is seen in the readings, however, is perhaps different from any of the usual concepts with which we have become familiar. It is a setting aside of our own concepts of how something should be done. It is casting out of our inner selves any thought of what we would have done, rather allowing ourselves to become channels through which God may work. It is a supplying of energy to the body which would allow coordination of organs and systems, which would bring about adequate assimilation and elimination. In purifying a mind which is in a state of mental confusion, fasting is a mechanism of the mind and not of the body or the diet. For prayer and fasting is not what man usually thinks of it—doing without food—but rather it is man bringing himself to low estate, abasing himself in order that the Creative Force of God might be made manifest.

The following four extracts may give us a more rounded commentary on this from the readings:

>. . .fasting. . .is as the Master gave: Laying aside our own concepts of *how* or *what* should be done at this period and let the *Spirit* guide. Get the *truth* of fasting!. . .to be sure, *overdone* brings shame to self, as overindulgence in anything—but the *true* fasting is casting out of self that as "*I* would have

done [replacing with] but as *Thou,* O Lord, seest fit. . ."   295-6

Hence, as the entity may ask, what about the spiritualizing of these? This is well, but this comes through direct reactions. As has been indicated, such are healed with fasting and prayer. But what does fasting and prayer mean here?

The supplying of those coordinations of the activities of the physical organs with the elements sufficient not only for producing the necessary forces, but for the carrying away and eliminating of the drosses that have already been created—and that find their reaction or manifestation in the depleted feeling that arises in the body forces.   3062-1

. . .purifying of mind is of the mind, not of the body. For, as the Master gave, it is not that which entereth in the body, but that which cometh out that causes sin. It is what one does with the purpose, for all things are pure in themselves, and are for the sustenance of man, body, mind, and soul, and remember—these must work together. . .   5401-1

. . .yet this must be approached with prayer and fasting. . .Not as man counts fasting—doing without *food;* but one that would abase himself that the Creative Force *might* be made manifest. This will be presented even as such is made known to those studying such phenomena, as physically called, in the process of operation.

Q-10. *Should we take this up with the Scientific Society of America?*
A-10. No! Take it up rather with God!   254-46

II. Arguments Against Fasting

There certainly are those conditions wherein fasting should not be attempted, because a variety of disturbances within the body might be produced. In 2684-1, for instance, a physical condition in addition to a disturbed mental condition was approached by a 43-year-old woman with a fast. In her case, it produced an unbalanced chemical condition within the body that prevented proper assimilation of foods and created gas in the duodenum, which in turn caused pain and irritation. An excess of acid was formed and the subsequent disturbances to the superficial and deep circulation brought about lesions in the sympathetic ganglia. These in turn reflected throughout the nervous system and produced a variety of different symptoms.

In another case, [2185], there was fear of cancer. The question was asked if there was any malignant growth in the man's body. The answer was that conditions of "plethora" existed in pockets of the lymphatic circulation throughout portions of the body which Cayce indicated were not yet malignant but which could be if there was not persistence in following the suggestions he had given. He stated that there should be no serious diets or activities because such create a strain on the body—and would occur in fasting or in following certain diets for a long period of time. He suggested that this person be well-balanced in his diets. Thus, fasting should be abstained from in cases where there are definite abnormalities of the body suggesting lack of proper substances.

In a different condition—uterine myoma—the woman had already fasted two weeks with nothing but orange and tomato juice and she complained of a coated tongue and indigestion. The rather obvious indication was that the fasting caused excessive amounts of poisons and wastes in the system which were detrimental rather than beneficial in this specific instance. Cayce's suggestion was to:

> Remove those *conditions* by the application of those properties as have been outlined, and by the manipulation necessary to cause the proper absorption of condition in system. We will find the growth (as is called) reducing, rather than that as is caused by poison in the system, and the *amount* as is seen that exists after fasting, as indicated, is that the condition is of the nature that may be removed by the absorption method, if there is the proper administration of conditions to cause, or produce, or bring about, those conditions in system where—through these may be accomplished. Hence, do as has been given for this, rather than that of the diet that weakens the vitality of the system. . .   283-3

There were still those who came rather consistently to Cayce for readings, almost insisting on fasting in the conventional manner. [2072] was like that and in his fifth reading he was put off in his attempt at a purifying fast until his body was more in proper balance and lesions had been removed from the ganglia.

There are many, then, who should not fast in the manner of abstaining from food. Cayce's concept of fasting mentioned earlier becomes more understandable and attractive here and emphasizes that mental conditions and disturbances cannot be made right through the mechanism of bodily fasting.

III. When Should We Fast, and How?

Certainly fasting in the traditional sense does have its place. In some situations and when the body is disturbed from certain causes, a fast can be beneficial. A 32-year-old woman, [1850], had a bad case of bronchitis with loss of voice and what Cayce described as a "super-acid" condition throughout her body. She was given adjunctive therapy in the way of stimulating the eliminations to remove congestion in the trachea and the bronchi, but interestingly was told to fast following an otherwise extreme regimen:

Keep away from foods! **Keep rather only water, milk and bread, for at least five to six days. This will be necessary if we are to eliminate the conditions from the body.** 1850-3

Then the young lady was instructed to go on a three-day apple diet with half a teacup of olive oil afterward, and then begin to eat a normal diet—not too rich nor too highly seasoned—after the cleansing was completed. Thus it can be seen that in this particular case cleansing of the physical body was the objective.

Obesity seems to be the most logical condition in which one should practice fasting. The readings substantiate this in one case of a woman, overweight and having trouble with vomiting, who was given some sharp advice:

When there is regurgitation, when there is the overloading in the system— no matter whether it's just plain water—the body wouldn't starve if it fasted for forty days! It would really be good for it! but be severe *for the body!* but overloading the system *overtaxes* the body. 5583-2

It must be noted, however, that not many of those individuals consulting Cayce for obesity ended up with advice to fast. They were instead directed to take Welch's grape juice, two ounces in one ounce of water 20 minutes before each meal. This is one condition, however, for which fasting was suggested and consequently might be considered.

Some other aspects of fasting from the readings indicate the subtlety of the fasting concept. For instance in homosexuality, a reading recommended physical hardships. Denying spending money on one's indulgences, sleeping on a hard bed, eating very little, taking no sweets, not going to movies or entertainment, and going "for days only on bread and water, but do it of thyself if ye would succeed, and ye may become even a greater pianist than Hofmann." (5056-1) This again becomes a fast for a specific purpose of denying the body when there has been an obvious history of lack of self-denial.

Fasting then is well in its place and perhaps its place is not nearly as common as practices throughout the world have led us to believe. We must keep in mind that it is also important to supply our bodies with the energies to build body forces so that life may continue normally as expressions of the Spirit within. (See 5326-1.)

For the body is indeed the temple of the living God. Therein ye may meet Him in prayer, in meditation, in psalm singing, yea in the activities of fasting, in not only the foods but in opening the mind, the consciousness, consciously to that which may flow in from music, from prayer, those influences which may flow in from deep meditation, which may be gained in having regular periods for this shutting out from self of the voices or the sounds of nature and listening to the still small voice within.   3620-2

Could we not say, then, that fasting physically may be needed for physical conditions and is the withholding of physical food; fasting mentally is that condition already described where we abase self—the ego—so that Creative Forces might be made manifest; and spiritual fasting is shutting out even the sounds of nature in listening to the still small voice within.

William A. McGarey, M.D.

Edgar Cayce readings referenced:

254-46	1850-3	3062-1	5326-1
283-3	2055-1	3630-2	5401-1
295-6	2072-5, 9	4008-1	5583-2
1553-15	2185-4	5056-1	
1779-4	2684-1	5257-1	

Extracts on Fasting

Yes, yes, we have the body here. There are disturbances, physical, as well as confusions, mental. In attempts at times to purify body forces, one may reach those extents, in the matter of custom or diet, as to cause hardships and to cause elements necessary for the better body-functioning to gradually be entirely eliminated from the body.

This, to be sure, is not an attempt to tell the body to go back to eating meat, but do supply, then, through the body forces, supplements, either in vitamins or in substitutes, for those who would hold to these influences—but purifying of mind is of the mind, not of the body. For, as the Master gave, it is not that which entereth in the body, but that which cometh out that causes sin. It is what one does with the purpose, for all things are pure in themselves, and are for the sustenance of man, body, mind and soul, and remember— these must work together, as should be indicated for the body in its interpretation of music. For music is of the soul, and one may become mind and soul-sick for music, or soul and mind-sick from certain kinds of music.

Physically, the strengthening of the organs of the sensory system are the more necessary. There are certain centers along the spine where there is greater coordination between the central nervous system and the sympathetic and those of the organs of sensory forces. So, as we would find, first, we would through hydrotherapy, thoroughly purify the body forces. Three to six, then, thorough fume baths; then thorough massages; including colonic baths. Do these at Reilly's. Thus we will purify the body by removing a great deal of the dross that is preventing better conditions. The massages— particular stress should be made in the 3rd cervical; 3rd, 4th, 5th, and 6th dorsal; the 9th dorsal and through the lumbar and sacral. Then use, in the massage, the oil rubs, combination of olive oil, peanut oil and lanolin. These will be most strengthening and invigorating for the body.

Do add to the diet about twice as many oranges, lemons and limes as is a part of the diet in the present. These also supplement with a great deal of carrots, especially as combined with gelatin, if we would aid and strengthen the optic nerves and the tensions between sympathetic and cerebrospinal systems.

...A great deal will depend upon the mental attitude of the body. Music is that realm between sublime and the ridiculous. Do practice the sublime. Not merely in thought but in what you think of and say about others, and how you treat them personally.   5401-1

Diet, fasting are well in their place; so is the application of that for supplying a need, for a supply of energies to build body-forces.

Q-2. Will more than one fast be necessary?

A-2. This depends upon what ye gain by the study and what is pointed out

to thee in thy meditation. Know God will speak with thee as ye speak with
Him in thy conscience, in thy soul-self, if ye really desire same.   5326-1

Q-4. Is there any malignant growth in my body?
A-4. Not in the present. There are conditions where plethora exists in
pockets of the lymph circulation through portions of the body, but not of the
malignant nature as yet—neither is it indicated that there would be, if there is
persistence in following the suggestions outlined and not attempting serious
diets or activities that cause such great strains on the body—as in fasting or
in following certain diets for a long period of time. Keep well balanced in the
diets.
Do that.   2185-4

Q-27. Spiritual foods?
A-27. These are needed by the body just as the body physical needs fuel in
the diet. The body mental and spiritual needs spiritual food—prayer,
meditation, thinking upon spiritual things. For thy body is indeed the temple
of the living God. Treat it as such, physically and mentally.   4008-1

Then, as to the diet:
During these periods when there is the tendency for cold and congestion,
and those activities in which there are sudden changes with the body-
temperature—we would use more of those vitamins as will be found in
Adiron—these would be the more beneficial. Take these with the meals; one
tablet at the morning meal, one at the evening meal, and two at the noon
meal, see?
Also keep a great deal of Vitamin B-1, especially. This as we find may be
obtained in the Knox gelatin or in steel-cut oats (cooked a long time). These
are the principal sources from which this may be obtained, in a manner that
would assimilate better with this body—if the other vitamins as found in
Adiron are taken in the manner indicated (as the A, B, G and D, and some C).
Do these, and we will find the better conditions, better resistance, better
strength built up for the body.
To be sure, keep the eliminations in good order. An aid to this would be
found in the use of a food prepared in this manner:
        1 cup black figs, chopped or ground very fine
        1 cup dates (not seeded)*
        ½ cup yellow corn meal (not too finely ground)
Cook this for twenty minutes in sufficient water (2 or 3 cups) for it to be the
consistency of mush, or cook until the meal is thoroughly cooked in same.

---

*Gladys Davis's note: I think the reference to dates "not seeded" means that you should use the
big dates that have not been packed, and take seeds out yourself just before preparing them.

Eat a tablespoonful of this mixture of an evening, not all at once but let it be taken slowly so as to be well assimilated as it is taken. This will be most helpful for the body.   1779-4

Q-4. Since babyhood, the mother has been perplexed as to what food is best for this entity. What caused this condition?
A-4. We haven't the physical condition, but feed the entity oft the foods which were the basis of the foods of the Atlanteans and the Egyptians—corn meals with figs and dates prepared together with goat's milk.   5257-1

An excellent food for the body of an afternoon and evening would be this combination:
    1 cup black figs, or packed figs, chopped or ground very fine
    1 cup dates, chopped or ground very fine
    ½ cup yellow corn meal (not too finely ground)
Cook this in sufficient water (2 or 3 cups) for 15 to 20 minutes, to make it the consistency of mush.   2055-1

Q-3. What bulk does she require that can be disguised in food or drink?
A-3. We would prepare a mixture to be taken as food, in this manner: Chop together a cupful each of black figs and dates. Put this on the stove in a cupful of milk (from which the cream has not been separated). Just before it comes to a boil, stir in same two tablespoonsful of corn meal. This will not only make bulk but will be the character of bulk as a food that will act with those properties for better eliminations, and give food values of a nature most helpful for the body in the present. This quantity might be used three or four meals, and this means it might be taken once or twice a day, dependent upon the ability to get the body to take same.   1553-15

GENERAL INTEREST EXTRACTS

In some of the readings, Cayce points out that life as we know it is a manifestation of spirit insistent on its being active in a manner determined by the nature of the mind and physical structure of the cells themselves—meaning that life is already present and active. He implies, then, that the disturbances which arise are disturbances of the ways in which this life force is manifesting in single structures and in systems throughout the body. Thus, his approach to etiology of diseases is a physiological one, but it assumes initially that the inner forces within the body are the spirit in action.

In analyzing the conditions here [muscular dystrophy], we find much of this prenatal, yet not that which might be called the sin of the fathers, nor of the entity itself, but rather that through which patience and consistency might be the lesson for the entity in this experience.   3681-1

Common cold

Bolting food or swallowing it by the use of liquids produces more colds than *any one* activity of a diet. . .   808-3

Vitamins are not as easily overcrowded in the system as most other boosters for a general activity.   902-1

Peyer's patches

There are to be sure, lacteal ducts. There are the strings or ducts all through the upper portion of the alimentary canal, or jejunum; but the larger patch or area is that lying just below the lower end of the duodenum, and where same *empties* into the jejunum, see? *This* patch is not only an *internal*

activity, but an *external*, that makes for the production of assimilation.
2153-4

There are basically three nervous systems: the cerebrospinal, which controls conscious movements and which includes in its makeup the frontal portion of the brain and the spinal cord; the autonomic nervous system (which Cayce calls the "sympathetic"), supplies various organs of the body functioning at an unconscious level—it may be understood as being the nervous system of the unconscious mind; and the sensory nervous system which involves the nerve supply associated with the organs of sense. These are considered collectively part of one unit.

These three nervous systems have contact with each other and maintain a balance and a coordination one with the other at all times within that state we call health. There are lymphatic patches, apparently within bursae, found in certain of the sympathetic ganglia paralleling the various levels of the spinal column. These patches of lymph tissue and fluid become the means by which proper synaptic relationship is maintained among the three nervous systems. Substances of a "globular" nature are manufactured in the Peyer's patches of the small intestine and carried by the lymphocytes to these patches, making it possible in that manner to maintain the coordination between the autonomic and the cerebrospinal nervous systems, and for these, in turn, to maintain a balance with the sensory forces of the body.

Peanut oil/Almonds

Q-21. Shall I resume peanut oil rubs?
A-21. There is nothing better. They supply energy in the body. And, just as a person who eats two or three almonds each day need never fear cancer, those who take a peanut oil rub each week need never fear arthritis.
1158-31

Constipation

There should be a warning to *all* bodies as to such conditions; for would the assimilations and the eliminations be kept nearer *normal* in the human family, the days might be extended to whatever period as was so desired; for the system is *builded* by the assimilations of that it takes within, and is able to bring resuscitation so long as the eliminations do not hinder. **311-4**

Cycles of therapy

It should always be kept in mind that a cycle of therapy is an important concept to be drawn from the Cayce readings. Thus any therapy should be given for a period of time, then a rest should be taken by the body. It is well to remember also that patience, consistency and perseverance are necessary elements for the patient and the doctor to observe and use as the body is being rebuilt and brought back to a normal balance.

GLYCO-THYMOLINE PACK

Use two to three thicknesses of cotton cloth well saturated with Glyco-Thymoline (purchased from your druggist). Apply this over affected areas or those areas specifically directed in your particular case. An electric pad may be used to keep the pack warm. The saturated cotton cloth should be applied first, then a piece of plastic to prevent soiling, and then the heating pad over that with perhaps a towel on top to hold it in place.

This should be applied for 20 to 30 minutes or longer if directed. Do not apply the pack when the Glyco-Thymoline is cold, as in chilly weather. Rather, you might place the bottle of Glyco-Thymoline in a pan of hot water to take the chill off before using it for the pack. Check the Circulating Files on specific ailment for length of days of application.

MASSAGE

Massage, of course, performs a number of functions, but the following rather specific function is even more interesting because it occurred in a patient who had acute leukemia, an 18-year-old boy. One who would give massages should bear the following information in mind at all times:

The massage is very well, but we would do this the more often, see? As long as there is an opportunity of it producing the effect to all areas of the better activity to the organs of the body. The "why" of the massage should be considered: Inactivity causes many of those portions along the spine from which impulses are received to the various organs to be lax, or taut, or to allow some to receive greater impulse than others. The massage aids the ganglia to receive impulse from nerve forces as it aids circulation through the various portions of the organism.   2456-4

PASSION FLOWER FUSION

Directions for preparation of the passion flower fusion (also known as mayblossom bitters): To one gallon of the fruit, flower, leaves and vine (including the bark) of the maypop plant add two gallons of distilled water. The container used should be made of enamel or crockware, and the lid of glass or the same. Reduce by slow boiling to one quart. Strain. Add nine ounces of 85% grain alcohol and one ounce of elixir of wild ginseng. It is most preferable to make the fusion from the fresh plant.

VENTRICULIN

Ventriculin and Ventriculin with iron were manufactured by Parke-Davis and Company until sometime in the mid or late 1950s. As listed in the 1953 issue of the *Physician's Desk Reference,* Ventriculin is described as a powder to be used orally, an antianemic substance derived from gastric tissue. The medical dictionary reference states that it is derived from the gastric tissue of hogs. Forty grams of the powder was described as one U.S.P. unit, and this was the daily suggested dosage. It was used as a stimulator of reticulocyte formation and as a specific for pernicious anemia. It was also used in atrophic gastritis. The Ventriculin with iron contained 12.5% naferon, which was iron and sodium citrate neutral. The latter was indicated for anemia due to iron deficiency states.

It is to be assumed that Cayce found the Ventriculin to be beneficial in a number of conditions since it was suggested not only in anemia but in conditions such as scleroderma, as an extreme example. Perhaps it was the enzymes which were present in the wall of the stomach from which the powder was derived that prompted the use of this particular substance in the readings. It may be that the readings saw this acting to promote better assimilation of foods and thus provide the substances within the bloodstream once assimilated, which would make for an ability to build red blood cells in the blood-forming organs.

Substances which might be to some extent equivalent in the 1967 P.D.R. are Converzyme (Ascher); Digestant (Canright); Accelerase (Organon); Entozyme (A.H. Robins). Entozyme has in it 250 mg. of N.F. equivalent pepsin; 300 mg. N.F. equivalent pancreatin; and 150 mg. biosalts. Converzyme tablets contain 5 mg. of cellulolytic enzyme; proteolytic enzyme 10 mg.; amylolytic enzyme 30 mg.; and lipolytic enzyme 800 Ascher units. This gives an idea of the relative difference between these more modern preparations and that which Cayce described in various places. It seems reasonable that these could be interchangeable.

WHY THE PATIENT'S CONDITION SEEMS TO WORSEN WHEN TREATMENT IS GIVEN

In some respects we find conditions appear to be more aggravated at times than aided, yet—as we will find—when it becomes necessary for a physical body to be builded. . .as of the brain cell's expansion itself, and where scar tissue. . .has formed. . .obstruction. . .in same—that. . .conditions [of retraction] must necessarily arise. . .that is, the system throwing out that as feelers, or as new lines of activity through that of the voluntary and involuntary nerve reactions from those plexuses in the system, that build for the resuscitating and regenerating of energies from within the system; for, as life is builded of each cell, by the multiplication of same, where tissue has been resuscitate or regenerate itself—[as do] the brain cells themselves, for the *life* of a brain *cell* is only according to the activity of a body physical and mental, and is *multipled* according to the *activities* of same as related to the assimilation of resuscitating forces. Then as the vibrations are made within the system, as break up the very cells in their electrical energy—as is seen in both white and gray nerve tissue, from the activity of those vibrations as come through from the applications of those vibratory forces that give off into the system those of the basic buildings of nerve energy itself, in that of the gold and the silver vibrations—these, as we find, *must* be shielded, guided, directed, prevented from those of the activities as would be from one that was being guided *in* that of the building up of *energy* as comes *from* the muscular reaction; for building brain cells is quite different from building that of muscular forces in an *organized* system—for this is as of a *re*organization. **161-3**

This boy had epilepsy quite severely with scarring apparently in the brain tissue. There is much to think about in regard to the suggestions made in this reading.

Glossary

abscess—a collection of pus formed by the disintegration of tissues

acidosis—a condition resulting from too much acid or too little alkaline reserve in blood and body tissues

adenoid—resemblance to a gland in appearance; in the plural: hypertrophied lymph tissue in the nasopharynx; known as the pharyngeal tonsil

adhesion—the stable joining of parts to each other, which may occur abnormally

alkalosis—a condition resulting from increase of base or decrease of acid without decreasing base in the body fluids

allergy—a hypersensitive state due to exposure to a particular allergen; classified as immediate or delayed; includes serum sickness, allergic drug reactions, contact dermatitis and anaphylactic shock; usually manifested in the gastrointestinal tract, the skin, and the respiratory tract

anemia (pernicious)—a decrease in the number of circulating red blood cells; called also *Addison's* or *addisonian a., Addison-Biermer a., cytogenic a.,* and *malignant a.*

aneurysm—a saclike swelling in the wall of a blood vessel, usually an artery

ankylosis—abnormal stiffness of a joint, often due to damage of joint membranes (in chronic rheumatoid arthritis), injury, or surgical procedure

anodyne—a medicine for relieving pain; e.g., opium, morphine, codeine, or aspirin

anorexia—loss of appetite

antigen—any substance which stimulates cells to produce antibodies

antispasmodic—an agent that relieves spasm

aphonia—loss of voice

apoplexy—the condition of having suffered a stroke; intracranial hemorrhage

arteriole—a small branch of an artery that communicates with a capillary network

assimilation—the absorption and transformation of food into living tissue

asthenia—loss of strength and energy; weakness

asthma—a disease involving the bronchus, characterized by paroxysmal attacks of dyspnea; usually due to an allergy

atrophy—a wasting away; failure of a cell, tissue, organ, or part to grow and develop

autonomic—self-controlling; functionally independent; automatic

autosomal—pertaining to any chromosome that is not a sex chromosome

axilla—the armpit; the small pyramidal space between the upper lateral part of the chest and the medial side of the arm

axon—that part of a nerve cell through which impulses travel away from the cell body

bacillus—any rod-shaped bacterium which produces spores

bifurcation—division into two branches; the site where a single structure divides into two

bronchi—plural of bronchus; any of the larger air passages of the lungs

bronchitis—inflammation of the bronchi

bursa—a sac or pouchlike cavity containing a viscid fluid that reduces friction

caecum—the first part of the large intestine

calculus—any abnormal stony mass or deposit formed within the body, usually composed of mineral salts

capsula—a general term for a cartilaginous, fatty, fibrous, or membranous structure enveloping another structure, organ, or part

carious—decayed; having bone decay, esp. of teeth

carotid—relating to either of the two principal arteries of the neck

cataract—an eye disease in which the crystalline lens or its capsule becomes opaque, causing partial or total blindness

catarrh—inflammation of a mucous membrane, causing an increased flow of mucus; inflammation of the air passages of the head and throat

cathartic—an agent that stimulates evacuation of the bowels by increasing bulk

cerebrospinal—pertaining to the brain and the spinal cord

cervical—pertaining to the neck

chancre—a venereal sore or ulcer; primary lesion of syphilis

chorioretinitis—inflammation of the choroid and retina

chromosome—rodlike structure that appears in the nucleus of a cell during mitosis; transmits genetic information

chyle—a milky fluid absorbed by the lacteals from the food in the intestine during digestion; composed of lymph and emulsified fats

cirrhosis—liver disease in which the hepatic cells degenerate and the surrounding connective tissues thicken

coccygeal—pertaining to the coccyx; four fused vertebrae at the base of the spine

colitis—inflammation of the colon

collagen—the protein substance of the white fibers of connective tissues and in the matrix of bone

colonic (irrigation)—a high enema; method of hydrotherapy used to cleanse the large intestine of accumulated toxins

congenital—existing at, and usually before, birth; referring to conditions that are present at birth, regardless of their causation

constipation—infrequent or difficult evacuation of the feces

consumption—a wasting away of the body, formerly applied especially to pulmonary tuberculosis

cortico-steroids—any of the steroids elaborated by the adrenal cortex (excluding the sex hormones of adrenal origin) in response to the release of corticotropin by the pituitary gland

coryza—an acute catarrhal condition of the nasal mucous membrane

costal margin—pertaining to a rib or ribs

cutaneous—pertaining to the skin

cyanose—a bluish coloration of skin due to decreased blood oxygen concentration

cystitis—inflammation of the urinary bladder

decubitus ulcer—an ulceration caused by prolonged pressure in a patient allowed to lie too still in bed for a long period of time; bedsore

demulcent—soothing; bland; allaying the irritation of inflamed or abraded surfaces

diabetes mellitus—a metabolic disorder characterized by a high blood glucose level and the appearance of glucose in the urine due to a deficiency of insulin

diaphoretic—pertaining to, or characterized by, or promoting diaphoresis (profuse perspiration)

diathermy—heating of body tissues by high-frequency electric current

diathesis—a predisposition to certain diseases

distal—farther from the midline or origin

diuretic—increasing the excretion of urine

diverticuli(tis)—inflammation of small pouches (diverticula) that sometimes form in the lining and wall of the colon

duodenum—the first portion of the small intestine that leads from the stomach to the jejunum

dypsnea—shortness of breath

dysuria—painful or difficult urination

edema—an excessive accumulation of fluid within the tissue spaces

effluvium—an outflowing, or shedding, especially of the hair; an exhalation or vapor or steam; disagreeable or noxious odor

electroencephalogram—a recording of the electrical activity of the brain

elimination—the act of expulsion, especially from the body

emphysema—a condition of the lung characterized by abnormal enlargement of air sacs

emulsion—a preparation of one liquid distributed in small globules throughout the body of a second liquid

emunctory—any excretory organ or duct

endemic—a disease restricted to and constantly present in a particular human community

endocrine—secreting internally; applied to organs and structures that secrete hormones directly into the blood or lymph

engorgement—local congestion; excessive fullness of any organ, vessel or tissue due to accumulation of fluids, especially of blood

enterovirus—a type of virus infecting the gastrointestinal tract and discharged in the excreta

enzyme—a protein that is produced in a cell and acts as a catalyst in a specific cellular reaction

epidermis—the outermost layer of skin

epilepsy—disturbance of the central nervous system manifested by temporary impairment or loss of consciousness, convulsive seizures, and sensory disturbances of the autonomic nervous system

etiology—the study or the theory of the factors that cause disease

fibrillary—pertaining to a fibril or fibrils (a minute fiber or filament)

fibrin—insoluble, fibrous protein formed from fibrinogen during blood coagulation

fibroblast—a connective tissue cell

fistula—an abnormal passage or communication, usually between two internal organs, or leading from an internal organ to the surface of the body

flocculation—a colloid phenomenon in which the disperse phase separates in particles rather than in a continuous mass, as in coagulation

fomite—an object, such as a book, wooden object, or an article of clothing that is not in itself harmful, but may serve as an agent of transmission of an infection

gallbladder—the pear-shaped reservoir for the bile

ganglia—a knot or knotlike mass; neuron cell bodies, usually outside the central nervous system

gastrin—a hormone secreted by the stomach lining that stimulates secretion of gastric juices

gastritis—inflammation of the stomach

gastroenterology—pain in the stomach and intestines

gestation—the period of development of the young in viviparous animals; the entire period of pregnancy

gland—an aggregation of cells, specialized to secrete or excrete materials not related to their ordinary metabolic needs

globulin—a type of protein characterized by being insoluble in water, but soluble in saline solutions or water soluble proteins; occurs in blood plasma

grand mal—a type of epilepsy, characterized by convulsions and loss of consciousness

gumma—a soft, gummy tumor, such as that occurring in tertiary syphilis

halitosis—offensive breath

hemianopsis—defective vision or blindness in half of the visual field

hemolysin—a substance which frees hemoglobin from red blood corpuscles by interrupting their structural integrity

hemorrhoid—a condition in which veins associated with the lining of the rectum become enlarged

herniation—the abnormal protrusion of an organ or other body structure through a defect or opening in a covering, membrane, muscle, or bone

herpes zoster—a viral infection of certain sensory nerves, causing pain and an eruption of blisters along the course of the affected nerve; shingles

homeostasis—a tendency to stability in the normal body states

hormone—a chemical substance secreted by an endocrine gland, which has a specific regulatory effect on the activity of a certain organ

hydrocephalus—a condition marked by enlargement of the cranium, accompanied by an accumulation of cerebrospinal fluid within the skull; "water on the brain"

hydrolysis—the splitting of a compound into fragments by the addition of water

hyperaldosteronism—an abnormality of electrolyte metabolism caused by excessive secretion of aldosterone

hypertrophic—pertaining to the enlargement or overgrowth of an organ or tissue

hypochondria—abnormal anxiety over one's health, often with imaginary illnesses and severe melancholy

hypoglycemia—an abnormally low concentration of blood glucose, which may lead to tremulousness, cold sweat, etc.

hypoprothrombinemia—deficiency of prothrombin (coagulation Factor II)

hysterectomy—the surgical removal of the uterus

idiopathic—self-originated; of unknown causation

ileum—a distal portion of the small intestine, extending from the jejunum to the caecum

impaction—the condition of being firmly lodged or wedged

impetigo—a streptococcal or staphylococcal infection of the skin, characterized by fragile, grouped, pinhead-sized vesicles or pustules

induration—the process of hardening

interstitial keratitis—a chronic variety of keratitis (inflammation of the cornea)

inulin—a vegetable starch

Islets of Langerhans—irregular microscopic structures scattered throughout the pancreas and comprising its endocrine portion

jejunum—that portion of the small intestine which extends from the deodenum to the ileum

keloid—a sharply elevated, irregularly shaped, progressively enlarging scar

ketosteroids—a steroid that possesses ketone groups on functional carbon atoms

lacteal—pertaining to milk

lesion—any pathological or traumatic discontinuity of tissue or loss of function of a part

leucocyte—any colorless, ameboid cell mass; white blood cell or corpuscle

levulose—fructose

lipiodial—resembling fat

lumbar—the part of the back between the thorax and the pelvis

lumen—cavity or channel within a tube or tubular organ

lymph—a transparent, lightly yellow liquid of alkaline reaction found in the lymphatic vessels and derived from tissue fluids

lymphocyte—a type of white blood cell produced in lympathetic tissue

lysis—destruction, as of cells, by a specific lysin (an antibody)

medulla oblongata—the portion of brain stem located between the pons and the spinal cord

menarche—the beginning of menstrual function

meningitis—inflammation of the meninges (the three membranes that envelop the brain and spinal cord)

metabolism—transformation by which energy is made available for uses of the organism

metabolites—substances produced by metabolism or metabolic processes

microglial—pertaining to the small, non-neural, interstitial cells that form part of the supporting structure of the central nervous system

multiple sclerosis—a disease of the central nervous system characterized by loss of myelin and the appearance of scarlike patches throughout the brain and/or spinal cord

myelin sheath—the sheath surrounding the axon of some (the myelinated) nerve cells

myelogenous leukemia—leukemia arising from myeloid tissue, resulting in abnormal production of granulocytes by cells in the red bone marrow

myopathy—any disease of a muscle

myotonia—increased muscular irritability with decreased power of relaxation; spasm of the muscle

myxovirus—general name for a large group of viruses

neonate—new-born infant

neuron—any of the conducting cells of the nervous system; a nerve cell

orthopedic—referring to correcting deformities of the musculoskeletal system

oxidation—the act or state of being oxidized; an increase of positive charges on an atom or the loss of negative charges

osseous—the nature or quality of bone; bony

pancreas—a large, elongated gland located behind the stomach, between the spleen and the duodenum

paresis—slight or incomplete paralysis

pathogenesis—the development of morbid conditions or of disease

paresthesia—an abnormal sensation, as burning, prickling, etc.

Parkinson's disease—the effect of a group of neurological disorders characterized by rhythmic tremor and muscular rigidity

paronychia—inflammation involving the folds of tissue surrounding the fingernail

patella—a triangular bone situated at the front of the knee

pathology—branch of medicine treating the essential nature of disease, especially the structural and functional changes in body tissues and organs causing or caused by disease

perineum—the region between the anus and the external reproduction organs

periostitis—inflammation of the periosteum (a connective tissue covering all bones of the body and having bone-forming properties)

peristalsis—the rhythmic waves by which organs provided with both longitudinal and circular muscle fibers propel their contents

peritoneal cavity—abdominal cavity lined by the serous membrane (peritoneum)

petit mal—type of elipsy in which there are attacks of momentary unconsciousness without convulsions

Peyer's patches—aggregations of nodules scattered throughout the mucosal lining of the ileum of the small intestine

pheochromocytoma—a type of tumor in the adrenal medulla and usually accompanied by hypertension

phlebitis—inflammation of a vein

phonation—the utterance of vocal sounds

photophobia—abnormal fear of light

pigmentation—coloration, esp. abnormally increased coloration

plasma—the fluid portion of circulating blood

platelet—a disc-shaped fragment found in the blood of all mammals; functions in blood coagulation

pleurisy—inflammation of the pleural membranes in the lungs

poultice—a soft, moist mass spread between layers of muslin, linen, gauze, or towels and applied hot to a given area

priapism—persistent abnormal erection of the penis, usually without sexual desire; accompanied by pain and tenderness

prognosis—a forecast as to the outcome of a disease

prolapsus—the falling down or sinking of an internal organ

purpurus—a group of disorders characterized by purplish or brownish red discoloration, caused by spontaneous bleeding into the tissue

pylorus—the lower end of the stomach through which digested food is emptied into the intestine

pyramidal tract—any of four columns of motor fibers that run in pairs on each side of the spinal cord and that are continuations of the pyramids of the medulla

reagin—a type of antibody in the blood associated with some allergic diseases

renal—pertaining to the kidney

rheumatic fever—an acute or chronic inflammatory disease occurring as a delayed infection, characterized by swelling, fever and pain

rhinitis—inflammation of the nasal mucous membrane

sacculate—pursed out with little pouches

sacrum—the triangular bone just below the lumbar vertebrae, formed usually by five fused vertebrae

sclerosis—a hardening of a part due to inflammation or disease

scotomas—dark areas of depressed vision or gap in the visual field

sebaceous—secreting a greasy, lubricating substance

sella turcica—a transverse depression along the midline within the cranial cavity; a portion of the sphenoid bone that rises up and forms a saddle-shaped mass ("Turk's saddle")

seminiferous—producing or conveying semen

serosal—pertaining or composed of serosa (any serous membrane)

serous membrane—any membrane that lines a cavity without an opening to the outside of the body

spasticity—an increase over the normal tone of a muscle, with heightened deep tendon reflexes

spirochete—a spiral bacterium

stasis—a stoppage or diminution of blood flow or other body fluid

sternocleidomastoid—a muscle attached to the sternum, clavicle, and mastoid process

"strep"—abbreviated form of streptococcus, a spherical-shaped bacterium occurring generally in chains

stupe—a cloth, sponge, etc., dipped in hot water, wrung dry, and applied to body as a compress

subluxation—an incomplete or partial dislocation

synapse—the site at which an impulse is transmitted from one neuron to another by electrical or chemical means

synovitis—inflammation of a synovial membrane which forms the inner lining of the capsule of a freely movable joint

thenar eminence—mound on the palm at the base of the thumb

thrombosis—formation, development, or presence of a blood clot that remains at its site of formation

titer—the quality of a substance required to produce a reaction with a given volume of another substance

trachea—a cartilaginous tube descending from the larynx and branching into the bronchi

treponeme—an organism of a genus of slender spirochetes, some of which are pathogenic to man

trigeminal nerve—pertaining to the fifth pair of cranial nerves

tubercle—any of the small, rounded lesions produced by infection (as in tuberculosis); a small, knoblike process

tubules—small tubes

ulceration—formation or development of an ulcer

urethra—the membranous canal which carries urine from the bladder to the exterior of the body

vagus—designating the tenth cranial nerve

varicella—chickenpox

varicose—unnaturally and permanently distended, as of a vein

vena cava—one of the two large veins located at the right atrium which returns low oxygenated blood to the heart

ventricle—a small cavity, such as of the brain or heart

vertebra—any of the 33 bones of the spinal column

vertigo—an illusion of movement; a sensation of dizziness as if the external world were revolving around an individual

villi—tiny fingerlike projections extending outward from the inner lining of the small intestine

viscid—glutinous or sticky

vitamin—an organic substance that occurs in many foods in small amounts and is necessary for normal metabolism

vitiligo—a disorder characterized by loss of pigment, resulting in white patches of skin

Index

abscess 122, 317

acid-alkaline balance 82, 89, 90, 101, 165, 305, 392

acidity 65, 81, 101, 107, 108, 150, 165, 360, 366-368, 382-384
  hyper- 185, 350
  stomach 17
  test for 112-113
  See also *superacidity*

acne 1-5, 315

aconite 29, 110, 114, 124

aconitine 110

adhesions 55, 64, 122, 134, 251, 315-321, 356

Adiron 404

adjustments, see *chiropractic* and *osteopathic manipulations*

adrenals 14, 15, 32, 60, 101, 134, 198, 215, 289, 322, 367

Adrex S.E.L. 201

Agorol 103

air, fresh 16, 37, 91

albumen 32

Alcaroid 74, 104, 156, 167

alcohol
  drinking 9, 74, 82, 85, 93, 307, 386
  grain 379, 381, 390
  rubbing 45

alkalinity 9, 82, 90, 108, 150, 326, 366-368, 382-384, 392
  test for 68, 112-113
  alkalizer 93

alkalosis 103, 367

Alka-Seltzer 150, 210

almonds 68, 369-372, 387, 407

Alophen 74

alum fusion 83, 84

ambergris 120, 202, 348

ammonia, muriate of 24

amyotrophic lateral sclerosis 6-13

analgesic 110

anemia 14-17, 39, 71, 74, 76, 154, 166, 412

aneurysm 27

angina pectoris 18-21

Anidex 66

ankylosis 39

anorexia 152

antibiotics 74, 150

antiphlogistine poultice 73

aorta 18

aphonia 22-25

apoplexy 26-30

appendectomy 122

apple diet 321, 401

apple brandy 73, 326

appliances 218
  radio-active (impedance device) 35, 38, 52, 63, 157, 202, 240, 251, 261, 356
  radium 356
  wet cell 7, 8, 20, 35, 44, 51, 88, 157, 166, 169, 187, 196, 228, 250, 283, 324-328, 334, 341

application 403

arsenic 340

arteriosclerosis 31-38

arthritis 39-54, 297-298, 303
  prevention of 407

ash, animated 65, 66, 74, 252

aspirin 74

assimilation 14, 16, 57, 74, 120, 283, 324, 384, 390, 407
  poor 6, 19, 40, 61, 80, 152, 224, 234, 265, 298-299, 351-353, 366

asthenia 233

asthma 55-59, 73, 126, 128

astringent 177

astrological effects 149

atmospheric pressure 72, 165

Atomidine 8, 17, 20, 35, 43, 58, 59, 61, 69, 75, 110, 114, 124, 156, 170, 177, 228, 251, 276, 283-286, 314, 326-327, 334, 342, 373, 392
  regimens 48-49, 61-62, 119, 130, 292
  definition 177
  douch 241

atrophy 6, 23

atropine 66, 190, 228

attitudes 237, 342

as cause of disease 4, 71, 76, 164, 302, 354
constructive 35, 67, 104, 219, 221, 242, 398
for healing 17, 28, 37, 38, 68, 125, 130-131, 334, 384
spiritual 166, 282, 283, 398-399, 402
autonomic nervous system 18, 22, 56, 127, 133, 138, 152, 169, 172, 189, 233, 237, 245, 298, 322, 367, 373
axilla 66

baking soda, see *bicarbonate of soda*
baldness 60-63
premature 279
balsam
of fir 72
of Peru 186
of tolu 120, 220, 379
bamboo 66
baths 28, 43, 47, 74, 241
Epsom salts 43, 47, 300
foot 94
fume 43, 47, 66, 94, 113, 167, 171
sitz 113
steam 94, 342, 343
See also *sweats*
battery, wet cell, see *appliances*
beef juice 374-376
benzoin 72, 325
compound tincture of 20, 59, 74, 113, 160, 177, 217, 325, 363-364, 379, 381
Benzosol 72, 129
Bible recommendations 25, 219, 251
bicarbonate of soda 47, 52, 78, 93, 150, 155, 219, 325, 377
biofeedback 68
birth 56, 343, 359
injury 246, 247
trauma 133
bismuth 340
See also *milk of bismuth*
BiSoDol 347
black root 220, 356
bladder 3, 32, 102, 106, 213, 367
blindness 331
color 87-89

blood 15, 18, 106, 195, 312, 383
building 412
clotting 168, 316, 322
pudding 170
red cells 158, 339
sugar 116-121, 199
white cells 154, 224, 232
body as the temple 402, 404
boil 317
bone
broken, see *fractures*
marrow 14, 15, 17
tissue 322
brace, stomach 356
brain 19, 28, 35, 134
cells 413
rebuilding 38
brandy 73
breast cancer 64-69
breath, bad 314
breathing 73
problems 35, 72, 126-131
bromide of soda 9
bromo quinine 74
bronchi 55, 70, 378, 379
bronchitis 70-75, 126, 148, 401
buchu leaves 220, 356
bulk, see *fiber*
burdock root 196, 356
burns 295
bursa 22, 40, 56
butter 176, 387, 388, 389
butterfat 176, 385

calamus oil 34
Calcidin 59, 73, 150, 196, 342
Calcios 58, 62, 242
calcium 39, 383, 385
insufficient 60
calculi renal, see *kidney stones*
Caldwell's syrup of pepsin 347, 396
calisaya 196, 356, 357
bark 220
callus formation 159
Calmol 177
camomile tea 306
camphor 166, 170, 317
gum 24, 84

spirits of 8, 48, 74, 93, 113, 176, 180, 186, 283, 327
camphorated oil 4, 83, 317-318
Canadian balsam 72, 129
cancer 64, 369, 399, 404
    breast 64-69, 371
    prevention 407
    prostate 297
    stomach 350
capsici
    elixir of 196
    tincture of 130, 166
carbohydrates 9, 289, 383, 386
carbolic acid 178
carbonation 360
cardiolipid 338
Carlsbad salts 180
carotid 127
cascara sagrada 186
Castoria 69, 74, 78, 82, 94, 103, 124, 139, 150, 155, 210, 356, 391, 394, 395, 396
castor oil 24, 103, 124
    See also *packs*
cataracts 76-79, 279
catarrh 14, 64
cathartics 33, 47, 65, 92, 347, 364
cedarwood, oil of 48
celerena, elixir of 130, 166, 196
celery, essence of 130
cells
    anterior horn 7
    blood 14, 17, 58
cerebrospinal system 18, 22, 56, 117, 134, 153, 159, 165, 169, 179, 189, 194, 233, 237, 260, 298, 367
chalk 186
charcoal 354
    See also *willow charcoal*
charred oak keg 326
chemical fumes 70
cherry, wild
    bark 130, 196, 220, 356
    syrup of 73, 378
chicken pox 185, 315
childbirth, see *birth*
chiropractic adjustments 3, 16, 37, 69, 191, 200, 201, 239, 333-335, 343

chloroform 73
choking 72, 380
cholesterol 31
chorioretinitis 336
chyle 133
cigarette smoking 70, 201
cinnamon 348, 354
circulation 20, 60, 78, 90, 392
    improper 64, 71, 76, 102, 149, 351, 358
    incoordination 1, 18, 26, 367
    to stimulate 309
    toxic 14, 19, 23, 32
cirrhosis 107
clary flower 120
clary water 202
climate, change recommended 59
coagulation 42, 168, 233, 316, 322, 368
coal oil, see *kerosene*
Coca-Cola syrup 3, 109, 292
coccyx 189, 195
cocoa butter 69, 285, 319
Codiron 74, 167, 261, 347
cold, common 70, 71, 80, 90-100, 379, 381, 392, 406
    causes of 96
    germ 148
    prevention of 97, 383
    treatment of 98-100, 392, 404
cold spot 137
colitis 80-86
collagen 315-316
colon 19, 33, 195, 392, 396
    congestion 258
    prolapsus 32, 65, 107, 153
colonics 16, 20, 34, 35, 44, 58, 61, 65, 69, 74, 78, 83, 103, 109, 124, 139, 149, 150, 167, 179, 187, 196, 202, 210, 261, 300, 306, 319, 347, 394
coma 26
congenital diseases 279, 337
congestion 60, 71, 80
connective tissue, collagenous 322
constipation 46, 50, 101-105, 122, 152, 172, 236, 366, 407
    relieving 3
consumptive condition 323
convulsions 132

copper sulfate 327
cortico-steriods 279
cortisone 199
coryza 90
cosmetics 60
cough 90, 378-381
  expectorant 378
  syrup 94
counseling 344
  spiritual 79, 344, 398-399, 402
cramps
  abdominal 152
cream of tartar 3, 187, 292, 306, 320
croup 73
crude oil 62
Cuticura ointment 307, 328
cycles of therapy 408
cystitis 106-115

debilitation 14, 60, 185
decubitus ulcer, see *ulcer*
desire 38
diabetes 116-121, 198, 279, 385-388
  in conjunction with prostatitis 298
diaphoretic 110
diarrhea 122, 152
diathermy 63, 180, 193, 218, 300, 334
  short-wave 3, 21, 167
diet 44, 393
  cleansing 24, 58, 393
  improper 1, 76, 101, 149, 175, 185
  light 29, 129
  liquid 93, 111
  recommendations 5, 9, 16, 20, 24,
    34, 46, 54, 62, 65-66, 68, 78, 82, 89,
    91-92, 103, 109, 112, 119, 125, 143,
    156, 182, 186, 201, 204, 211, 218,
    228, 229, 239, 243, 251, 261, 262,
    272, 286, 291, 295-296, 299, 307,
    310, 327, 355, 369, 374, 382-389,
    391, 403-405
  See also *fasting* and *foods to avoid*
Dilantin 139
diuretic 110
diverticulitis 122-125
dizziness 56, 353
  See also *vertigo*

DNA 169
dock root, yellow 220
  tincture of 130
dogwood bark 356
douching 110, 114, 241
dreams 68, 202
  bad 102
duodenum 76, 200, 208, 289, 303, 306,
  375, 406
  stasis 258
  ulcers of 352
dust 70
dypsnea 33
dystrophia myotonica 278
dysynergy 123

eczema 389
edema 363
  cerebral 258
egg 386, 389
  and whiskey 305
  enema 355
  white 94, 150
elder flower 357
electrical treatments 66
eliminants 46, 390-396
eliminations 1, 14, 15, 19, 28, 57, 69, 78,
  120, 144, 159, 201, 286, 307-308,
  373, 390-396, 407
  improper 1, 14, 19, 20, 23, 27, 40, 61,
    64, 70, 76, 107, 108, 123, 134, 139,
    148, 152, 185, 234, 289, 299, 333,
    345, 351, 360
  See also *fasting*
Elliott machine 300, 301
elm 155, 209, 306, 308
  slippery 306
emaciation 39
emotions 154, 200, 215, 302, 357, 403
  caused by physical 117, 154, 236
  disturbed 107
  harmful 1, 22, 91, 101, 104
emphysema 126-131
emunctory 22, 23, 41, 81, 120
endocrine system 134, 200, 258, 288,
  322
enema 28, 44, 58, 82, 92, 103, 109, 218,

306, 347, 364, 393
   egg 355
   salt and soda 104, 392, 393
Eno salts 46, 78, 150, 180, 356, 391,
   394
enterovirus 152
environment, disease
   affected by 38
enzyme preparations 412
epilepsy 127, 132-147
Epsom salts 187, 319, 326, 397
   See also *baths* and *packs*
estrogen 236
eucalyptol 72, 73, 129, 176, 219
eucalyptus
   oil of 59, 325, 379, 381
excitement, avoid 37
exercise 16, 19, 37, 45, 140, 220, 238,
   384, 393
   head and neck 187
   mild 83
   specific 34, 37, 74, 178, 197
expectorant 73, 150
eyes 76, 87, 102
   watery 90

fainting 132
fasting 133, 398-405
fatigue 165, 233, 236
   See also *tiredness*
fear 23, 215, 329
   suppression of 1
feet
   cold 241
   heaviness in 102
   swelling of 102
   wet 320
fermentation, gastric 19
fever 81, 90, 133, 404
fiber 69, 122
fibrin 315
figs, syrup of 69, 395, 396
Fleet's Phospho Soda 155, 157
Fletcher's Castoria, see *Castoria*
flocculation test 338
flu 56, 80, 148-151, 185
   aftereffects 152-157, 396

food
   how to eat 91
   to avoid 29-30, 34, 37, 46, 54, 58, 65,
      75, 78, 82-83, 89, 93, 109, 112, 119,
      139, 143, 156, 180, 186, 195, 201,
      204, 218, 220, 261, 286, 385, 389
   See also *diet, recommendations*
Fowler's solution 75
fractures 127, 158-163
fruits of the spirit 183

gall
   bladder 41, 215
   duct 268, 394
gargle 94
gastritis 208-212, 412
   in conjunction with prostatitis 298
gastroenterology 122, 152
gastrointestinal disturbances 258
gelatin 54, 69
gestation 56, 383
ginger
   essence 85, 156
   fusion of 301
   tincture of 83
ginseng
   elixir 85, 378, 411
   essence of 156
   fusion of 85, 301
glands, see specific names
glandular extracts 61, 202, 242
glass, green 66, 342
globulin 226
glucokinin 119
glucose 119, 369, 386
   tolerance test 198
glycerine 94, 150, 178, 186, 378
glycosuria 116
Glyco-Thymoline 65, 78, 82, 94, 110,
   112, 114, 156, 167, 180, 241, 348,
   382, 395
   enema 326
   See also *douching, packs*
gold 6, 7, 8, 13, 166, 170, 265
   chloride 8, 47, 51, 88, 186, 250, 284,
      326
gonads 134

gonorrhea 297
gout 40
grand mal, see *epilepsy* and *seizures*
grape juice 401
grapes 382
   See also *poultices*
gumma 336
gums 312-314

habits 298
   contributing to disease 33-34
hair 60, 379
   color 63
   See also *baldness*
halitosis 102
hallucinations 102
hands, cold 102
hapten 338
hay fever 55
headache 70, 102, 164-167, 236, 353,
   379
   migraine 258-263
head noises 299, 332, 333
healing
   laying on of hands 68
   mental 67
   physical 68
   spiritual 67, 202
hearing 23
heart 18, 19, 36, 65, 117, 153, 236, 350
   attack 31
   burn 64
   disease 74
hemianopsia 258
hemolysin 339
hemophilia 168-171
hemorrhage 26, 27, 361
hemorrhoids 172-184
hepatic circulation 23, 24, 36, 40,
   106, 134, 172, 185, 234, 298, 396
   See also *liver*
heredity 61, 87, 194, 248
herniation 123
heroin 73
herpes zoster 185-188
hiccough 378-381
hog lard 62

homosexuality 401
honey 73, 94, 112, 150, 156, 354, 378,
   385, 388, 389, 390
horehound, syrup of 73, 378
hormones 158, 242, 367
   crystallization of 41
   imbalance 265
   male 64, 66
hydrocephalus 189-193
hydrolysis 119, 386
hydrotherapy 24, 37, 44, 63, 69, 74,
   149, 167, 300, 306, 403
   See also *baths, sweats, colonics*
hyperaldosteronism 194
hypertension 37, 71, 194-197
hypnosis 25
hypnotics 67
hypochondria 237
hypoglycemia 119, 198-207, 386

ice 179
   packs 186
Ichthyol 328
ideals 166, 183
idiopathic 137
ileum 134
   plexus 367
immunization 383
impedance device, see *appliances*
impetigo 315
impotence 266
Indian turnip, essence of 156
indigestion 208-212, 234, 237, 392
infection 60, 104, 152, 315, 382
infertility 153
inflammation 23, 71, 80, 81, 122, 152,
   319
   chronic 320
influenza, see *flu*
infrared lamp 17, 228
inhalants 150, 325, 380
   formulas for 59, 72-73, 129-130,
   305, 326, 381
Innerclean 69, 144
insanity 245
insomnia 236
insulin 118, 386, 387

inulin (inulides) 119, 386
Iodex 66
iodine 14, 41, 169, 225, 340, 383
    See also *Atomidine*
Ipecac 73
Ipsab 313, 314
iron 383, 412
    muriated 84
itching 303

jejunum 66, 134, 303, 392, 396, 406
Jesus 31
juniper, oil 120, 219

Kaldak 196
karma 6, 8, 41, 87, 190, 215, 248, 279
keloid 316
kelp 46
kerosene 48, 160, 285
kidneys 3, 15, 19, 32, 35, 36, 40, 92,
    102, 106, 113, 153, 195, 298, 331,
    348, 367, 382, 394, 396
    stones 213-222, 234

lacteals 2, 14, 15, 19, 66, 80, 133, 152,
    375, 406
    See also *Peyer's patches*
Laetrile 369
lanolin 8, 48, 159, 274, 284, 318, 356
lard 62
larynx 23, 55, 71, 378
laudanum 29, 110, 114, 124
    tincture of 186
Lavoris 112, 167
    See also *packs*
laxatives 61, 74, 110, 150, 306, 364,
    391, 390-396
    dietary 47
    fruit 46, 110, 181
    vegetable 69, 391
lemon 94, 150, 387, 403
lemonade 93
leptandrin 111
lesions 22, 37, 55, 81, 107, 122, 350
    brain 247, 251
    lacteal 56, 133, 247
    skin 5, 185, 303-311

spinal 19, 60, 71, 76, 133, 165, 173,
    185, 195, 354
leukemia 223-231
    leukocyte 58, 65
    leukocytosis 232-235
leukopenia 232-235
levulose 119, 386
light, green 66
lime water 354
lipiodial 338
lisping 333
Listerine 94
litmus paper 112
liver 3, 18, 27, 32, 36, 40, 41, 56, 65, 80,
    102, 103, 106, 116-117, 134, 155,
    208, 215, 226, 259, 266, 322, 331,
    348, 367, 379, 392, 394, 396
    See also *hepatic circulation*
lobelia, oil of 166
locomotion 27, 65
lues 336-344
lung 14, 19, 36, 55, 102, 126-131, 227,
    259, 382
lymphatics 14, 23, 40, 55, 80-82, 91,
    189, 303, 374, 407
    circulation 404
    drainage 347, 361
    inflammation 323
    nodes 190
lymphocytes 14, 22, 58, 117, 169, 226,
    232, 367
lysis 339

macrophage 267
mammary glands 64
mandrake root 196, 220
manipulations, see *massage* and
    osteopathic manipulations
massage 4, 8, 28, 34, 37, 43-45, 47-48,
    62-63, 66, 74, 78, 94, 113, 128, 130,
    142, 150, 157, 167, 171, 177, 187,
    192, 217, 228, 239, 271, 283, 284,
    334, 355, 371, 403
    abdominal 103, 137, 138, 142, 283,
    379
    alcohol 326
    chest 74, 94

deep 20
foot 20, 93
fractures and sprains 159, 160, 161
gum 313
reasons for 410
scalp 62
See also *oils for massage*
masturbation 248
mayblossom bitters 411
measles 148
meditation 25, 68, 79, 202, 221, 260,
402, 404
meeting self 41
See also *karma*
meningitis 336
menopause 236-243
surgical 236
menses 1
menstral problems 153
mental
as healer 33, 403
balance 37
illness 35, 244-257
strain 164
mentholatum 176
mercury 340
metabolites 117
microglial cells 267
milk 383
milk of bismuth 17, 156, 167, 301, 355,
391
Milk of Magnesia 17, 210, 355, 392
mineral imbalances 62
Minit-Rub 379
morphia, sulphate of 84
mouth, dry 102
mucosa 122, 126, 198, 304, 396
mucus 66, 72, 81, 122
mullein 362-363
poultice 363
stupes 218
tea 218, 308, 363, 389
multiple sclerosis 6, 8, 137, 264-277
mummy food 405
mumps 148
muscles 6, 30, 278, 287
atrophy 6-7

music 403
muscular dystrophy 278-287, 406
muscularis 122
mustard, oil of 20, 48
musterole 74
mutton
suet 74, 113
tallow 92, 180
myelin 267
myelogenous leukemia 227
myocarditis 37
myrrh 82
tincture of 34, 48, 142, 159, 217, 251,
285, 317, 355
myxovirus 148

nails, finger 60
naferon 412
narcotics, avoiding 29, 67
nausea 81, 102, 152, 164, 258, 353, 401
treatment for 354
nephritis 218
nerve
rebuilding 38, 88, 283
reflexes 42
sheaths 11-12, 267
nervous
breakdown 19
systems 22, 65, 81, 102, 164, 236,
283, 331, 403, 407
See also *autonomic, cerebrospinal,*
and *sensory*
neuritis, in conjunction with prostatitis 298
neurologist 25
neuropathy 25
Nitrazine paper 68
nitre 109
sweet spirits of 92, 187
nose
discharge 90
spray 150, 379
Nujol 4, 48, 177
Nurses Brand 177

obesity 117, 288, 296, 359, 401
oils

for massage 4, 8, 20, 28-29, 31, 47-48, 78, 82, 83, 113, 159, 160, 179, 187, 217-218, 250, 271, 284, 294, 317-319
oil cap 62
olive oil 8, 20, 29, 34, 48
enema 355, 393
for massage 82, 113, 142, 160, 217, 253, 274, 284, 317, 355, 363, 364
internal 65, 82, 89, 103, 124, 137, 142, 167, 180, 354, 377, 393, 401
shampoo 63
Oneness 200
onion juice 92
See also poultices
opium 110
optic centers 87
weakness 65
orthopedics 158
osteopathic manipulations 3, 16, 20, 24, 29, 34, 44, 50, 58, 61, 62, 69, 74, 78, 88, 94, 103, 109, 118, 124, 130, 138, 141, 142, 150, 157, 171, 179, 191, 217, 228, 251, 261, 300, 333, 347, 361, 378
oxygen 324

packs 239
baking soda 219
castor oil 24, 44, 69, 103, 124, 131, 137, 138, 142, 156, 167, 180, 219, 251, 325, 354, 355, 377, 392
Epsom salts 24, 29, 78, 180, 300, 319, 397
Glyco-Thymoline 78, 82, 110, 197, 300, 354, 409
hot and cold 179
ice 186
Lavoris 354
salt 47, 114, 300
pancreas 19, 27, 56, 116, 134, 198, 208, 266, 348, 350, 351, 386, 394
paralysis 27
agitans 35
paresis 342
paresthesia 258
Parkinson's disease 35

paronychia 320
passion flower fusion 139, 142-143
recipe 411
patience and consistency 406, 408
Pazo 177
peanut oil 8, 28-29, 45, 47, 78, 159, 187, 196, 250, 274, 284, 318, 327, 334, 356, 364, 371, 407
penicillin 340
peppermint
essence of 314
oil 196
pepsin
elixir of lactated 85, 156, 167, 301, 355, 378, 391
syrup of 347
periostitis 336
peristalsis 65, 123, 373, 393
perspiration 1
Peruvian bark 356
petit mal, see epilepsy and seizures
Petrolagar 144
Peyer's patches 14, 16, 22, 56, 80, 81, 101, 117, 128, 153, 164, 169, 195, 208, 233, 345, 406
See also lacteals
phenobarbital 139
pheochromocytoma 194
phonation 279
See also stuttering
phosphate of soda 104, 219, 347
photophobia 258
pigmentation, abnormal 60
piles, see hemorrhoids
pineal 134, 241, 246, 289, 367
pine
oil 29, 47, 113, 159, 325, 381
woods 251
pituitary 134, 246, 258, 288
plaque 31
plantain tea 371
See also poultices
plaster 74
pneumonia 148
podophyllin 47, 111, 186, 356
poke root 356
possession 246

potassium
  bromide 166, 196, 357
  excess 60
  iodide 130, 166, 196, 357
potato 89
  poultice 78
poultices
  antiphlogistine 73
  grape 83, 84, 156, 354
  mullein 363
  plaintain 66
  potato 78
  onion 73, 150
prayer 68, 79, 221, 255, 282, 398-399,
  402, 404
pregnancy 174, 215, 236, 359, 394
prenatal influences 61, 64, 280, 337,
  406
Preparation H 177
prevention 13, 36-38, 91
priapism 266
prickly ash bark 314, 356
prostatitis 35, 297-302
protein 58, 106, 383, 385
psoriasis 289, 303-311, 320
psychosis 245
pumpkin seed 390
purification 401, 403
purpuric 19
pus 106, 312
pylorus 19
pyorrhea 312-314

quartz light, mercury 66

radio-active appliance, see *appliances*
radium 67
rash 336
reagin 338-339
Rectal Medicone 177
regeneration 413
renal 102, 298
Resinol 307
respiratory system 70, 72, 90, 148
rest 81, 93, 125, 177, 201, 243, 347, 357
retardation, mental 137
rheumatic fever 40, 345

rhinitis 90
rhubarb, syrup of 73, 186, 378
Rochelle salts 3, 187, 292, 306, 320,
  390
rubs, see *massage*
Russian white oil 160, 219
  See also *Usoline* and *Nujol*

saffron tea 210
  yellow 82, 155, 210, 306
sage 120, 348
  See also *clary*
Sal Hepatica 94, 391, 396
salt 194, 196, 314
  bile 74
  in combination 3, 187, 292, 306, 320
  in enema 29, 392, 393
  packs 47, 159
  rub 294
  sea 46
  soda and 186, 313
  See also *Epsom salts, Eno salts,
  Rochelle salts*
sanguinaria 47, 111
sarsaparilla 104
  compound 130
  root 196, 220
  syrup of 219, 357
sassafras
  oil 48, 82, 160, 186
  root oil 48, 159
scalp 60, 258
scar 315-321
  on brain 147
  tissue 71, 413
sciatic center 8
scleroderma 322-328, 412
sclerosis 6-13, 264-277
sebaceous glands 1
sedative 43, 110, 139, 387
sedentary life 36
seizures 132, 135
senna 47, 110, 364, 390, 394, 396
sensory nervous system 22, 164, 194
serosal layers 122
serous membranes 319
serum, for breast cancer 66

Serutan 124
shampoo 63
shingles 185
short-wave treatments, see *diathermy*
silver nitrate 284, 286
sinus 70
   sinusitis 347
skin 40, 60, 102, 303-311, 322-328
   eruptions 1-5, 102
sleep 93
   loss 91, 102, 173
   See also *insomnia*
sneezing 90
snuff 177
soap, castile 176
soda
   and gold 286
   in enema 29, 392, 393
sodium bicarbonate
   chloride 314
   See also *bicarbonate of soda*
   and *salt*
spasticity, of colon 122
speech
   as high vibration 23
   impairment 22-25, 329-335
sperm 13, 266
spinal misalignments, see also *chiro-*
   practic adjustments and *osteopathic*
   manipulations
sphincter
   muscle 32, 172, 178, 182, 391
   pyloric 351
spirits frumenti 93
   See also *alcohol, drinking*
spiritual healing 67, 398-399, 402
spirochete 336-344
spleen 27, 36, 65, 116, 120, 200, 208,
   266, 331, 350, 394
sports 140
sprains 158-163
starches 288-289, 382, 383
steam bath 94, 342
   See also *baths, steam*
sterility, see *infertility*
steroid 350
stillingia, tincture of 73, 85, 156

stockings, elastic 362
stomach 16, 18, 19, 65, 101, 208, 348,
   366, 382, 394
   ulcers 350-357
strep 149
stress 60, 101, 165, 172, 183, 345, 350
stroke 26-31
stupes 217, 218, 363
stuttering 329-335
sugar 382
   beet 120, 202, 348
   blood 116-121, 198, 385
suggestive therapy 24
sulfate morphia 24
Sulflax 124
sulphur 3, 187, 292, 306, 320
sulphuric acid 327
sunshine 16, 356
superacidity 71, 172, 174, 175, 399, 401
surgery 67, 158, 174, 220, 341
sweats 28, 44, 113, 157
   See also *steam bath*
sweet oil, see *olive oil*
sympathetic nervous system 18, 22, 27,
   127, 159, 165, 248, 258
   See also *autonomic*
synapse 22
   dysfunction 249
synovitis 341
syphilis 336-344

tachycardia 236
teas, see *camomile, mullein, saffron,*
   watermelon seed
teeth 312-314
tension 101, 236
   nervous 1, 194
   relief of 345
testicle, atrophy 279
throat 23, 70
   prescription for 73
   problems 35, 345-349
thymus 60, 367
thyroid 14, 60, 200, 266, 288, 322, 367
   extract 124
Tim 174, 175, 176, 179, 181
tiredness 35, 91, 102, 113, 367

tobacco 177
tolu 130, 381
  balsam of 120, 379
  tincture of 72
tonic, chill 74
Tonicine 242
tonsillitis 104, 345-349
toxicity 358
toxins 32, 37, 40-41, 46, 60, 64, 70, 80, 102, 104, 109, 122, 152, 164, 214, 234, 258, 305, 345, 392, 400
trachea 70
treponeme 336
tuberculosis 233, 382
turpentine 72
  oil of 59, 72, 379, 381
  rectified 72, 129, 130, 219
  spirits of 93, 113, 180, 217, 218
  See also *packs, stupes*
twitching, fibrillary 6

ulcer 315, 350-357, 361
  duodenal 208, 350-357
  peptic 208
  stomach 350-357
ultraviolet
  light 342, 356
  ray 52, 66, 125, 150, 227
  See also *violet ray*
underfeeding 82
Unguentine 328
Upjohn's Citrocarbonate 392
ureter 213
uretha 32, 106, 108
urine, test for acidity 112-113
Usoline 48
  See also *Nujol*
uterine myoma 400
uterus 107

vaccine 148
vagus center 71, 87
valerian, tincture of 83, 166, 196, 356
varicose veins
  internal 172
  legs 358-365
vascular system 27, 31
Vaseline 62

vena cava, see *venereal disease, syphilis*
Ventriculin 17, 228, 412
vertigo 165, 331
  See also *dizziness*
vibrator
  electric 44, 63, 74, 167, 196, 239, 285, 334, 356
  vibratory treatment 79
vinegar 382
  apple 159
  massage 47
violet ray 63, 74, 78, 88, 124, 157, 160, 166, 179, 241, 272, 293, 306
  See also *ultraviolet ray*
vision 23
vitamins 92, 164, 169, 369, 403, 404, 406
  deficiencies 164, 200
  not recommended 120
vitiligo 60
vocal cords 23
vomiting 152, 164, 258

walking, recommended exercise 34, 140, 239, 361
water 93, 109, 111, 209, 392
  cinnamon and lime 354
  sea 314
watermelon seed tea 109-113, 187, 218
wet cell battery, see *appliances*
whiskey, rye 378
White's Codliver Oil Tablets 394
willow charcoal 327
wine, red 326, 375
wintergreen oil 196, 343
witch hazel 4, 47-48, 160, 167, 187, 250, 318

x-ray 66, 261, 321

yeast, to relieve constipation 3, 393

Zilatone 104, 157, 292, 394
zinc 327
  stearate of 186
Zollinger-Ellison Syndrome 350

THE WORK OF EDGAR CAYCE TODAY

The Association for Research and Enlightenment, Inc. (A.R.E.®), is a membership organization founded by Edgar Cayce in 1931.

- 14,256 Cayce readings, the largest body of documented psychic information anywhere in the world, are housed in the A.R.E. Library/Conference Center in Virginia Beach, Virginia. These readings have been indexed under 10,000 different topics and are open to the public.

- An attractive package of membership benefits is available for modest yearly dues. Benefits include: a journal and newsletter; lessons for home study; a lending library through the mail, which offers collections of the actual readings as well as one of the world's best parapsychological book collections, names of doctors or health care professionals in your area.

- As an organization on the leading edge in exciting new fields, A.R.E. presents a selection of publications and seminars by prominent authorities in the fields covered, exploring such areas as parapsychology, dreams, meditation, world religions, holistic health, reincarnation and life after death, and personal growth.

- The unique path to personal growth outlined in the Cayce readings is developed through a worldwide program of study groups. These informal groups meet weekly in private homes.

- A.R.E. maintains a visitors' center where a bookstore, exhibits, classes, a movie, and audiovisual presentations introduce inquirers to concepts from the Cayce readings.

- A.R.E. conducts research into the helpfulness of both the medical and nonmedical readings, often giving members the opportunity to participate in the studies.

For more information and a color brochure, write or phone:

A.R.E., Dept. C., P.O. Box 595
Virginia Beach, VA 23451, (804) 428-3588